Also by **Ashgate**

LAWRENCE I. CONRAD and DOMINIK WUJASTYK
Contagion: Perspectives from Pre-Modern Societies

ROGER FRENCH, JON ARRIZABALAGA, ANDREW CUNNINGHAM and LUIS GARCÍA-BALLESTER
Medicine from the Black Death to the French Disease

PENELOPE GOUK
Musical Healing in Cultural Contexts

PEREGRINE HORDEN
Music as Medicine: The History of Music Therapy Since Antiquity

NAOMI J. MILLER and NAOMI YAVNEH
Maternal Measures: Figuring Caregiving in the Early Modern Period

and in the Collected Studies Series

PHILIP D. CURTIN
Migration and Mortality in Africa and the Atlantic World, 1700–1900

MONICA H. GREEN
Women's Healthcare in the Medieval West: Texts and Contexts

JERRY STANNARD
Herbs and Herbalism in the Middle Ages and Renaissance

JERRY STANNARD
Pristina Medicamenta: Ancient and Medieval Medical Botany

VIVIAN NUTTON
From Democedes to Harvey: Studies in the History of Medicine

WALTER PAGEL, edited by MARIANNE WINDER
Religion and Neoplatonism in Renaissance Medicine

NATHAN SIVIN
Medicine, Philosophy and Religion in Ancient China: Researches and Reflections

ANDREW WEAR
Health and Healing in Early Modern England: Studies in Social and Intellectual History

VARIORUM COLLECTED STUDIES SERIES

Medicine in a Multicultural Society

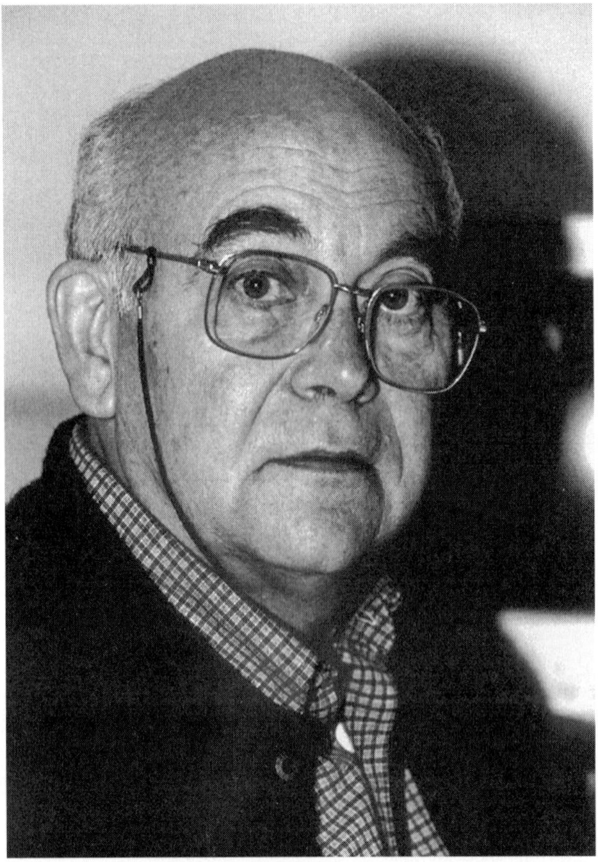

Professor Luis García-Ballester
(1936–2000)

Luis García-Ballester

Medicine in a Multicultural Society

Christian, Jewish and Muslim Practitioners in the Spanish Kingdoms, 1222–1610

Ashgate
VARIORUM

Aldershot · Burlington USA · Singapore · Sydney

Published in the Variorum Collected Studies Series by

Ashgate Publishing Limited
Gower House, Croft Road,
Aldershot, Hampshire GU11 3HR
Great Britain

Ashgate Publishing Company
131 Main Street,
Burlington, Vermont 05401–5600
USA

Ashgate website: http://www.ashgate.com

ISBN 0–86078–845–8

British Library Cataloguing-in-Publication Data
García-Ballester, Luis
Medicine in a Multicultural Society: Christian, Jewish and Muslim Practitioners in the Spanish Kingdoms, 1222–1610. (Variorum Collected Studies Series: CS702).
1. Medicine – Spain – History. 2. Medicine, Medieval – Spain. 3. Medicine – Spain – Religious Aspects.
I. Title.
610.9'46'0902

US Library of Congress Cataloging-in-Publication Data

The Library of Congress Control Number has been preassigned as:
00–108966

The paper used in this publication meets the minimum requirements of the American National Standard for Information Sciences – Permanence of Paper for Printed Library Materials, ANSI Z39.48–1984. ∞ ™

Printed by St Edmundsbury Press, Bury St Edmunds, Suffolk

VARIORUM COLLECTED STUDIES SERIES CS702

CONTENTS

This volume contains xii + 374 pages

PREFACE

The papers collected here reflect one side of my research covering a span of over twenty years. They all focus on medicine and science (natural philosophy) in the multicultural societies of the Spanish kingdoms of Castile and Aragon bertween the thirteenth and the seventeenth centuries. Medicine cannot be divorced from the political, religious, economic and scientific forces which inform every society at any time. The study of Galen's thought and Galenism in medieval and early modern European medicine has been another of my major concerns over the years. Some of the results of my efforts in this area will be offered in another volume of the *Variorum* series under the title *Galen and Galenism: Theory and Practice from Antiquity to Renaissance*.

All but one of the articles in this first volume were originally published in English. John Smedley, publisher of the collection *Variorum*, suggested me that all the collected papers in this volume appear in an English version. Therefore, I offer here a revised and shortened version of my article on the Franciscan and Dominican *studia* of Santiago de Compostela and their commited interest for the 'natural books' (*libri naturales*), originally published in Spanish. Some of these articles are complemented by other published studies which could not be included in this selection due to their lenght. Thus the article on 'Nature and Science in Thirteenth-Century Castile' is complemented by the long introductory study to my edition (in collaboration with Avelino Domínguez) of the *Historia naturalis*, a scientific encyclopaedia by the Franciscan Juan Gil de Zamora (3 vols., Valladolid: Junta de Castilla y León, 1994). The complex situation of medicine in the *mudéjar* and *morisco* minorities in widely discussed in two of my books, *Historia social de la medicina en la España de los siglos XIII al XVI* (Madrid: Akal Editores, 1976) and *Los moriscos y la medicina* (first edition, Granada: Universidad de Granada, 1976; a revised and enlarged version was published in Barcelona by Editorial Labor in 1984).

Moreover, during the last four years I have further studied the problems posed by medical teaching and practice, as well as the perceptions of health and disease among Christian, Jewish, Muslim and *Converso* practitioners in the late medieval and renaissance Crown of Castile. As a result, I have recently finished a new book on medicine in medieval Castile (until c. 1525) which draws upon a great deal of new sources, *La búsqueda de la salud. Sanadores y enfermos en la Corona de Castilla, siglos XIII al XVI* (Barcelona: Península Ediciones, in press). The eager reader willing to broaden the views offered in this collection may turn to this book, whose publication excuses me of including a cumbersome 'Addenda et Corrigenda' in this present selection. I have enriched my historical analysis with new sources and only changed my general views on minor points.

I am grateful to my former students Jon Arrizabalaga, Montserrat Cabré and Fernando Salmón, who suggested this selection to John Smedley, whose kindness and technical advice have improved it. I am also indebted to Mati Pardo, the secretary of the Unit of the History of Medicine at the University of Cantabria for her technical assistance. I should also like to thank the owners of the copyrights of the original publications for their kind permission to reprint the works reproduced in this collection.

LUIS GARCÍA-BALLESTER

Puente Arce, Cantabria,
June 2000

FOREWORD

Doctrina est actio doctoris in discipulum, reads Ali ibn Ridwan's commentary on Galen's *Tegni*, and it is followed by a description of this 'action': it takes an oral or written form, and it happens in the master's presence or in his absence. We can vouch for the fact that Luis García-Ballester's teaching has taken all these forms, as the three of us have experienced from the time we first met Luis as medical or history of medicine students.

Academic celebrations can often convey melancholic feelings for what has been left behind. This collection of studies by Luis García-Ballester was conceived as such a celebration, but one far removed from such feelings. Luis, the doyen of Spanish historians of medicine still on active service, has no plans to limit his curiosity and he gives every sign of that to all those who are in touch with him. An infectious enthusiasm surrounds him when discussing a paper, when gently pressing archivists to allow him to consult materials at their closing hours, or when persuading a not-so-convinced student about the rewarding fascination of working on the most dreary-seeming subjects.

Luis' vitality and optimism, together with an incessant and ever-growing output of work made it difficult for us to remember that he was soon going to be 65 years old. In the summer of 1997, when we began to think about paying homage to him, we thought that our best tribute could be facilitating the publication of selected studies from his own work by a celebrated international press. He has always looked north towards the best international academic traditions and we have witnessed how deeply moved he has been by the *Festschriften* devoted to those senior scholars he admires. Time is ripe to reverse these emotions and place Luis García-Ballester's work and persona at the centre of an academic celebration.

Our original one-volume proposal of selected studies found an enthusiastic ally, John Smedley, who in his capacity as publisher of the Variorum Collected Studies Series not only welcomed it but suggested its expansion to a second volume, so that Luis's long-term research on Galen and Galenism may be given the platform it deserves.

By taking this initiative, we know that we are expressing not only our own gratitude, but also that of many historians of medicine from several generations who have had the privilege of interacting with Luis García-Ballester as pupils and colleagues during his fruitful academic career.

JON ARRIZABALAGA
MONTSERRAT CABRÉ
FERNANDO SALMÓN

Barcelona-Santander, June 2000

Post scriptum. On the 10 October 2000, while this volume was already in press, Luis García-Ballester died from cancer first diagnosed in 1999.

ACKNOWLEDGEMENTS

Grateful acknowledgement is given to the following for permission to reproduce the articles in this volume: *Bulletin of the History of Medicine*, Baltimore (I); *Arbor*, Madrid (II); the American Philosophical Society, Philadelphia (III); The University of Chicago Press (IV); Macmillan Press Ltd, Basingstoke (V); Editions Rodopi BV, Amsterdam (VI); Cambridge University (VII; VIII); ITPS Ltd, Andover (IX).

PUBLISHER'S NOTE

The articles in this volume, as in all others in the Collected Studies Series, have not been given a new, continuous pagination. In order to avoid confusion, and to facilitate their use where these same studies have been referred to elsewhere, the original pagination has been maintained wherever possible.

Each article has been given a Roman numeral in order of appearance, as listed in the Contents. This number is repeated on each page and quoted in the index entries.

MEDICAL SCIENCE IN THIRTEENTH-CENTURY CASTILE: PROBLEMS AND PROSPECTS*

In his classic *Introduction to the History of Science,* George Sarton stated: "The importance of Alfonso X el Sabio's activity as a promoter of translation and scientific research can hardly be exaggerated. He might be called the founder of Spanish science; he was one of the greatest intermediaries between Arabic and European knowledge."[1] This sequence of assertions was based on research into the astronomical work of the scientific circle around the king[2] and on the fact that Alfonso was "the founder of the Spanish scientific language and literature,"[3] but it disregarded gaps in our knowledge of the nature of science in the "Wise King's" reign, gaps that still have not been closed. For example, our knowledge of the medical science available in Castile at the time is incomplete. This society, which had a fascinating ruler and existed during a decisive century, has nevertheless failed to attract the attention of historians of medicine, in Spain and abroad. No work has been done on the development of medical science in Alfonso's reign (1252–84), or indeed on any aspect of medicine in thirteenth-century Castile.[4] I am not going to be so bold as to try to fill, in only a few pages, this historiographical void; I shall simply raise a number of questions and provide foundations for their answers.

13th

The French historian of science and Hispanicist Guy Beaujouan has

* Revised version of a paper presented at the fifty-eighth annual meeting of the American Association for the History of Medicine, Durham and Chapel Hill, North Carolina, 17 May 1985. I am indebted to Michael R. McVaugh for helpful comments and text corrections, and two anonymous *Bulletin* reviewers for useful criticism.

[1] George Sarton, *Introduction to the History of Science,* 3 vols. in 5 (1931; reprint, New York: Krieger, 1975), 2(2): 835.

[2] Manuel Rico y Sinobas, ed., *Libros del saber de astronomía del rey d. Alfonso X de Castilla,* 5 vols. (Madrid: Tip. de Don E. Aguado, 1863–67). A new microfiche version edited by Lloyd A. Kasten and John Nitti is *Concordances and Texts of the Royal Scriptorium Manuscripts of Alfonso X el Sabio* (Madison, Wisconsin: Hispanic Seminary of Medieval Studies, 1978). A group at Barcelona University led by professors Juan Vernet and Julio Samsó is currently studying the whole of Alfonso X's astronomical works; see Juan Vernet, ed., *Nuevos estudios sobre astronomía española en el siglo de Alfonso X* (Barcelona: Consejo Superior de Investigaciones Científicas [hereafter C.S.I.C.], 1983).

[3] "The translation ordered by him required the building up of a new vocabulary," Sarton, *Introduction,* 2(2): 839.

[4] We have only found Luis Barcia-Merayo's brief paper, "La medicina en el *Lapidario* de Alfonso el Sabio," *Medicamenta,* 1969, *52:* 221–22, which is of little value. The recent monograph by Luis Sánchez Granjel, *La medicina española antigua y medieval* (Salamanca: Universidad de Salamanca, 1981), adds nothing to the little that was already known about medicine in Castile in the thirteenth century.

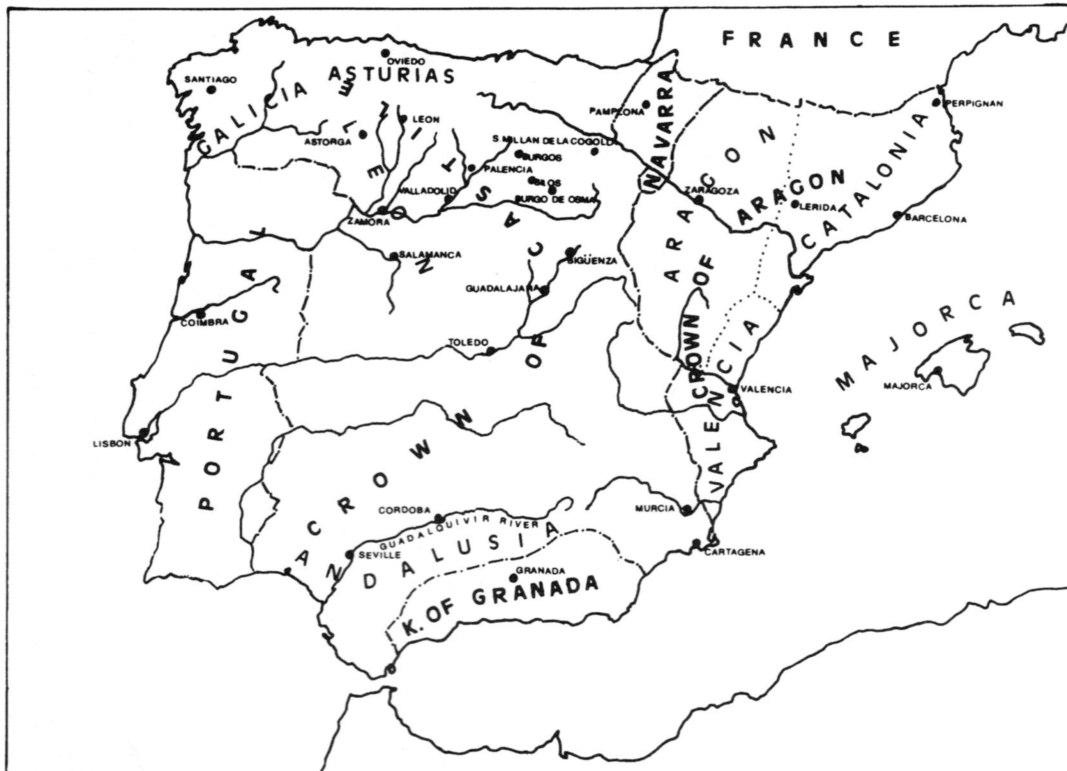

The Iberian peninsula in the thirteenth century. The kingdoms that occupy the territory of present-day Spain are those of Aragon, Castile, Navarre and Granada.

pointed to four factors that conditioned the formation of science in Spain in the late Middle Ages: the Muslim presence, the outstanding role played by the Jews, the precocious maturity of the Peninsular languages, and the weakness of Spanish universities.[5] These four factors were also operative in the field of medical science, in what we might term the dynamics of the assimilation, elaboration, and transmission of medical ideas. Specifically, they acted upon the book, the manuscript: this was the vehicle for science, which in the medical field extended from what we today call medical sciences (anatomy and physiology together in the widest sense of the terms) to theoretical and general therapeutics, passing through the complete range of pathology.

The complexities of medical practice, though intricately interwoven with the world of medical science, present another order of problems. These complexities included the practical dimensions in which the medical act was performed; the doctor's training and his performance as a professional; and the description of specific healing techniques. Furthermore, we must never lose sight of the fact that all this was carried out in a complex web involving the obvious interplay of scientific, economic, political, philosophical, religious, and other elements. An important part of this web, again, was composed of the four factors indicated by Beaujouan. Neither the level of medical ideas nor the different aspects of medical practice in thirteenth-century Castile has been studied.[6]

We must acknowledge one major obstacle to such a study, especially to the clarification of medical practice in those territories covered by the Crown of Castile in Spain in the late Middle Ages (and particularly the thirteenth century): our lack of documentary evidence. This deficiency provides perhaps the greatest contrast between Castile and the other part of Spain during this period, the Crown of Aragon (Catalonia, Aragon, Valencia, Majorca). One small detail will suffice to illustrate this point: the magnificent archives in Barcelona and Valencia enable us, for the years of the fourteenth century, to know the names of perhaps two thousand professional healers (Christians, Jews, Moors) who were practicing in a population of some eight hundred thousand inhabitants;[7] in contrast, we know the names of scarcely more than two dozen healers for the same period for the whole of the Crown of Castile (from Galicia, Asturias, Leon, to Seville and Murcia), which had a population of approximately four million. We cannot be sure how far this lack of evidence for Castile distorts our conclusions, but if we were to take the ratio between healing or medical attention and population size as

[5] Guy Beaujouan, *La science en Espagne aux XIVe et XVe siècles* (Paris: Université de Paris, Palais de la Découverte, 1967), p. 7.

[6] I have elsewhere considered the role played by the Muslim minority in Christian medicine in Spain in the late Middle Ages. See Luis García-Ballester, *Historia social de la medicina en la España de los siglos XIII al XVI*, vol. 1, *La minoría musulmana y morisca* (Madrid: Akal, 1976-).

[7] Michael R. McVaugh and I are currently working on medicine as a medical system or organization in the Crown of Aragon during the fourteenth century.

an indicator, we might well ask ourselves if there was any medicine at all in Castile. Did scientific research, one of the things that has led to King Alfonso X being called "The Wise," not affect medicine?

In the second half of the twelfth century, Toledo and some other parts of Castile (to which the extensive Guadalquivir valley and Murcia had not yet been added) witnessed a decisive chapter in the history of European medicine, the production of numerous translations into Latin from Arabic of the most important works in Greek and Arabic biology and scientific methodology as well as medicine. Why then is it that, barely one hundred years later, we can find no trace in Castile of the rich medical corpus translated in Toledo?[8] Here the scarcity of documents is insufficient to explain the lack of a satisfactory response.

In my current investigations into the medicine of thirteenth-century Castile, I have noticed a number of circumstances and facts that seem to me to begin to answer these questions. Let me offer some of the conclusions that I have reached.

First, the Castilian universities show no signs of scholastic medicine, while the other medieval institutions that had earlier transmitted scientific and medical knowledge (the monasteries and cathedral schools) now display interests that are old fashioned and out of date.[9] Second, the mendicant orders—the Dominicans and the Franciscans in particular—became leaders in the scientific and medical world (though not on the practical level) during the second half of the thirteenth century. Both the scanty scholastic medical literature existing at the time and the limited translation into Latin of Arabic writers on medicine are due to members of these orders.[10] Third, the medical works that would later constitute the doctrinal corpus of thirteenth-century scholastic medicine, a great many of which had been translated into Latin in Toledo during the last thirty years of the twelfth century,[11] were totally absent from the scientific circles of Alfonso X, although in Arabic they circulated within the Jewish and Moorish communities of Castile. A fourth fact, very important in comparison with the translation activity in Castile around 1175, is the reduction in quantity and the decline in scientific quality of the medical contents of the works translated, as can be observed from their astrological character.[12] Fifth, the systematic

[8] For the medical translations of Toledo during the twelfth century, see Heinrich Schipperges, *Die Assimilation der Arabischen Medizin durch das Lateinische Mittelalter*, suppl. no. 3 to *Sudhoff's Archiv* (Wiesbaden: Franz Steiner Verlag, 1964).

[9] See Luis García-Ballester, "El papel de las instituciones de consumo y difusión de ciencia médica en la Castilla del siglo XIII: el monasterio, la catedral y la universidad," *Dynamis*, 1984, *4*: 33–63.

[10] Avelino Domínguez García and Luis García-Ballester, "El tratado *de anathomia* (c. 1280) de Juan Gil de Zamora (c. 1241–1320)," *Dynamis*, 1983, *3*: 341–71. We will return to this topic of limited translations from Arabic into Latin.

[11] García-Ballester, *Historia social de la medicina en la España*, 1: 31–42, and later in this paper.

[12] We refer to the medical content of the following works written at the *Scriptorium* of Alfonso X: *Lapidario*, ed. Sagrario Rodríguez M. Montalvo (Madrid: Editorial Gredos, 1981); *Libro de las Cruzes*, ed. Lloyd A. Kasten and Lawrence B. Kiddle (Madrid: C.S.I.C., 1961); and *Picatrix*, studied by David Pingree in "Between the *Ghāya* and *Picatrix*: I. The Spanish version," *J. Warburg Courtauld Institutes*, 1981, *44*: 27–56.

revision of the legislative corpus that either belongs to or is attributed to the reign of Alfonso X[13] raises the interesting problem of the status of medicine as a profession in the Castile of the second half of the thirteenth century. For at this very time Castile established procedures that made possible social control over professional medical activity and thus joined a process that had been initiated toward the middle of the twelfth century in the Kingdom of Sicily and had spread north during the thirteenth and early fourteenth centuries.[14] Finally, the scientific circles close to Alfonso X, and Alfonso himself, attributed more importance to faith than to science in matters of health and sickness, as if, faced with these problems, natural science could offer no satisfactory answers.[15]

I shall not attempt in this paper to analyze all these problems in depth, though I will allude to many of them in passing. Instead, I shall dwell on the four elements in thirteenth-century Castile whose contributions (or failure to contribute) had important consequences for medicine: the universities; the cathedrals and monasteries; the Jews; and the mendicant orders.

I

The university is undoubtedly the most important and lasting scientific institution of the late Middle Ages. Throughout Europe from the thirteenth century onward, it developed into the preeminent location for the conduct of the processes of scientific assimilation, elaboration, and transmission. This institution is crucial to our understanding of the development of medical science in the late Middle Ages, and it is a fundamental part of our effort to explain certain sociomedical phenomena, such as the status of the medical profession and its subjugation to social controls.[16]

[13] *Las siete partidas del rey don Alfonso el Sabio,* 3 vols. (Madrid: Real Academia de la Historia [hereafter R.A.H.], 1807); *Opúsculos legales del rey don Alfonso el Sabio,* 2 vols. (Madrid: R.A.H., 1836); Rafael Muñoz Garrido and Carmen Muñíz Fernandez, *Fuentes legales de la medicina española, siglos XIII-XIX* (Salamanca: Universidad de Salamanca, 1969).

[14] See Paul O. Kristeller, "The school of Salerno: its development and its contribution to the history of learning," *Bull. Hist. Med.,* 1945, *17:* 138–94; Vern L. Bullough, *The Development of Medicine as a Profession: The Contribution of the Medieval University to Modern Medicine* (Basel: S. Karger; New York: Hafner, 1966); Ronald J. Doviak, "The University of Naples and the Study and Practice of Medicine in the Thirteenth and Fourteenth Centuries" (Ph.D. diss., City University of New York, 1974); Danielle Jacquart, *Le milieu médical en France du XIIe au XVe siècle* (Geneva: Librairie Droz, 1981); Luis García-Ballester, "Los origenes de la profesion médica en Cataluña: el *collegium* de médicos de Barcelona (1342)," in *Estudios dedicados a Juan Peset Aleixandre,* 2 vols. (Valencia: Universidad de Valencia, 1982), 1: 129–149; Robert S. Gottfried, "English medical practitioners, 1340–1530," *Bull. Hist. Med.,* 1984, *58:* 164–82; Katharine Park, *Doctors and Medicine in Early Renaissance Florence* (Princeton, New Jersey: Princeton University Press, 1985); Luis García-Ballester, Michael R. McVaugh and Agustín Rubio, "Licensing, learning and the control of medical practice in fourteenth-century Valencia" (forthcoming).

[15] I am studying the medical aspect of the *Cantigas* using both the text and the miniatures of MS. Escorial T.I.I.

[16] "Thus one of the purposes of the university was to initiate the professional into a set of attitudes and controls, to give him a professional conscience, and to develop a feeling of group solidarity." Vern L. Bullough, "Achievement, Professionalization, and the University," in *The Universities in the Late Middle Ages,* ed. Jozef Ilsewijn and Jacques Paquet (Louvain, Belgium: Leuven University Press, 1978), p. 508.

During the thirteenth century, faculties of medicine were being formed within the universities around an academic syllabus that would prove to be extremely sensitive to innovations arriving in the form of works by Greek and Arab doctors. These contributions shaped the curriculum, but at the same time they caused important changes in the scientific production of the faculty members.[17] Generally, we can assert that the final years of the thirteenth century and the first decade of the fourteenth marked the high point of medical scholasticism, which was full of such freshness and vigor and which proved to be so efficient at providing answers to the medical problems raised by the ruling minorities of the age that it was highly attractive to non-Christian scientific minorities like the Jews.[18] Now, in spite of the legal documents of Alfonso X's period, it does not seem that there was any medical instruction or even medical scholarship in any of the universities or *studia generales* in the territories covered by the Crown of Castile. It is not surprising that the outstanding medical figure in thirteenth-century Spain, Arnald of Villanova (c. 1240–1311), was not from the Crown of Castile but from the Crown of Aragon; moreover, he was able to receive scholastic medical training at a *studium* (Montpellier) in the Crown of Aragon.[19]

In his classic work *The Universities of Europe in the Middle Ages,* Hastings Rashdall indicates three general characteristics of the thirteenth-century Castilian *studia* or universities: their close relationship with the crown; the strong influence exerted on them by the cathedral chapter; and their economic system of maintenance based on ecclesiastical tithes. In addition, Rashdall notes that each realm had to have its own university.[20] Alfonso X's kingdom (the Crown of Castile) comprised, unified under the person of the king, the former kingdoms of Castile and Leon, as well as extensive new territories in Andalusia and the kingdom of Murcia; these last two came under the sovereignty of the Crown of Castile between 1243 (capitulation of the kingdom of Murcia) and 1248 (conquest of Seville).

In what had formerly been the kingdom of Castile, two universities existed in the thirteenth century, in Palencia and in Valladolid. It may be that medicine was discussed at Palencia in its golden years (1215–20), when a

[17] Luke Demaitre, *Doctor Bernard de Gordon: Professor and Practitioner* (Toronto: Pontifical Institute of Mediaeval Studies, 1980); Nancy G. Siraisi, *Taddeo Alderotti and His Pupils: Two Generations of Italian Medical Learning* (Princeton, New Jersey: Princeton University Press, 1981); Luis García-Ballester, "Arnau de Vilanova (c. 1240–1311) y la reforma de los estudios médicos en Montpellier (1309): el Hipócrates latino y la introducción del nuevo Galeno," *Dynamis,* 1982, *2:* 97–158.

[18] This phenomenon, which I have termed "the reflux of scholasticism" ("Aproximación a la historia social de la medicina bajomedieval en Valencia," *Cuadernos de Historia de la Medicina Española,* 1969, *8:* 45–78), is being analyzed from the viewpoint of the Hebrew language by Dolores Ferre in her doctoral thesis on the Hebrew translations of Arnald of Villanova's medical works. The first results are to be found in her master's thesis "La traducción hebrea de las 'Parabole medicationis' de Arnau de Vilanova" (Universidad de Granada, 1983).

[19] Michael R. McVaugh, "Arnald of Villanova," in *DSB,* ed. Charles C. Gillispie, 16 vols. (New York: Charles Scribner's Sons, 1970), 1: 289–91.

[20] Hastings Rashdall, *The Universities of Europe in the Middle Ages,* new edition by Frederick M. Powicke and Alfred B. Emden, 3 vols. (Oxford: At the Clarendon Press, 1936), 2: 64–65.

clear connection existed between this *studium* and the cathedral school at Chartres in matters related to the trivium and the quadrivium,[21] and may have extended to *libri naturales* and *medicinalis scientia*. But the *studium* of Palencia had disappeared by 1250, while there is no evidence for the teaching of medicine at Valladolid in this century.

The university of Salamanca, in the kingdom of Leon, had had a rather precarious existence from its foundation shortly before 1230 by Alfonso IX. It was revitalized by Ferdinand III (1217–52) and by Alfonso X (1252–84). Indeed, it was by the latter's action in 1254 that, for the first time in either Castile or Leon, a *studium generale* was given an endowment for two chairs for the teaching of medicine. But the endowment that these chairs received was scanty, to say the least—on a par with that given the humble disciplines that constituted Leon's so-called arts faculty, and five times smaller than that given the chairs in law.[22]

We should also note that Alfonso X's obvious personal interest in academic and sociomedical matters cannot be shown to have been translated into established institutions. The king's preoccupation with such matters is clear in the second and seventh *Partidas*;[23] in the second book of *El Espéculo*;[24] and in the famous law of book 4 of the *Fuero Real*, which provides for social control of the medical profession.[25]

But as a whole these texts reveal a lack of coherence—or even a contradiction. In some, university chairs are referred to; in others, no mention of them is made. Some texts seem to presuppose the circulation of scientific and medical ideas, which can only be explained by the existence of academic institutions, while others follow prescholastic patterns typical of the early Middle Ages. Unfortunately, we still have no critical editions of either the *Fuero Real* (whose very existence is proven only for the 1290s) or the second and seventh *Partidas*; for that matter, we do not yet have a full historical analysis of these legal texts.[26]

It is not in the thirteenth, not even in the fourteenth, but in the fifteenth century that we first find convincing evidence of a functioning medical faculty at Salamanca. The first professor in medicine we can identify there is

[21] Francisco Rico, "La clerecía del mester," *Hispanic Rev.*, 1985, *53*: 1–23. Rico's article is of great interest since it offers us a clue to understanding the attitudes, which we shall discuss later, of the Castilian Franciscans Pedro Gallego (c. 1200–1267) and Juan Gil of Zamora.

[22] Rashdall, *Universities of Europe*, 2: 65–90; Enrique Esperabé Arteaga, *Historia pragmática e interna de la universidad de Salamanca*, 2 vols. (Salamanca: F. Núñez Izquierdo, 1914–17), 1: 22; Vicente de la Fuente, *Historia de la universidades, colegios, y demás establecimientos de enseñanza en España*, 3 vols. (Madrid, 1884–89), 1: 295.

[23] The titles of these laws are: "Who shall be physicians of the king, and what they must do" (*Part.* 2, tit. 9, law 10) and "How the physicians or spicemerchant who offers or sells herbs knowingly in order to kill another shall receive the penalty due to murder" (*Part.* 7, tit. 8, law 7).

[24] *Espéculo*, ed. Gonzalo Martínez Díez (Avila: Fundación Sánchez Albornoz, 1985), pp. 152–53: book 2, tit. 12, law 4.

[25] *Fuero Real*, book 4, tit. 16, law 1, in *Opúsculos legales del rey don Alfonso el Sabio*, 2: 146.

[26] Alfonso García Gallo, "Nuevas observaciones sobre la obra legislativa de Alfonso X," *Anuario de Historia del Derecho Español*, 1976, *46*: 609–70.

Joan Ruis,[27] teaching in 1406—a century and a half after Alfonso X had decreed "I see fit to order that there shall be ... two professors in medicine" (1254).[28] Significantly, it is in this century, in 1468, that we first have proof of the presence of scientific texts in Salamanca's library:[29] Aristotle's *Libri naturales,* which were already currency in most European universities after 1250 and provided a methodological and biological basis for a science of medicine,[30] and the writings of Hippocrates and Galen, many of which had been translated into Latin at Toledo in the second half of the twelfth century and had become the basis for a profound renovation of scholastic medicine at, for example, Bologna and Montpellier about 1300.[31] The clearest indication of the weakness of thirteenth-century Castilian university institutions is the fact that it seems to have taken nearly two hundred years for the University of Salamanca to attain the levels achieved by, and discover the material characteristics of, scholastic medical institutions elsewhere in Europe. It would seem, in fact, as if the Castile of Alfonso X were indifferent to the upheaval caused in European intellectual circles by the collection of works we have mentioned, even though many of them had come into existence at Castilian Toledo.

II

In addition to the university, two other medieval institutions played an important role in the circulation of medical ideas: the monastery and the cathedral chapters. The latter were closely linked to the universities.

There has not yet been any systematic research into the contents of Castilian monastic libraries from the thirteenth century (or, for that matter, from previous ones) which would enable us to draw definite conclusions, but the little information that is available lets us state quite firmly that the economic stability achieved by the monasteries in this century was accompanied neither by intellectual growth nor by an interest in the new methods

[27] The first proof we have that the two chairs in medicine were actually functioning comes in 1406, when Joan Ruis was professor. See Vicente Beltrán de Heredia, *Cartulario de la universidad de Salamanca, 1218–1600* (Salamanca: Universidad de Salamanca, 1970), p. 659; Salamanca, *Archivo universitario,* book 1647, fols. 35–36.

[28] Esperabé Arteaga, *Historia de la universidad de Salamanca,* 1: 22.

[29] At this date appearing for the first time we find Aristotle and Albert the Great's writings on biology and natural philosophy; the medical works of Salerno; Hippocratic and Galenic writings which entered university circles at Paris, Bologna, and Montpellier in the 1280s and the works of medieval doctors like Johannes de Sancto Amando and Arnald of Villanova (Salamanca, *Archivo universitario,* book 1, fols. 126, 166v, 187v, and 229; book 3, fol. 110v). See also Julio González, *El maestro Juan de Segovia y su biblioteca* (Madrid: C.S.I.C., 1944); Ottokar Bonmann, "De testamento librorum johannis de Segovia," *Antonianum,* 1954, *29:* 209–16; Guy Beaujouan, *Manuscrits scientifiques médiévaux de l'université de Salamanque et de ses "Colegios Mayores"* (Bordeaux: Feret et Fils, 1962), pp. 2–3.

[30] James A. Weisheipl, "The Life and Works of St. Albert the Great," in *Albertus Magnus and the Sciences: Commemorative Essays 1980,* ed. James A. Weisheipl (Toronto: Pontifical Institute of Mediaeval Studies, 1980), pp. 13–51; David Lindberg, *Roger Bacon's Philosophy of Nature: A Critical Edition* (Oxford: Oxford University Press, 1983), p. xvii.

[31] See n. 17.

of learning and scientific production associated with the universities.[32] If we compare the bibliographical resources of two great Castilian monasteries—San Millán de la Cogolla[33] and Silos[34]—with those of the chapters of the most dynamic Castilian cathedrals (e.g., Burgo de Osma and Toledo), our attention is drawn by the intellectual inertia and poverty shown by the Castilian monastic communities, which isolated themselves from the new scholastic science (including medicine) of the thirteenth century.[35] During the thirteenth century, we know only of the interest for astronomy shown by Martín Gil, abbot of the Cistercian monastery of Moreruela (Zamora), to whom Pedro Gallego, bishop of Cartagena, dedicated, between 1260 and 1267, his abbreviated Latin translation of the *Elementa astronomica* of Al-Fārgānī.[36] As we see, Gil's interest was not focused on Latin scholastic science or medicine, but on Arabic astronomy, an interest that was shared by Alfonso X and his court.

Guy Beaujouan remarked that science in the period that concerns us was still carried out in Castile halfway between the Jewish community and the cathedral,[37] and it is indeed in these two places that we find partial answers to the questions being formulated in this paper. I shall not stress here the decisive role played by the cathedral chapters and schools in the cultural and scientific change that took place in Europe during the twelfth century, except to point out that the Spanish cathedrals in Toledo, Leon, Segovia, and the Ebro valley area played an important part in what has been termed with a certain impropriety the cultural and scientific renaissance of Christian Europe in the twelfth century.[38] Did they remain attentive to the world of medical science in the thirteenth century? Or did they close themselves in, thus abandoning this earlier intellectual and scientific leadership? This is something that has not been studied, certainly not for the field of medicine. Now we can offer a kind of answer, at least for the age under

[32] Manuel Díaz y Díaz, "Notas de bibliotecas de Castilla en el siglo XIII," in *Livre et lecture en Espagne et en France sous l'Ancien Régime: Colloque de la Casa de Velázquez* (Paris: Editions A.D.P.F., 1981).

[33] Rudolf Beer, *Handschriftensätze Spaniens* (Vienna, 1894), p. 367.

[34] The manuscript, which lists the bibliographical references, is in the Bibliothèque Nationale, Paris, nouv. acq. lat. 2169, fol. 16v. See also Léopold Delisle, *Nouvelles mélanges de paléographie et de bibliographie* (Paris, 1880), pp. 105–7; Marius Ferotin, *Histoire de l'abbaye de Silos* (Paris, 1897), pp. 262–63.

[35] García-Ballester, "El papel de las instituciones," pp. 36–37.

[36] "Frater P[etrus] divina miseracione cartaginensis episcopus fratri Martini egidii (*marg.* abbati) de Morelola salutem et pacen ..." (fol. 49rb), in Biblioteca Nacional, Madrid (M), 8918, fols. 49rb-56vb (*Incipit* [hereafter *Inc.*]: Quoniam artificum operantis ...). It is listed in Manuel de Castro, *Manuscritos franciscanos de la Biblioteca Nacional de Madrid* (Valencia: Ministerio de E. y C., 1973). This MS has never been used. The only MS known was a fragment: Biblioteca comunale, Sarnano (S) [Macerata], E. 108, fols. 46r-49r, encountered by Gaudenzio Melani, "Un frammento inedito della 'Summa astronomica' del Viscovo francescano Pietro Gallego," *Studi Francescani,* 1943, *15:* 79–89. Melani did not identify Martinus Egidius (Martín Gil) with the abbot of the monastery of Moreruela (Morelola *M,* Merola *S*). María I. Alfonso Antón, *La colonización cisterciense en la meseta del Duero: El ejemplo de Moreruela,* 2 vols. (Madrid: Universidad Complutense, 1983). Neither of these MSS is in Lynn Thorndike and Pearl Kibre, *A Catalogue of Incipits of Mediaeval Scientific Writings in Latin,* rev. ed. (Cambridge, Massachusetts: Medieval Academy of America, 1963).

[37] "à mi-chemin, si l'on peut dire, entre *l'aljama* et la cathédrale." Beaujouan, *La science en Espagne,* p. 21.

[38] See Charles H. Haskins's classic work *Studies in the History of Mediaeval Science* (Cambridge, Massachusetts: Harvard University Press, 1924).

discussion, by focusing again upon the book, the vehicle for disseminating medical science in the medieval world.

By studying the Castilian cathedral libraries that have been conserved or by gathering information about what they contained, we can begin to evaluate their role in the complex processes of scientific communication and transmission. Unfortunately, here once again we are faced with a paucity of material. Only one trustworthy thirteenth-century inventory remains for what must have been the rich contents of Galician cathedral libraries.[39] I have not found catalogues from the cathedrals of Astorga or Palencia; in Burgos there is nothing for the thirteenth century;[40] what there is for Sigüenza is lacking in medical significance,[41] and the same is true for Cordoba;[42] nor is there anything in Seville or in Cartagena-Murcia. So it is not at all surprising that what we know of the library resources of thirteenth-century Salamanca[43] should not give us the slightest hint of any interest in medical literature, scholastic or prescholastic, despite the formal provision of two chairs in medicine there. Yet this is in keeping with what we have already concluded about the unimportance and perhaps even the absence of medical instruction at Salamanca in this period.

Nevertheless, the material that existed in the libraries of four Castilian cathedrals—Zamora,[44] Oviedo,[45] Burgo de Osma,[46] and Toledo[47]—allows

[39] It was published by Henri Omont, "Catalogue de la bibliothèque de Bernard II, Archévêque de Saint-Jacques-de-Compostelle (1226)," *Bibliothèque de l'Ecole des Chartres,* 1893, *54:* 327–33. There are no medical works, although among the borrowed books (which for that reason are not included in the inventory) is "Totum Avizennemum in tribus corporibus." Bernard II was archbishop of Santiago between 1224 and 1237; it would seem that he studied at Paris. The library is rich in books on law and the Scriptures, as well as on the subjects studied at the so-called arts faculties. The "Totum Avizennemum" would have fallen into this last category, since it no doubt belonged to the group of Avicenna's works translated into Latin by Domingo Gundisalvo in Toledo in the second half of the twelfth century (whose nucleus is the *Sufficientia* or *Kitāb al-Shifā',* an encyclopedia in four parts: logic, physics, mathematics, and metaphysics). Avicenna's Aristotelianism dominated the arts faculties until the arrival of the new version by Averroës of Aristotle's writings on natural philosophy. See Georges C. Anawati, "Ibn Sīnā," in *DSB* (suppl. 1), 15: 494. On Archbishop Bernard II and his library, see the opinions of Antonio García y García, *La canonística medieval en Galicia* (Santiago de Compostela: Universidad de Santiago, 1981), pp. 21–25. Unfortunately, owing to lack of chronological data, the work of José Vill-Amil y Castro, "Los códices de las iglesias de Galicia," *Revista de Archivos, Bibliotecas y Museos,* 1873, *3:* 283–85, 297–99, 309–11, 328–31, 346–51, 363–67, 370–73; 1874, *4:* 141–42, 152–56, 170–72, 218–20 and 348–51, cannot be used for our purposes.

[40] The earliest inventories of the Burgos cathedral library belong to the late fourteenth and early fifteenth centuries, and correspond to donations and legacies from canons and bishops. Archivo de la catedral, Burgos, MS no. 53, fols. 619–49; Demetrio Mansilla, *Catálogo de los códices de la catedral de Burgos* (Madrid: Instituto Enrique Flórez, 1952), pp. 15, 155–73, and 175.

[41] José Rius Serra, "Inventario de los manuscritos de la catedral de Sigüenza," *Hispania Sacra,* 1950, *3:* 431–65.

[42] Antonio García y García, Francisco Cantelar Rodríguez and Manuel Nieto Cumplido, *Catálogo de los manuscritos e incunables de la catedral de Córdoba* (Salamanca: Universidad Pontificia de Salamanca, 1976).

[43] Manuel Gómez Moreno, "Inventario de la catedral de Salamanca (año 1275)," *Revista de Archivos, Bibliotecas y Museos,* 1902, *7:* 175–80; Florencio Marcos Rodríguez, "La antigua biblioteca de la universidad de Salamanca," *Hispania Sacra,* 1961, *14:* 281–319.

[44] Maria L. Guadalupe, "El tesoro del cabildo zamorano: aproximación a una biblioteca del siglo XIII," *Studia Historica* (*Historia Medieval*), 1983, *1:* 167–80.

[45] Juan I. Ruiz de la Peña, "Alfonso Nicolás, burgués de Oviedo y alcalde del Rey," *Asturiensia Medievalia,* 1975, *2:* 113–76.

[46] Tomás Rojo Orcajo, "Catálogo descriptivo de los códices que se conservan en la Santa Iglesia Catedral de Burgo de Osma," *Boletín de la Real Academia de la Historia,* 1929, *94:* 655–792; *95:* 152–314.

[47] José M. Millás Vallicrosa, *Las traducciones orientales en los manuscritos de la biblioteca de la catedral de Toledo* (Madrid: C.S.I.C., 1942).

us to identify a number of interesting developments in the transmission of scientific and medical ideas in thirteenth-century Castile, developments that were basically concentrated in the period of Alfonso X's reign. Having studied this material, I have been able to establish the following points:

1. What Beccaria has called "pre-Salernitan medical literature"[48] was still circulating in Castile in the thirteenth century. This literature was composed of a limited legacy from classical Greek medicine, and literature of a lesser order, of poor scientific quality, even including superstitious elements, which was written between the fifth and eleventh centuries. These short works of a practical nature gave advice in the form of remedies using medicinal herbs.[49] This literature had enjoyed a wide diffusion elsewhere in Europe but only up to the eleventh century.

2. In the second half of the thirteenth century, virtually the entire corpus of Salernitan literature arrived in Castile, including both the medical works written before Constantine[50] and the first translations by Constantine and Johannes Afflacius, as well as the elaborations carried out throughout the twelfth century. This corpus contained two different kinds of medical texts. First, a number of general treatises that eventually fused into an academic syllabus—the *Articella*—around which the early teaching of the faculties of medicine revolved until late in the Middle Ages; the core of this syllabus included the *Ysagoge* of Johannitius, the *Aphorismi* and *Pronostica* by Hippocrates, short semiological works on the pulse and urine, and, later, the *Tegni* by Galen.[51] Second, a variety of specialized and solidly elaborated treatises concerning three subjects fundamental to medicine: *dieta* (establishing the foundations of what was to become a rich tradition in the Western world), *pharmacia* (the famous *Antidotaria*), and *chirurgia* (a rich production that would continue to be published in the sixteenth century).[52]

3. For the Castilian cathedral chapters, the raw material of Salernitan medical science was material for use and consumption rather than a basis

[48] Augusto Beccaria, *I codici di medicina del periodo presalernitano, secoli IX, X, e XI* (Rome: Edizioni di Storia e Letteratura, 1956), p. 9.

[49] At Zamora cathedral we have identified the *Epistola ad Maecenatem* (*Inc.*: Libellum quam roganti tibi . . .). See Thorndike and Kibre, *Catalogue of Incipits*, col. 817 [hereafter TK]. The *Epistola ad Maecenatem*, which was circulated in the medieval world under the name of Hippocrates, appears in all the manuscripts accompanying other herbaria, such as the *De herba vettonica* of Antonio Musa and the Pseudo-Apuleius. Beccaria, *I codici di medicina*, pp. 143, 144–45, 210, 268–71, 324, 340, 373, 386. In the library of the Bishop of Oviedo, Don Miguel (1289–92), was the *Therapeutica* or *Practica* (*Inc.*: De alopecia et ophyasy. Contingit hec duplex passio . . .) of Alexander of Tralles (c. 525–c. 605), which was probably translated in Ravenna in the seventh century and forms part of the medical writings which link the classical tradition to the Christian scientific world of the early Middle Ages (TK, 259 and 364). Beccaria, *I codici di medicina*, pp. 25, 27, and 409.

[50] The most significant of these, also found in the library of the Bishop of Oviedo, is the *Practica* of Petrocellus (*Inc.*: Medicinalis tractatus specialiter secundum philosophorum . . .), TK, 859.

[51] We have discovered the *Ysagoge* of Johannitius in the cathedral at Burgo de Osma (Rojo Orcajo, "Catálogo descriptivo," pp. 658–63), and a collection of the *Articella* (*Ysagoge, Pronostica, Liber pulsuum* of Philaretus and *De urinis* of Theophilus) in the library of Toledo cathedral, MS 97–25, fols. 1–52v (Millás Vallicrosa, *Las traducciones orientales*, pp. 125–27).

[52] In a thirteenth-century inventory of the cathedral at Burgo de Osma we have found the *Liber urinarum* of Ishāq b. Sulaymān al-Isrā'īlī [Isaac Judaeus] (*Inc.*: In latinis quidem libris . . .); the *Megategni* of Galen (*Inc.*: Quoniam intentio gloriosissimi . . .); the *Liber pantegni* of 'Alī b. al-'Abbās al-Mağūsī [Haly Abbas]; the *Viaticum of Abū Ğa'far Abū b. Ibrāhīm b. Abī Ḥālid al Ğazzār (Inc.*: Quoniam ut ait tallius . . .); and the commentary of

for original scientific creation.[53] There is not the slightest trace in Castile of the scientific and medical production that Salernitan literature generated as it spread through the rest of Europe during the thirteenth century—and no hint, significantly, of any academic assimilation of the *Articella*.[54]

4. The so-called medical corpus of Toledo cannot be found in the Christian scientific institutions of thirteenth-century Castile. This corpus is the complex of medical works both Greek (basically the famous pathology and therapeutics of Galen) and Arabic (at the head of which we find Avicenna's *Canon,* the authentic key to interpretation, on which traditional Galenic medicine was based until the seventeenth century).[55] Its systematic introduction into European universities did not begin until the 1280s, but it was already being used by scholastic authors fifty years earlier.[56] In Castile, however, where the university was not functioning properly in this period, the corpus could not be absorbed.

Yet, if we have managed to detect the raw material of Salernitan medi-

---

Matthaeus Olatearius on the *Antidotarium Nicolai* (*Inc.*: Liber iste quem in presentia[rum] legendum . . .). For the inventory, see Rojo Orcajo, "Catalogo descriptivo," pp. 658–63.

The thirteenth-century medical manuscripts preserved in the library at Toledo cathedral are nos. 98-3 and 98-4. The medical works from Salerno are: *Liber dietarum* (*Dieta particulares*) (*Inc.*: Complevimus in libro primo universalem significationem granis . . .), MS 98-3, fols. 4r-28vb; *De stomacho* (*Inc.*: Oportet nos intelligere quia prima actio nature . . .), MS 98-4, fols. 75r-83r (TK, 1012); *Pantegni,* trans. Johannes Afflacius, MS 98-4, fols. 46r-59v (TK, 1447); *Antidotarium* (=*Pantegni,* lib. X) (*Inc.*: Antiqui medici bifariam intendunt medicine compositionem in experimentis . . .), MS 98-4, fols. 1r-46r (TK, 110); *Liber de modo medendi et opurgandi tribus modis* (*Inc.*: In medendis corporibus et maxime purgandis variis sepe . . .), MS 98-4, fols. 110r-119v (TK, 691); *Liber pauperum, de capillis cadentibus* (*Inc.*: Capillis ex raritate cadentibus cutis inspissetur . . .), MS 98-4, fols. 59v-72r (TK, 186); *Practica magistri Bartolomei Bituriensis* (*Inc.*: Practica dividitur in duo, in scientiam conservativam sanitatis et curativam egritudinis . . .), MS 98-3, fols. 69v-87va (TK, 1080); *Circa instans,* MS 98-3, fols. 88ra-111ra; MS 98-4, fols. 90rss.; *Rogerina major* (*Inc.*: Sicut ab antiquis habemus auctoribus et eorundem . . .), MS 98-3, fols. 29r-65vb (TK, 1479); *De urinis* de Maurus Salernitanus (*Inc.*: Quoniam de urinarum scientis tractaturi sumus . . .), MS 98-3, fols. 118ra-124ra (TK, 591). For the description of the Toledo manuscripts, see Millás Vallicrosa, *Las traducciones orientales,* pp. 141–44 and 145–47.

[53] The only scholastic activity we have detected at the cathedral school of Toledo during the second half of the thirteenth century was that of Alvaro of Toledo between 1270 and 1300. His work revolved around astrological, astronomical, and cosmological works by Johannes Hispanus, Gerard of Cremona, Alpetragius, Abraham ibn Ezra, and Averroës (*De substantia orbis*). See MSS 47-15 and 98-21 (323-Inv. 1727). Manuel Alonso, *Comentario al "De substantia orbis" de Averroës (Aristotelismo y averroismo) por Alvaro de Toledo* (Madrid: C.S.I.C., 1941); Millás Vallicrosa, *Las traducciones orientales,* pp. 64, 156–66 and 180–202.

[54] We should remember that the first commentaries at Montpellier on Salernitan literature appear at the end of the first third of the thirteenth century, with the commentaries on the *Ysagoge* by Henry of Winchester (*fl.* 1239) and that the definitive introduction of the *Articella* into the curriculum at the University of Montpellier took place in the middle of this century (c. 1240). Michael R. McVaugh, "The 'Humidum radicale' in thirteenth-century medicine," *Traditio,* 1974, *30*: 259–83; and *idem,* "An early discussion of medicinal degrees at Montpellier by Henry of Winchester," *Bull. Hist. Med.,* 1975, *49*: 57–71; García-Ballester, "Arnau de Vilanova," pp. 99–104.

[55] If we widen the scope of our investigation to include the fourteenth-century medical manuscripts that have been preserved at Toledo cathedral, we find two copies of Gerard of Cremona's version of the *Canon* (MSS 47-19 and 47-20). I do not think that their presence in Toledo can be interpreted as proof of a link with the medical tradition of the *corpus toletanum* of the twelfth century. Remember that the *Canon* was first used in medical circles at European universities around 1240. (Danielle Jacquart, "La réception du *Canon* d'Avicenne: comparaison entre Montpellier et Paris aux XIIIe et XIVe siècles," *110ème Congrès Nationale des Sociétés Savantes,* Sect. d'Hist. des Sciences et des Tech., Montpellier, 1–5 April 1985 (in press). I think they are here, not because they had been copied *in situ Toleti,* but, like the rest of the Salernitan literature mentioned, because they were brought and circulated by Castilian clerics educated in Europe. Unfortunately, they have not been studied from a codicological point of view, and therefore I cannot give further details.

[56] For this process at Montpellier and Paris, see my article "Arnau de Vilanova," pp. 109–46; see also Jacquart, "La réception du *Canon.*" For the same process in the north of Italy, see Siraisi, *Taddeo Alderotti and His Pupils.*

cine (from the second half of the eleventh and the twelfth centuries), why have we found none of the raw material of Toledan medicine? To what can we attribute Castile's break with and/or ignorance of its own medical tradition?[57] Why was this rich medical corpus from Toledo not assimilated in Castile, when it was so readily transmitted and creatively elaborated in European universities (Montpellier, Bologna, Paris, and so on)? Only at the end of the thirteenth century do we find an indication of the presence of this corpus in Castile—and then as a re-importation from the universities of Italy and northern Europe—in the career of the Franciscan Juan Gil of Zamora (c. 1240–c. 1320). Juan Gil had studied in Paris and traveled across Italy, England, and France and returned to Castile, not to a university setting, but to the court of Alfonso X, where the king named him tutor to his rebel son and successor, Sancho. Gil wrote a medical work on the poisons and projected a scientific encyclopedia that would describe (in alphabetical order) the contents of the microcosm and macrocosm. The extant portion of his encyclopedia shows a good knowledge of the new scientific and medical texts, but as far as we know, the work never went beyond the letter *A;* nor did that fragment arouse any interest in Castile.[58]

III

We have used Guy Beaujouan's image of the situation of science between the Jewish community and the cathedral to help us explore these most fertile territories for the development of scientific and medical material in Castile in the second half of the thirteenth century. We began by looking at the cathedral. We now turn to the Jewish community's use of medical science.

The first thing we must say is that this subject goes beyond the study of the introduction and transmission of scientific ideas produced in Europe.

[57] I believe that to speak of a medical tradition at Toledo in the twelfth century and those that followed is inappropriate. Everything seems to indicate that Toledo was the place where medical works were translated, but that the work of translation was not followed up by one of copying and elaboration. European scientists came and went. Christian Toledo was a scientific market rather than a place of medical study.

[58] His intention was similar to that of the Dominican Thomas of Cantimpré (c. 1204–c. 1280). Luis García-Ballester, ed., *De natura rerum (lib. IV-XII) por Tomás de Cantimpré . . . Estudio preliminar, transcripción y traducción . . .*, 2 vols. (Granada: Universidad de Granada, 1974), 1: 18–34. The work has been preserved in two manuscripts: Staatsbibliothek Preussischer Kulturbesitz, Berlin, lat. 934, fols. 62–304 (Valentin Rose, *Verzeichnis der lateinischen Handschriften der königlichen Bibliotheke zu Berlin,* 2 vols. [Berlin, 1901–5], 2(3): 1147–51), and Biblioteca de El Escorial, Madrid, P.I. 10, fols. 1–73 (Guillermo Antolin, *Catálogo de códices latinos de la Real Biblioteca de El Escorial,* 5 vols. [Madrid: Imprenta helenica, 1910–16], 3: 263–64). The letter *A* deals with 167 items in more than 1,200 typed pages. Together with Dr. Avelino Domínguez García, I am editing this important scientific encyclopedia, which has rich and interesting medical material and has remained unpublished to date. Domínguez García and García-Ballester, "El tratado *de anathomia* (c. 1280) de Juan Gil de Zamora (c. 1241–c. 1320), " (n. 10). I speak of the little interest in the work in Castile because only two manuscripts have been found. Juan Gil's work on poisons has been edited by Manuel de Castro ("Iohannes Aegidii Zamorensis, OFM, *Contra venena at animalia venenosa:* Introducción, edición y notas," *Archivo Ibero-Americano,* 1976, *36:* 3–116). This edition is based on a Vatican MS (*Urbinates latini* 1404, fols. 1r-99v). I encountered another manuscript copy of the *Contra venena* in Palma de Mallorca (Fundación Bartolomé March. Biblioteca, MSS s.a., 14th c., fols. 1r-107r), which is slightly different from that of the Vatican.

The Jewish communities in Castile during the thirteenth century were still centers that maintained and produced original medical science. Unfortunately, here again there is a paucity of material; there is, however, sufficient material to allow me to make a few statements that, I believe, will help, if not to explain, at least to complicate a little more the picture presented by medicine in thirteenth-century Castile, and, of course, raise a few more questions.

The Christian reconquest of the twelfth and thirteenth centuries led to the flight of most Muslim scholars (including philosophers and physicians) from Castile, and those Muslims who chose to remain encountered increasingly difficult social conditions. Under these circumstances, the learning and the importance of the Muslim or *Mudejar* doctor in Christian Spain was bound to suffer a decline.[59] This does not mean that Greco-Arabic medical literature disappeared from the territories conquered by Christians during the eleventh, twelfth, and thirteenth centuries, from Madrid-Toledo to Seville-Murcia, for it is still to be found there. We are not referring to the persistence of an Arabism expressed in Latin medical literature; we have already seen that the only Latin Arabism in circulation in thirteenth-century Castile was Salernitan. We are referring to the persistence, in thirteenth-century Christian Castile, of medical literature—both by classical Greek authors, especially Galen, and by Arabs, especially Rhazes—written in Arabic.

For while the scientific language for the Christian scientific community elsewhere in Europe was Latin, in the thirteenth century Arabic was still the undisputed language for science in large areas of the Spanish Christian kingdoms, and was used in the Jewish communities and even by such Christian doctors as Arnald of Villanova, who had received a scholastic university training.[60]

This persistence of Arabic-language scientific and medical literature in thirteenth-century Castile had a number of features that should be stressed: (1) It was not at all medical writing of a secondary nature, that is, short, minor treatises; on the contrary, it included the most important and extensive medical writings of Galen and the classical Arabs. (2) This literature was circulated and used in urban centers—because medical science was an urban phenomenon—basically by members of the Jewish minority, though the Christian Mozarabic and the Muslim or *Mudejar* minorities may well have been involved. (3) It was taught and perpetuated in the midst of these communities and was subjected to a limited degree of scholastic elaboration written in Arabic. (4) There is no evidence that these medical writings in Arabic were used by members of the Christian majority in the second half of the thirteenth century in academic centers like the weak university of Sala-

[59] García-Ballester, *Historia social de la medicina,* 1: 29–75; *idem, Los moriscos y la medicina: un capítulo de la medicina y la ciencia marginadas en la España del siglo XVI* (Barcelona: Editorial Labor, 1984).

[60] See n. 19.

manca, or the mixed schools (*studia*) (Arabic-Spanish-Latin-Hebrew) created at this time in Seville and Murcia.[61]

By analyzing the resources in Arabic manuscripts from several libraries,[62] I have been able to establish the existence of a wealth of medical literature in Arabic that was being read and copied in various Castilian cities within the Jewish (and perhaps Muslim) community, and outside the university and the Christian majority. The complex of works in circulation is impressive not only for its diversity but also for its importance.

If we organize this material, we find that the Hippocratic corpus is represented, but only by the *Aphorisms* and books from the *Epidemics* and *On Prognostics*;[63] that is to say, by books that were eminently didactic and clinical in character. On the other hand, it includes the most interesting of Galen's extensive medical production, ranging from his treatises on anatomy and physiology (*De usu partium* and *De facultatibus naturalibus*)[64] to his semiological writings (*De symptomatum differentiis, De differentiis febrium*),[65] writings on pathology (*De locis affectis, De crisibus, De diebus criticis, De differentiis morborum*),[66] on therapeutics and dietetics (*De compositione medicamentorum, De alimentorum facultatibus*),[67] and on hygiene (*De sanitate tuenda*).[68] One of the manuscripts contains, grouped together, the collection of Galen's most important medical works (pathological and clinical) which in Latin scholastic medicine would go under the title *De morbo et accidenti*,[69] and would be the nucleus of the important commentaries on general pathology in the freshest and most attractive scholastic writing during the transition from the thirteenth to the fourteenth century.[70] Together with this impressive sample from the Galenic corpus, works of the great masters of Jewish and Arabic medicine were also in circulation; the writings of Rhazes, Avicenna, Haly Abbas, Avenzoar, and Maimonides were copied frequently and assiduously.[71] Many of these writings had not been translated from Arabic into Latin in the Toledo of the end of the twelfth century, and some of them, by both Greeks (Galen) and Arabs (Rhazes,

[61] Sarton, *Introduction*, 2(2): 834; Beaujouan, *La science en Espagne*, pp. 21–22.

[62] The most interesting data are to be found in the Arabic manuscripts of the Escorial (Hartwig Derenbourg and H.-P.-J. Renaud, *Les manuscrits arabes de l'Escurial*, book 2, fascicle 2, *Médécine et Histoire Naturelle* [Paris: Librairie orientaliste Paul Geuthner, 1911]). My conclusions are based on an analysis of the reading and transmission certificates existing in the manuscripts themselves. On the usefulness of these certificates, see Georges Vajda, *Les certificats de lecture et de transmission dans les manuscrits arabes de la Bibliothèque Nationale de Paris* (Paris: C.N.R.S., 1957).

[63] Derenbourg and Renaud, *Les manuscrits arabes*, p. 83 (no. 873–8).

[64] *Ibid.*, pp. 57 (no. 850), 54 (no. 846).

[65] *Ibid.*, pp. 12 (no. 799-1), 29 (no. 818-2), 56 (no. 849-3).

[66] *Ibid.*, pp. 12 (no. 799-2), 56 (no. 849-2), 55 (no. 849-1), 29 (no. 818-2), 12 (no. 799-1).

[67] *Ibid.*, pp. 14 (no. 801-2), 15 (no. 802-1).

[68] *Ibid.*, p. 16 (no. 802-3).

[69] *Ibid.*, p. 91 (no. 880).

[70] For the commentaries at Montpellier, see García-Ballester, "Arnau de Vilanova," pp. 131–34; for the commentaries at Bologna, see Siraisi, *Taddeo Alderotti and His Pupils*, p. 102.

[71] Derenbourg and Renaud, *Les manuscrits arabes*, pp. 20–84 (nos. 806, 807, 810, 814, 816, 817, 823, 833, 870, 873).

Avenzoar), would not appear in Latin until the 1270s or 1280s, when they contributed in a decisive way to the renovation of scholastic medicine in European university circles[72]—outside of Castile.

The presence and circulation of these works among the Jewish and Muslim communities in thirteenth-century Castile tells us of the vitality and originality of medical science in these minorities, whose knowledge of Arabic guaranteed them access to the most authentic sources of medical science. However, their own medical writings do not yet possess a creative dimension, and tend to be of the nature of medico-scientific *florilegia.* Truly creative elaborations made their appearance among the Jewish community of Castile a century later. They were Arabic manuscripts copied at Toledo in 1376 and at Guadalajara in 1387 using texts of Hippocrates, Galen, Paul Aegineta, Rhazes, Maimonides, ibn Māsawayhi, and others. They were usually in the form of questions and answers, but one extremely important work in essay form has survived.[73] It is interesting to note that the text that was most frequently used to structure this scholastic medical production was the *Ḥāwī* (*Continens*) of Rhazes, and not the *Canon* of Avicenna, the latter a work that was not as well received in Al-Andalus as it was in the Latin Western world.[74] Is this apparent absence of medical creativity in the Jewish communities of the thirteenth century real, or might it be a product of our current very limited knowledge? Scholars today have only a small fraction of these Arabic-Jewish medical writings left to study. The increasing repression and eventual expulsion of the minorities from Spain in the later Middle Ages resulted in the destruction of much of their literature,[75] and cultural factors have continued up to the present to obstruct our knowledge of the portion that has survived.[76]

[72] For example, the Latin version, translated from Arabic, of Galen's work *De interioribus* began to circulate at Montpellier between 1250 and 1300 (Luis García-Ballester and Eustaquio Sánchez Salor, eds., *Arnaldi de Villanova Opera Medica Omnia (AVOMO),* vol. 15, *Commentum supra tractatum Galieni de malicia complexionis diverse* [Barcelona: Universidad de Barcelona, 1985], pp. 31–33; Richard Durling, ed., *AVOMO,* vol. 15, *Doctrina Galieni de interioribus,* pp. 299–302. The *Continens* of Rhazes was not translated into Latin until 1279 (Sarton, *Introduction,* 2(2): 833), and the Latin version of Averroës' *Colliget* did not begin to circulate until 1285 (MS, Biblioteca Malatestiana, Cesena [Italy], D. XXV.4, fol. 28r). On the debate concerning the other possible dates for the translation of the *Colliget* proposed by Steinschneider, see Michael R. McVaugh, ed., *AVOMO,* vol. 2, *Aphorismi de gradibus* (Granada: Universidad de Barcelona, 1975), pp. 61–62.

[73] The most important systematic medical treatise written in Arabic by a Castilian Jewish physician was the *Kitāb al-ṭibb al-qăsṭalī al-malūkī* (*Book of Regal Castilian Medicine*). It was probably written in the first two decades of the fourteenth century; the author was physician to Ferdinand IV, king of Castile (1295–1312). The work is still unpublished. There are two copies, one was finished in Toledo on 10 February 1414 (Christian era). (Biblioteca Nacional, Madrid, Arabic manuscripts, D.C.I., fols. 1r-38v); the other one was copied from the former in 1782 by Mariani Pizzi and has survived in the British Museum (William Cureton, *Catalogus codicum manuscriptorum Orientalium qui in Museo Britannico asservantur,* 3 vols. (London: Imprensis curatorum Musei Britannici, 1838–71), vol. 2, *Codices arabici,* Supplementum, p. 458. Codex DCCCCXXXVI, Add. 11,272). We are preparing a critical edition with Spanish translation and commentaries in collaboration with Professor Concepción Vázquez (University of Salamanca) and Professor Pedro Gil (University of Navarra at Pamplona).

[74] Roger Arnaldez and Albert Z. Iskandar, "Ibn Rushd [Averroës]," in *DSB,* 12: 7b[*sic*]-8. See Derenbourg and Renaud, *Les manuscrits arabes,* pp. 82–84 (nos. 873–8 and 873–11).

[75] García-Ballester, *Historia social de la medicina,* pp. 50–53 and 59–64.

[76] As an example we could cite the interesting Muslim-Spanish manuscripts which have survived in the library of the al-Qārawīyīn at Fez (Morocco) and have not yet been catalogued. For socioreligious reasons these manuscripts were not moved away to Rabat, the capital.

IV

In the field of medicine, therefore, there was a double omission in Castile in the relationship between the Christian Latin world and the Arabic-speaking minorities. In the first place, the translation program from Arabic into Latin or from Arabic into Castilian in thirteenth-century Castile (and in the reign of Alfonso X in particular) did not include any of the medical works that were circulating in Arabic among the Jewish and Muslim minorities in the cities. In the second place, Castilian scientists with Latin scholastic training received in European university circles (men who held ecclesiastical positions in Zamora, Santiago, Salamanca, Cordoba, Burgo de Osma, Sigüenza, and Toledo, as well as some doctors at the court), together with the Castilian university institutions themselves, chose to ignore the flourishing medical knowledge in the Jewish communities of their own cities, knowledge that was used by Jewish or Muslim doctors with whom they must have shared their daily lives.

The only exception to this double omission is to be found in the kingdom of Murcia, which became part of the kingdom of Castile after being conquered from the Moors in 1251–55.[77] There, members of the mendicant orders (Dominicans and Franciscans) showed enough curiosity about Arabic medical science to maintain a small program of translation and study. This program appears to have been limited and localized, yet it is very interesting, for it reveals to us the survival of a pattern of relations between the Latin and Arab scientific and cultural worlds; it suggests that it may have been possible, at the end of the thirteenth century, to renew the process of transmission of medical works from Arabic into Latin in the territories in the south of Castile. These territories were unique in bordering territories of Arab culture (the Muslim kingdom of Granada, North Africa)—which, in fact, was still the dominant culture among the population of the newly won lands—as well as the Mediterranean Sea (which meant that intense commercial and cultural relations were quickly established with northern and southern Italy after the Christian conquest).[78]

The first translations from Arabic to Latin in these territories were made by the Franciscan Pedro Gallego (c. 1200–1267), who was named first bishop of Cartagena (Murcia) in 1250.[79] During the seventeen years of his bishopric he completed translations of four works with implications for medicine: an abridgement (with personal touches) of the *Liber de animalibus* (*Historia animalium,* books 1–9) of Aristotle,[80] an abridgement of

[77] Julio González, *Reinado y diplomas de Fernando III,* vol. 1, *Estudio* (Cordoba: Publicaciones del Monte de Piedad y Caja de Ahorros de Córdoba, 1980), pp. 340–54.

[78] Juan Torres Fontes, "El obispado de Cartagena en el siglo XIII," *Hispania,* 1953, *13:* 339–580.

[79] A. Pelzer, "Un traducteur inconnu: Pierre Gallego, franciscain et premier evêque de Carthagène (1250–1267)," in Franz Ehrle, *Scritti di storia e paleografia: miscellanea Francesco Ehrle,* 5 vols. (Rome: Biblioteca Apostolica Vaticana, 1924), 1: 408–56; Atanasio López, "Fr. Pedro Gallego, primer obispo de Cartagena (1250–1267)," *Archivo Ibero-Americano,* 1925, *12:* 65–91.

[80] Vatican, *Vat. lat.* MS 1288, fols. 131r–155r. Georgius Lacombe, *Aristoteles latinus.* Codices. Pars prior (Rome: La libreria dello Stato, 1939), p. 226; Pelzer, "Un traducteur inconnu," pp. 435–44.

Averroës' compendium to the *De partibus animalium* (*Historia animalium,* books 1–2, chapter 2) of Aristotle,[81] and a text on *Oeconomia* (*in regitiva domus*), probably based on the pseudo-Galenic work.[82] He also wrote a *Summa astronomica,* in which he appears to summarize the treatise of Al-Fārgānī, *Elementa astronomica.*[83] We do not know if he had carried out any scientific activity before his arrival in Murcia, but we have to remember that he had a strong friendship with Alfonso X and belonged in the court of the king before his appointment as bishop of Cartagena;[84] it is also perfectly possible that the peculiar socioeconomic and socioscientific situation of Murcia provided him with a scientifically stimulating atmosphere.

The second place in Murcia where medical works were translated was the school of Arabic and Hebrew languages (*studium arabicum et hebraicum*) founded by the Dominicans in 1266 for missionary and apologetical purposes. This school was similar to others created in the thirteenth century in the territories on the borders of Christendom ("Germania," "Hungria," "Hispania").[85] For reasons unknown to us, Rufino Alejandrino (from Alessandria in Italy, to the north of Genoa) arrived in Murcia to learn Arabic. He was taught the language there by a Dominican, Dominiscus Marrochinus.[86] With the latter's help he translated at least two works: the first was an ophthalmic work, which he finished in 1271;[87] the second was a group of works collected in a manual like those used in teaching medicine and entitled *Liber quaestionum medicinalium discentibus in medicina,* attributed to "Huneyn filius Ysaac medici qui latine dicitur Johannicius."[88]

This second item is an authentic student textbook, very similar to the *Articella* elaborated in the Latin Christian world of Salerno.[89] It consists of three clearly differentiated parts (*particule*): the first (*theorica seu sciencia*)

[81] Vatican, *Vat. lat.* MS 1288, fols. 159r–161r. Lacombe, *Aristoteles latinus,* p. 227; Pelzer, "Un traducteur inconnu," pp. 446–47.

[82] Vatican, *Barb. lat.* MS 52, fols. 22r–24r; Bibliothèque Nationale, Paris, *lat.* MS 6818, fols. 28r-30v. Pelzer, "Un traducteur inconnu," pp. 423–28.

[83] See n. 36. Professor Julio Samsó of the University of Barcelona is studying the work.

[84] López, "Fr. Pedro Gallego," pp. 68–71.

[85] Ugo Monneret de Villard, *Lo studio dell'Islam in Europa nel XII e nel XIII sècolo* (Vatican City: Biblioteca Vaticana, 1944), pp. 35–37; José M. Coll, "Escuelas de lenguas orientales en los siglos XIII y XIV," *Analecta Sacra Tarraconensia,* 1944, *17:* 132–35; Angel Cortabarría Beitia, "San Ramón de Penyafort y las escuelas dominicanas de lenguas," *Escritos del Vedat,* 1977, *7:* 125–54.

[86] Thomas Kaeppelli, *Scriptores Ordinis Praedicatorum Medii Aevi* (Rome: S. Sabinae, 1970), vol. 1 (A–F), pp. 328–29.

[87] "Explicit libri de egritudinibus oculorum [Iesu filii Haly] translatus Murcie per magistrum Dominicum fratrum predicatorum rogatu magistri Rufini de Alexandria scolaris eius in arabico et sociorum, gracias del alto et vero. Anno domini MCCLXXI." Burgerbibliothek, Bern, 216, fols. 1ra–43vb. This copy dates from 1279 (fol. 43vb).

[88] "Explicit Johannicius translatus a Rufino Alexandrino cum adiutorio magistri sui in arabico fratris Dominici Marrochini de oridine fratrum predicatorum in Murcia de arabico ad latinum. Deo gracias." Staatsbibliothek Amploniana, Erfurt, F 271, fols. 11ra–25rb. In the manuscript (fol. 18vb) there is a mention of "Huneyn filius Ysaac medici qui latine dicitur Johannicius." The first news of this work was given by Moritz Steinschneider, *Die hebraeischen Übersetzungen des Mittelalters und die Juden als Dolmetscher* (Berlin, 1893; reprint, Graz: Akademische-u. Verlagsenstalt, 1956), pp. 710–11.

[89] Paul O. Kristeller, "Bartholomaeus, Musandinus, and Maurus of Salerno and other commentators of the 'Articella,' with a tentative list of texts and manuscripts," *Italia Medioevale e Umanistica,* 1976, *19:* 57–87.

has a question-and-answer format and largely coincides with the original Arabic of the *Isagoge* of Ḥunain b. Ishāq;[90] the second part (*practica*) is devoted to remedies and concludes with a chapter on the pulse (*de pulsu*);[91] and the third part, after a brief chapter on ages (*de etatibus*), is composed of brief writings (*de exercicio, de febribus, de apostema, de urina*).[92] This type of work, with simple contents and a schematic or erotetic (question-and-answer) presentation, often aroused greater interest among Christian, Jewish, and Arab doctors in the late Middle Ages than the extensive and complex works of the Greek and Arab masters. That this Arabic-language students' manual should have been current in Murcia between the years 1270 and 1280 is of great interest, and tells us of the presence and circulation among the Muslim and Christian population of a medical literature elaborated and prepared for didactic purpose, in addition to telling us of the existence of another Latin version of the *Isagoge* and "another" *Articella* overlooked by scholars.

V

> Medicine, as the learned Ancients showed, means both the knowledge to recognise things as they are according to nature and to know the influence of each thing on the others; thus those who possess this skill in abundance can do much good and cure many ills, especially by looking after men's lives and health, ridding them of illnesses in which they suffer great injury or come close to death. And those who do this are called physicians, who not only fight to cure men's illnesses but also keep them in health so that they may not become ill.[93]

This text from the second *Partida* makes it clear that the Castile of Alfonso X accepted the importance of medicine as a social activity and of physicians as a peculiarly skilled group. What emerges from the rest of the scanty information available to us, as I have tried to show, is that this acceptance does not seem to have entailed an interest in the new medical science becoming available in the thirteenth century. In Christian Castile, neither the institutions that had traditionally been the means of preserving and communicating knowledge in the earlier Middle Ages—the monasteries and the cathedrals—nor the emerging universities that would take their place, give any evidence of paying attention to the new translations of Greco-Arabic texts that had been produced in their very midst, in twelfth-century Toledo. While Castilian Jews (and perhaps Muslims) assimilated this scientific literature, there remained a gulf between their medicine and that of the Christian community. Christian Castile finally became acquainted with

[90] Erfurt, F 271, fols. 11ra–13vb.

[91] *Ibid.*, fols. 13vb–20rb.

[92] *Ibid.*, fols. 20rb–vb (*de etatibus*), 20vb–21va (*de exercicio*), 21va–23rb (*de febribus*), 23rb–va (*de apostemate*), 23va–25rb (*de urina*).

[93] *Part.* 2, tit. 9, law 10.

Salernitan medicine in the early thirteenth century, and went no further for a long time.

These circumstances pose a difficult question for future historians to answer. Castile possessed cultures in which sophisticated medical learning was very much alive; it was the source from which most of that new learning made its way, in Latin, to the rest of Christian Europe; it had a monarch apparently supportive of scientific inquiry; and it shared in the new university movement of the thirteenth century. It would seem, therefore, to have been even more progressive in these ways than its neighboring kingdom in the Iberian peninsula, the Crown of Aragon—yet Aragon shows plainly the powerful effect of the new knowledge, and Castile does not.

What lines of interpretation may eventually prove to be useful in explaining this anomaly? It may be that the mood of the *reconquista* in Castile was harsher, less willing to profit from a pagan culture than was the case in Aragon; or that Castile had a generally less developed urban society, in which the new medicine could flourish; or that the personal interests of Alfonso X were fixed upon astronomy to the detriment of medicine, while those of Jaime II of Aragon (1291–1327) were markedly in the new scholastic medicine; or that Castilian universities were too weak to be able to sustain the new learning. Other factors could be suggested. But at the moment we are still too poorly informed to be able to decide which, if any, of these factors played a part. All we can do for now is acknowledge the paradox that Christian Castile, which gave so much Greco-Arabic medical learning to the Latin West, showed no interest in making use of it.

Nature and Science in Thirteenth-Century Castile.
The Origins of a Tradition: the Franciscan and Dominican *Studia* at Santiago de Compostela (1222-1230)*

To José Mª López Piñero, who has opened up new frontiers as regards research and teaching within the fields of the history of medicine and the history of science, and who knows how to teach one to conquer them.

I

One of the periods in the history of Spain most neglected by researchers within the field of the history of science, and, perhaps for that same reason, one of the least well-known, is the first half of the thirteenth century. And our lack of knowledge is most acute as regards the scientific activity that might have been undertaken during that period in the lands that, from the 1230s onwards, were known as Castile, stretching from Galicia and the Cantabrian coastline in the north to the distant southern frontier of the kingdom, which by the middle of that century reached as far as both the Atlantic and the Mediterranean, following the conquest of the Guadalquivir valley and the Kingdom of Murcia.[1] The aim of this article is to carry out a preliminary analysis of three hitherto unknown centres of scientific activity in the city of Santiago de Compostela in the first third of the thirteenth century. This will enable us to pose certain questions as

---

* I would like to thank Jaume Riera (ACA, Barcelona) for correcting my first draft of the transcription of the document, some of whose suggestions have been included in this version. Without the help of Pedro Cátedra (University of Salamanca) and of Adeline Rucquoi (CNRS, Paris) I would have been unable to identify *items* 26, 46 and 47. Guy Beaujouan (Paris) pointed out some interesting clues for *item* 34, for the identification of which I am in debt to André Allard (University of Brussels). I would also like to thank Fr Antonio García y García (Pontifical University of Salamanca) and Fr Isaac Vázquez Janeiro (Pontifical University of Salamanca) for their corrections and suggestions concerning both the article itself and the transcription of the document, as well as Fr José Mª Alonso del Val (Santander), Fr Cándido Zubizarreta (Sanctuary of Aránzazu) and Andrew Cunningham (Cambridge) for their assistance in the search for bibliography, and Michael R. McVaugh for reading the English version.

[1] See, for example, the recent chapter written by J. SAMSÓ, 'Las ciencias exactas y físico-naturales', in García de Cortázar, J. A. (coordinator), *La época del gótico en la cultura española (ca.1220-ca.1480)* volume XVI of Jover Zamora, J. M. (ed.), *Historia de España Menéndez Pidal*. Madrid, 1994, pp. 553-593, in which no scientific activity is mentioned in Castile prior to the second half of the thirteenth century (p. 556).

regards the promotion of science (natural philosophy) in Castile in the first half of the thirteenth century.

The recent publication of an important document,[2] written in Santiago de Compostela and dated to the 1220s and 1230s, now in the Vatican Library (Vat. Lat. 659, fol. 1r), enables us to reconsider the origins of the tradition of natural philosophy studies in the Hispanic kingdoms (Galicia, Kingdom of León and Kingdom of Castile) and to give these studies their proper place as part of the attention paid to the study of nature, both in the Hispanic kingdoms and in the rest of Europe, by members of the recently founded Franciscan and Dominican orders. The above-mentioned document, hitherto unstudied from the point of view of the history of science, not only confirms the leading role of Galician Franciscans and Dominicans in this intellectual achievement, but also enables us to trace the roots in the Iberian Peninsula of the scientific activity carried out by members of these orders in Castile during the second half of the thirteenth century. This activity included that promoted by the Franciscan bishop Pedro Gallego and a group of Dominicans in the frontier lands of Murcia in the period between 1250 and 1280,[3] and that carried out around 1280 by Juan Gil at the Franciscan *Studium* of Zamora, which was brought together in his *Historia Naturalis*.[4]

The document, of considerable significance for the intellectual history of southern Europe, sheds lights on the intellectual activity of the Franciscans and Dominicans in their recently founded *Studia* in their respective Santiago de Compostela communities (dating from the year 1220, and certainly prior to 1222, at least as far as the Franciscans are concerned). These dates coincide with the earliest records of similar activity on the part of the Grey Friars in their Oxford house, founded in 1224 under the protection of Robert Grosseteste, and the activity undertaken by the Black Friars at Saint Jacques in Paris (1218). The contents of the document provide the key that enables us to explain why a number of Franciscans and Dominicans in the lands of Castile devoted themselves to the study of the natural things (from metaphysics, geometry, astronomy-astrology, physics and medicine, to the whole series of subjects now

[2] DE CASTRO, M., 'La biblioteca de los franciscanos de Val de Dios, de Santiago (1222-1230)', *Archivo Ibero-Americano*, 53 (1993) 151-162. This article corrects the one by D. DE BRUYNE, 'Une liste de manuscrits pretés au XIII siècle à des frères mineurs', *Antonianum*, 5 (1930) 229-232. De Bruyne confused 'Vallis Dei' with 'Vallis viridis', a Franciscan house that was moved to the vicinity of the University of Paris in 1230; neither did he take into account the fact that the document was dated according to the Era of Spain, and he thus attributed it to the year 1260.

[3] GARCÍA BALLESTER, L., 'Medical Science in thirteenth-century Castile: problems and prospects', *Bull. Hist. Med.*, 61 (1987) 183-202, at pp. 199-200.

[4] *Johannes Aegidius Zamorensis. Historia Naturalis.* Introducción, edición crítica, traducción castellana e índices by A.Domínguez and L. García Ballester, 3 vols. Valladolid, 1994.

known as biology) in the thirteenth century. In the case of the Franciscans, this process was to culminate at the end of the century in the partially successful attempt to put together a monumental scientific encyclopaedia which aimed to place the whole range of knowledge related to nature at the disposition of those who did not frequent university circles. On reading the contents of the above-mentioned document, a wide range of pieces of information dating from different moments of the thirteenth century, relating to the attention paid by certain Franciscan and Dominican friars towards questions connected with mathematics (astronomy, astrology) and the natural sciences, started to fall into place. This led me to study the document and to focus this article on trying to follow up the lead that finally takes us to the scientific encyclopaedia drawn up by Juan Gil, who sought to emulate the achievement of his fellow Friar Minor, Bartholomew the Englishman, a younger contemporary of his and the author of the lengthy *De proprietatibus rerum*, a work which, whether read in the original Latin or vernacular versions, introduced generations of Europeans from the thirteenth until well into the sixteenth century to rational knowledge of nature. However, I must confess that I did not even suspect the existence of this lead during the more than ten years that, in collaboration with Avelino Domínguez, I devoted to editing and translating Juan Gil of Zamora's *Historia naturalis*. Indeed, the scarcity of documentary evidence for intellectual life in the early thirteenth-century Iberian peninsula is one of the main reasons for emphasising the importance of the document in question.

However, why were the Franciscans and Dominicans in particular involved, and why at such an early date as the 1220s? Why was it in Santiago de Compostela that a centre of intellectual activity that paid attention to the most recently produced works of the seats of learning of Latin Christendom was created? Allow me to digress for a moment in order to consider certain very specific episodes within the activity carried out by Francis of Assisi and Dominic Guzmán, the founders of the Friars Minor and the Friars Preacher respectively.

II

In the little more than twenty years that elapsed between 1205, when Francis of Assisi (born in 1181) embarked upon a new life, and his death in October 1226, he strove to remind the southern European society of his time of the advisability of living in accordance with the advice and rules to be found in the Gospels.[5] A

---

[5] I have used the edition by GUERRA, J. A., *San Francisco de Asís. Escritos, biografías, documentos de la época,* 5th ed., Madrid, 1993. English edition by HABIG, M.A., ed., *St. Francis of Assisi. Writings and Early Biographics.* English Omnibus of the Sources for the life of St. Francis, 3rd ed., Chicago, 1973.

very similar decision was taken in Montpellier in 1206 by the already mature Dominic (born *ca.*1175), subprior of the cathedral chapter of Osma, when, in the company of his bishop, Diego, he stated that only the exemplary nature of one's own life, together with poverty and austerity, would make preaching efficacious.[6] This was not a new development within the contemporary panorama of deeply-felt spiritual currents that affected the whole of Europe and which demanded that Christianity should be reformed on the basis of evangelical poverty and simplicity. Such movements were of an extremely popular nature, often proclaiming the need for spiritual reforms together with a demand for social reforms. Nevertheless, some of these movements, such as Catharism, linked their spirituality with rejecting the material world and preached a form of Manichaeanism in which a return to evangelical roots was incompatible with the beauty of the world; in which the material nature of all bodies, both heavenly and earthly ones, including the human body, had to be rejected and associated with the idea of sin; in which any intellectual activity oriented towards investigating the material world that surrounds us and in which we are immersed was considered to be highly suspect.[7]

At all times Dominic Guzmán, a cleric who formed part of circles that experienced the intellectual renewal of the second half of the twelfth century with a certain degree of intensity (we should remember that he had received his training in the liberal arts in the Palencia *Studium*, which was intellectually linked to the Chartres circle,[8] and that he himself belonged to the intellectually aware Osma chapter), insisted that preaching should be based on full knowledge of the Scriptures and that preachers should be intellectually prepared for their task.[9] In 1233 Juan of Navarre, one of the young intellectuals who followed Dominic Guzmán and the founder of the house of Saint Jacques in Paris, recalled Dominic's insistence when 'he would advise and exhort the brothers of the order, both by word of mouth and by means of letters, to study the New Testament and

---

[6] I have used the edition by GALMES, L., GÓMEZ, V. T. *et al.*, *Santo Domingo de Guzmán. Fuentes para su conocimiento.* Madrid, 1987.

[7] BAZELL, DIANNE M., *Christian diet: a case study using Arnald of Villanova's De esu carnium*, Cambridge, Mass., 1991 (PhD dissertation, Harvard University). See, among others, DONDAINE, A., (editor), *Le liber de duobus principiis*, Rome, 1939; THOUZELLIER, CH., *Catharisme et Valdéisme en Languedoc à la fin du XIIe siècle et au début du XIIIe,* Paris, 1966; DUVERNOY, J., *Le Catharisme. La réligion des cathares,* Toulouse, 1976.

[8] RICO, F., 'La clerecía del mester', *Hispanic Rev.*, 53 (1985) 1-23.

[9] GALMES, L., GÓMEZ, V. T. *et al.*, (note 6), General introduction to *Santo Domingo de Guzmán*, pp. 3-74. On the meaning of the intellectual renovation of the Church, and the consequent new vision of nature, man and the cosmos, as well as the rise of the new theology and the dream of a new Christianity, see the still indispensable work by M.-D. CHENU, *La théologie au douzième siècle,* Paris, 1957 (2nd ed., Paris, 1966).

the Old constantly...; to concentrate on their study with great diligence'.[10] Francis of Assisi, who did not belong to intellectually aware clerical circles,[11] insistently proclaimed the value of the beauty of material things; in fact, not only did he not demonise the creatures that surround man or man himself, the material component of the human being, but he even made the world a positive element in his reform programme for Christianity, which was none other than a return to the simplicity of the Gospels. Making use of an old tradition within Christian writings, not only did he insist that nothing associated with human beings should be rejected by Christians, but also that all the goodness and beauty that there is in the world should be taken into account by Christians. Moreover, even illness itself and the biological fact of death were stripped of their hideousness and adversity. It is significant that the famous 'The Song of Brother Sun' (or 'Praises of God in this Creatures') was written by Francis of Assisi when his body was in a feeble state, much weakened by a painful illness that was to cause his death.; it is also significant that it was written in a state of intense mysticism (after the well-known episode of the stigmata),[12] and that the latter did not cut him off from the world, but rather produced in him a greater attention for everyday material things that define the very concept of life. In this work, there is a review of each and every one of the components of what in medieval culture was known by the names of 'macrocosmos' and 'microcosmos', which brought all creatures together in one unity, from the heavens to the earth, from the stars to the blade of grass, illness and bodily death itself. 'The Song... ' is a call to humankind, to all human beings, to make them understand that Christianity is a call for the total salvation of the world, of which all the elements that make it up form part; it is a commitment to comprehensive salvation among all the natural beings that comprise the cosmos.

> Be praised, my Lord, with all Your creatures,/ especially brother Sun,/... he is beautiful and radiant.../ Be praised, my Lord, by sister moon and the stars/ in heaven You made them, bright, precious and beautiful /... by brother wind, / and the air..., and any weather,/ ... by sister water,/ which is very useful.., and precious, .../, by brother fire,/... it is ... vigorous and strong./... by sister our mother earth,/ which sustains...us,/ And produces various fruits with colourful flowers and grass./ illness

[10] GALMES, L., GÓMEZ, V. T. *et al.*, (note 6), pp. 159-160.

[11] His studies did not go beyond the elementary ones offered by the grammar school of his city of origin, GUERRA, J. A., Introduction to *San Francisco de Asís* (note 5), p. 7.

[12] *Ibid.*, p. 48-49.

> and tribulation.../ by sister our bodily death.../ May my Lord be praised and blessed.[13]

The movement inspired by Dominic and Francis was particularly successful among young men belonging to the intellectual circles of the new towns and cities, as well as among young monks (for instance Cistercians) who were keen to live the adventure of a renewed form of Christianity to the full; these young men knew how to make the message of evangelical life centred upon poverty compatible with their intellectual calling.[14] Francis himself, when drawing up his first Rule (1221), which synthesised his thoughts and acted as a guide for those who followed them, insisted that 'the brothers who know how to work should work and exercise the craft that they know... Each one should remain in the art and craft to which he has been called', and he encouraged them and authorised them 'to have the utensils and means necessary for their crafts'.[15] Work, which for Francis was not a punishment but an instrument of salvation, should be well done (*fideliter*), carried out with joy and make us particularly pleasant, for it is something positive that God sends us.[16] The industriousness of the new urban middle class was identified with this spirituality that offered such a positive view of daily work (whether intellectual or manual) and made it compatible with the message of salvation and spiritual and social reform that was demanded by the new Christianity, which was based on the message contained in the Gospels in

---

[13] *Ibid.*, p. 49-50. English translation by CUNNINGHAM, A., Science and Religion in the Thirteenth Century Revisited: The Making of St. Francis the Proto-Ecologist, *Studies in History and Philosophy of Science*, (2000), in press. The last three verses have been translated by me.

[14] For the first disciples of the Friars Minor, CELANO, T. DE, *Vida primera*, chap.X, and the notes of GUERRA, J. A., *San Francisco de Asís* (note 5), pp. 155-157, can be consulted; for the early followers of Dominic, see the statements made by witnesses in his canonisation process; GALMES, L., GÓMEZ, V. T. *et al.*, *Santo Domingo de Guzmán* (note 6), pp. 145-176. ECCLESTON tells us that no sooner had the Franciscans opened a house in Oxford (1224) than, 'intraverunt ordinem multi probi bachelarii' (*Fratris Thomae vulgo dicti de Eccleston Tractatus De Adventu Fratrum Minorum ad Angliam...*, edidit A. G. Little, Manchester, 1951, p. 27). See the chapter entitled 'Moines, Clercs, Laïcs. Au carrefour de la vie évangélique', in CHENU, *La théologie au douzième siècle* (note 9), pp. 225-273.

[15] First Rule, 7,3-9, in GUERRA, J. A., *San Francisco de Asís* (note 5), pp. 96-97. 'Ferramenta et instrumenta suis artibus opportuna', *Opuscula sancti Patris Francisci Assisiensis...*, edidit C. Esser, Grottaferrata, 1978 (Bibliotheca Franciscana Ascetica Medii Aevi, 12).

[16] In the Second Rule (1223), Francis deals with the subject of work more explicitly and positively: 'Fratres illi, quibus *gratiam* dedit Dominus laborandi, *laborent fideliter et devote*' (critical edition by C. Esser, 5.1 (see note 15). The italics are mine). Work is a form of prayer: 'Ita quod (by means of work), excluso otio animae inimico, sanctae orationis et devotionis spiritum non extinguant, cui debent cetera temporalia deservire' (*ibid.* 5,2). I would like to thank Fr Isaac Vázquez Janeiro (Pontifical University of Salamanca) for having made known to me these texts of the Second Rule, which help to stress the positive evaluation of human labour, a fundamental aspect of the *novus homo* advocated by Francis of Assisi.

its purest form.[17] It is true, however, that both Dominic and Francis told those who devoted themselves to intellectual tasks to be on their guard against the temptation to cloak themselves in seriousness and to walk 'frowning hypocritically'.[18] Francis warned them that "study does not extinguish the spirit of prayer and devotion" (1223-24. Letter to Antonio, the first professor of theology at the Franciscan *Studium* of Bologna);[19] Dominic reminded them that intellectual tasks should never be a screen that prevents one from noticing poverty, or from expressing solidarity with those who suffer it and trying to find a solution to it. This is what Brother Esteban, a law student at Bologna in his youth and a companion of Dominic Guzmán, tells us, when he recalls the anecdote about the young canon of Osma who, when he saw the famine that afflicted Castile after the disaster of the Battle of Alarcos (1195), 'sold his books glossed in his own hand; he gave the value of the same and other things that he possessed to the poor, saying: 'I do not want to study on dead skins while men die of hunger'.[20]

The positive contemplation of the natural world as something that was necessary for the rational foundations of the Christian faith (one of the concerns of Christian intellectuals in these centuries) was common currency in certain ecclesiastical and lay intellectual circles throughout the twelfth century; what is more, the conviction that the study and rational knowledge of nature were indispensable to prepare for the study of the creation and even of the Deity (and, as a result, the construction of a theology) did not come from members of these mendicant orders, or from their founders. It was a conviction that already had deep roots among a certain mid-twelfth century European intellectual minority who were in close contact with both the Greek and the Arabic sources of the natural books. One of these intellectuals, Hermann of Carinthia (Hermann of Dalmatia), had intellectual ties with the Chartres School and was enthusiastic about the new Arab science; he knew both Arabic and Greek and lived the intellectual life of the Ebro valley, southern Italy and Castile to the full. In the Prologue to his version of Ptolemy's *Almagest,* translated from the Greek in Sicily in about 1150 (one of the great intellectual achievements of the Medieval Latin West, repeated a few years later by Gerard of Cremona in Toledo, although on that occasion from the Arabic), he wondered:

---

[17] LE GOFF, J., 'Franciscanisme et modèles culturels du XIIIe siècle': *Atti dell'VIII Convegno Intern.* Assisi, 1981 (Società Internazionale di Studi Francescani), p. 95 *et seq.*

[18] First Rule 7,16. GUERRA, J. A., *San Francisco de Asís* (note 5), p. 97.

[19] *Ibid.*, p.74.

[20] Canonisation process: Acts of the witnesses of Bologna, Witness VII, in GALMES, L., GÓMEZ, V. T. et al.: (note 6), p.166. On the new *vita apostolica*, see the section entitled 'La théologie évangélique', in CHENU, *La théologie au douzième siècle* (note 9), pp. 257-273.

> Is it not true that the invisible realities of the Godhead are perceived in intellectual terms through the creature? Is it not equally true that human intellect is not able to perceive imperceptible realities if it has not first created an access route by means of the study of the perceptible realities?.[21]

One of the innovations of early thirteenth-century Europe was the great vitality and optimism of its intellectual circles, which were experiencing the great commotion caused by the arrival of large numbers of Graeco-Arabic scientific works (largely translated in the course of the previous century) and, as a result, of the rational method of enquiry, which enabled man to find out about the realities of the entire cosmos, both of the macrocosmos and the microcosmos. That is to say, just as they read in Aristotle's works and saw expressed in the geometry to be found in Euclid's *Elements*, these texts taught them something fundamental: that the purpose of rational enquiry about natural things, and also of those which lay outside the perceptible world (ranging from a mathematical theorem to God Himself and His mysteries, the latter being revealed by means of the Scriptures), was to discover the premises upon which an already known fact could be demonstrated or deduced. From that moment onwards, any investigator (the intellectual, whether he was a member of the clergy or a layman) was not only aware of the fact that was in existence (a star, a planet, the liver, the human or divine nature of the Son of God), but also the reasons for this same fact. These two ways or stages in the process of acquiring knowledge of reality (*scientia*) were known to the Latin intellectuals of the period under consideration by the names of *demonstratio quia* and *demonstratio propter quid* (or *quare*) respectively.[22]

---

[21] 'A creatura siquidem mundi invisibilia Dei intellecta conspiciuntur (*Rom* I, 20), nec satis insensibilium veritatem percipere potest mens humana si ad eam preludio sensibilium sibi via facultatemque preexcuderit'. I follow the Latin text reproduced by R. Lemay (which does not differ from that given by HASKINS, C. H., *Studies in the History of Mediaeval Science*. Cambridge, Mass, 1924, pp. 191-93, at p. 192: for Hermann of Carinthia, see *ibidem,* pp. 43-66), as well as Lemay's hypothesis attributing this translation the Hermann of Carinthia, a theory that Haskins would not accept (*Ibid*., p. 54). See, LEMAY, R., 'De la scholastique à l'histoire par le truchement de la philologie: Itinéraire d'un médiéviste entre Europe et islam' in *La diffusione delle scienze islamiche nel medio evo europeo* (Convegno Internazionale, Rome, 2-4 ottobre 1984), Rome 1987, pp. 399-538, fragment at p. 437 and notes on p. 457.

[22] See CROMBIE, A. C., *Robert Grosseteste and the Origins of Experimental Science*. Oxford, 1953 (3rd ed., 1971), and the excellent summary to be found in his chapter, 'Grosseteste's Position in the History of Science' in Callus, D. A. (ed.), *Robert Grosseteste, Scholar and Bishop. Essays in Commemoration of the Seventh Centenary of his Death*. Oxford, 1955 (repr. 1969), pp. 98-120. For the intellectual minority, rational knowledge of nature, man and the universe in which he lived (with its consequent desacralisation) became the very justification of human dignity. Adelard of Bath did not hesitate to proclaim this in the Prologue of his treatise 'On the astrolabe' (*Astrolabium*), dedicated to the young King Henry II Plantagenet: 'Dicis enim ut in domo habitans quilibet, si

Ptolemy's cosmological works and those of the Arabic writers, Alfarabi and Algazel, which provided a commentary on these same works, Aristotle's methodological, cosmological and biological works, known via Avicenna and Averroes, together with Greek geometry (Euclid) commented on by the Arabs, offered the intellectual tools necessary to enable Christian intellectuals to launch their own studies of the natural things.[23] Brother sun, sister moon and the stars, the air, brother fire, sister water, mother earth, the rain, the seasons, the minerals, the animals, the flowers and the trees, reproduction and growth, sleep, ageing, illness and sister bodily death herself were all natural phenomena that might be discovered, understood and thus dominated by man with the new tool of a form of reasoning suitably enhanced by the new methods of Aristotelian logic, of the new mathematical sciences (astronomy-astrology), of the 'new Aristotle' that, either directly from the Greek world or via the Arabs, gave access to the complex yet fascinating world that was hidden behind the adjective 'natural'. What were known as the 'natural questions' (ranging from the rainbow to the rain, from the origin of life to the reasons for illness and death, from the process of biological generation to the size of the cosmos) were to be offered as a new frontier of knowledge to twelfth- and thirteenth-century European intellectuals. Human relationships themselves could be improved and socially ordered if Aristotle's books on ethics, to which the same author's *Politics* and *Economics* were soon to be added, were read in addition to the Gospels.[24]

The cosmological vitalism that pervades the 'Canticle' was to be perfectly compatible with that dominating Aristotle's writings on natural philosophy; his very teleologism was a comfortable path along which medieval intellectuals might proceed: they were to use it as a point of reference in their determination to make the Gospels' message of salvation known through creatures, even incorporating the latter in the same process of salvation alongside humankind. This may well be one of the greatest innovations in Francis of Assisi's message of Christian renewal, since he reconsidered the traditional relationship, which contemplated man's dominance of nature, an approach that is so much a feature of Judaeo-Christian cosmogony. This was but one aspect of the *novus homo*

---

materiam eius et compositionem, quantitatem et qualitatem sive districtionem ignoret, talis hospicis dignus non est, ita si qui in aula mundi natus atque educatus est, tam mirande pulchritudinis rationem scire negligat, post discretionis annos indignus, atque si fieri posset ejiciendus est' (Manuscript in the Fitzwilliam Museum, Cambridge, McClean 165, fol. 81. Cited by HASKINS, *Studies in the History of Mediaeval Science* (note 21) p. 29).

[23] See, for example, DRONKE, P. (ed.), *A history of twelfth-century western philosophy*, Cambridge, 1988.

[24] MINIO-PALUELLO, L., 'Aristotle: tradition and influence', in Ch. C. Gillispie, *Dictionary of Scientific Biography* (DSB), New York, 1970, vol. I, pp. 267-281.

preached and practised by Francis of Assisi.[25] Francis introduced an alternative way of perceiving nature on the part of the new Christian, an approach that was the fruit of his personal situation in the world. His insistence on the virtue of humility went beyond individual practice, since it also committed man, as a species, in his attitude towards nature: creatures are more than just signs or symbols that reveal God unto us or animals that man uses, they are humankind's brothers and sisters and protagonists in their own right of a process of salvation and dialogue with God. The fishes and the birds converse with God and the wolf of Gubbio dies a saint.[26] This is not incompatible with the study of the Aristotelian biological corpus (hierarchy of nature, teleology); on the contrary, it was to stimulate knowledge of their condition as living beings. When the Portuguese Anthony of Padua (died 1231), Francis of Assisi's companion, wanted to refute the Cathar doctrines that had attracted many people in northern Italy, he preached to the freshwater and saltwater fishes, which, in order to listen to him, lined themselves up according to their size. The main theme of the sermon, which is preserved in the *Little Flowers*, is a reflection based on the teleologism that the Maker has placed in creatures, in this case in fish:

> 'My fish brothers, you should give as many thanks as you can- Anthony reminded them- to your Creator who has granted you such a noble element as your dwelling place, so that you have fresh and salt water, just as you please. Moreover He has given you many refuges to escape from storms...You were chosen as food for ... Jesus Christ, before His Resurrection and in a mysterious way afterwards'... .
> At these and similar words and preaching of St. Anthony, some of the fishes began to open their mouths, and all of them nodded their heads, and by these and other signs of reverence they praised God as much as

---

[25] This innovation in the man-nature relationship in Western Latin Christianity was emphasised by WHITE, L. Jr., 'The historical roots of our ecologic crisis', *Science*, 155 (3767) (1967) 1203-1207. White's opinion has been severely criticised by CUNNINGHAM, A., Science and Religion in the Thirteenth Century Revisited: The Making of St. Francis the Proto-Ecologist (note 13). On the *novus homo*, see D. V. LAPSANSKI, *Perfectio evangelica. Eine begriffsgeschichtliche Untersuchung im früfranziskanischen Schrifttum*, Munich, 1974, pp. 46 *et seq*.; similarly MICCOLI, G., 'La proposta cristiana di Francesco d'Assisi', *Studi Medievali*. Serie Terza, 24 (1983) 17-73, and the works cited in both of these publications.

[26] The anecdote that his biographer, Thomas of Celano, told should be recalled by way of example: 'He also burnt with ardent love for worms, for he had read that it was said of the Saviour: 'But I am a worm and no man' (Psalms 21,7). And, for this reason, he would pick them up from the way and place them in a safe place so that passers-by would not crush them with their feet' (chap. XXIX, 80; GUERRA, J. A., *San Francisco de Asís* (note 5), p. 190). Such anecdotes make us think about panpsychic doctrines and the idea of reincarnation, which were so widespread among the Cathars. See the article by L. WHITE, Jr., mentioned above (in note 25) and the works referred to in note 7 of this article.

> they could. Then St. Anthony, seeing how reverent the fishes were toward God the Creator, rejoiced in spirit and cried out in a loud voice: 'Blessed be the Eternal God because the fishes of the waters give God more honor than heretical men (the Cathars), and animals lacking reason listen to this word better than faithless men'.
> At this miracle the people of the city, including the above-mentioned heretics, ... all of them felt remorse in their hearts.[27]

Nature and its living beings became new subjects about which to preach.[28] The beauty of the world and that of all the creatures that make it up was interpreted in terms of salvation. The novelty of the Franciscans' new message in part lay in the way it presented man's salvation as a commitment to the salvation of the entire cosmos, of which all creatures form part, from the heavens and the stars to the earth. Understanding this not only depended on a mystic sympathy for all created things, but it also made the new natural philosophy, the complex structure of which was formed by the new cosmological and natural sciences, possible.

Sixty years after Brother Anthony's sermon, his fellow Franciscan, Juan Gil of Zamora, emphasised the need for an order (in this case, an alphabetical order) which would enable one 'to understand visible things..., their properties..., so that anyone, in the midst of such a great variety of things, might more easily find what he might wish'.[29] Teleologism pervades his vision of nature. In the Prologue to his scientific encyclopaedia, he wrote:

> ... bark protects trees, as feathers and beaks protect birds and scales fish. In this way, the providence of the Creator has endowed each thing according to its natural function.
> It produces admiration (to observe) circular movements in the sky, rectilinear movements in the elements, the movement from the centre to the periphery in plants, the contraction and stretching of worms, the progressive movement of animals, the rational movement of men... All this is governed by divine wisdom, ... Consider what is more admirable, the wild boar's teeth or those of the moth..., the pig's snout or the sparrow-hawk's beak, the horse's head or that of the locust, the elephant's bones or those of the mosquito, the eagle or the ant, the lion or the flea, the tiger or the tortoise... Who gave the hedgehog its spines and taught it to roll like a top on scattered fruits, so that with this load it

[27] *Little Flowers of St. Francis*. A modern English translation from the Latin and the Italian..., by R. Brown, New York, 1958, pp. 1392-3.

[28] SCHMITT, J. C., 'Recueils Franciscains d'*Exempla* et perfectionnement des techniques intellectuelles du XIIIe au XVe siècle', *Bibliothèque de l'École des Chartes*, 135 (1977), 5-22.

[29] *Historia naturalis*, ed. A.Domínguez and L. García Ballester (note 4), vol. I, p. 112, 25-36.

> creaks like a cart when it goes forward...? All these (examples) are evidence of God's wisdom... The leaves and their shapes... All the limbs of the human body... The colours of things... The earth and the flowers encourage love... The pleasure of the sense of smell produces admiration... Through visible things that which is invisible in the Lord is manifested... It is necessary to know the visible things first... That is why I wrote this book, which I entitle *Natural history* or *The nature of things.*[30]

Juan Gil, who had already shaken off the original approach made by Francis of Assisi and the earliest brethren, as reflected in the *Canticle* or the *Little Flowers*,[31] quite openly admitted the alliance between Aristotelianism and Christianity which characterised twelfth- and thirteenth-century Christian intellectuals, and which endowed their programme for the intellectual renovation of Christianity with such vigour. For this purpose, he chose a specific passage from the book *De partibus animalium* in the translation from Arabic into Latin by Michael Scott, to be more precise from Book XI:

> We should contemplate the shapes and be joyful for the craftsman who made them.[32]

This Aristotelian fragment became a commonplace for medieval natural philosophers in the thirteenth century, who saw in it the legitimisation of their constant enquiries concerning the natural things.

III

Elsewhere I have recalled how the new Aristotelian and Arabic natural books first became available to Christian intellectual circles from the late eleventh and early twelfth centuries onwards and far more widely known as from the mid-twelfth century, thanks to the Latin versions that were translated both from Arabic and Greek.[33] This made it possible to introduce a new type of relationship

---

[30] *Ibid.*, vol I, pp. 111,5-112,36.

[31] For Juan Gil, who returned to the traditional approach of Latin Christianity to the man-nature relationship, the only reason for the existence of nature was the fact that it might be of service to man. This Franciscan expressed such a view very clearly in his *Historia naturalis:* 'To attend man, the upper, middle and lower things have been created; that is to say, the angels, the heavens and the elements, and *all the things that are born from the earth*' [HN (note 4), p. 112]. The italics are mine.

[32] *De part. anim.* I, 5. 645a 15-30

[33] GARCÍA BALLESTER, L., 'Medicina y filosofía natural en la Europa latina de los siglos XII y XIII: un debate abierto', *Arbor*, 142 (1992) 119-145; *idem* 'The construction of a new form of

in Christian intellectual circles, the relationship between religious knowledge, acquired through faith (*fide tantum*), and human reasoning (*ratione*), acquired by means of secular sciences such as arithmetic, geometry, astronomy, medicine and natural philosophy in general, which had been borrowed from Arab intellectuals.[34]

Recent studies on the corpus of natural philosophy and medical works translated from Arabic into Latin by the Franciscan Pedro Gallego and the friars of the recently founded Dominican *Studium* in Murcia, as well on Juan Gil's scientific encyclopaedia,[35] have endeavoured to explain this intellectual activity as the consequence of a twofold phenomenon. Firstly, there were the results of the contact between, on the one hand, certain Christian intellectuals (the Franciscan Pedro Gallego and the Dominicans in Murcia), who still paid great attention to Arab natural philosophy and who were still convinced of its potential intellectual fruits, and, on the other, the scientists belonging to the Muslim minority that remained in Murcia until the 1267 revolt; in the later thirteenth century such a phenomenon could only take place in the frontier regions of southern Europe (and the presence of Italian Dominicans in the *Studium* of Murcia only reinforced this model). Secondly, one must take into account the consequences of the return to the Kingdom of Castile in the last third of the thirteenth century of a generation of Franciscan and Dominican students who had graduated from European universities, where they had become familiar with a model of diffusion of the natural questions (that is to say scientific encyclopaedias), which had proved to be of great use for endowing preaching with new vigour and subjects (as was the case with Juan Gil himself).

However, although the document which was made known by Manuel de Castro and which has not yet been studied from the point of view of the history of science does not invalidate either of these two explanations, it does provide decisive new information (and gives rise to certain conjectures) for the intellectual history of the Hispanic Kingdoms, as well as for an understanding of the diffusion of the new intellectual currents that shook southern Europe in the

---

learning and practising medicine in medieval Latin Europe', *Science in Context*, 8 (1995) 75-102. See HASKINS' *Studies* (note 21).

[34] See JOLIVET, J., 'The Arabic inheritance', in DRONKE, P. ed.: *A history of twelfth-century western philosophy* (cited in note 23), pp. 113-148.

[35] MARTÍNEZ GÁZQUEZ, J., 'La *Summa de astronomia*, de Pedro Gallego, y el *Liber aggregationibus scientiae stellarum*, de Al-Fargani', *Actas del Simposio sobre 'Astronomia Alphonsi'* (Berkeley, 1985), Barcelona, 1987, pp. 153-179; *Petri Galleci Opera omnia quae extant. Summa de astronomia. Liber de animalibus. Regitiva domus*. Ed. J. Martínez Gázquez, Firenze, 2000 (Millennio Medievale. Testi); L.GARCÍA BALLESTER, 'Medical science in thirteenth-century Castile: problems and prospects' (cited in note 3); L. GARCÍA BALLESTER and A. DOMÍNGUEZ, Introductory study to the *Historia naturalis* , by Juan Gil de Zamora (*ca*. 1240-*ca*. 1320), in *Johannes Aegidius Zamorensis. Historia Naturalis*. Vol. I, pp. 17-98.

first third of the thirteenth century. In the first place, it enables us to detect three hitherto unknown centres of scientific activity (intellectual activity related to the *libri naturales*) in medieval Spain, all of which were located in Santiago de Compostela: namely, the episcopal see itself and the Franciscan and Dominican *Studia*. Secondly, it makes it possible to reconstruct the first link in an intellectual chain between the *Studia* of the new houses of Val de Dios (*Vallis Dei*, of the Friars Minor) and Bonaval (*Bona vallis*, of the Friars Preacher), founded in Santiago around 1220, and certainly no later (the importance of this chronological detail will be discussed below), and the intellectual activity of the first bishop of Cartagena, the Franciscan Pedro Gallego, between 1250 and 1267, and that of the Dominicans of the recently founded *Studium* of Murcia (1266). In the last third of the thirteenth century, this intellectual activity also incorporated the literary form of the 'scientific encyclopaedia' (Juan Gil's *Historia naturalis, ca.* 1280), which in turn cannot be separated from the activity of the Dominicans Thomas of Cantimpré (*De naturis rerum*, written between 1228 and 1248) and Vincent of Beauvais (*Speculum naturale*, finished in 1250) or that of the Franciscan Bartholomew the Englishman (*De proprietatibus rerum*, finished in about 1245). All these works helped to spread the natural questions and a rational approach to all the problems related to nature, both of man himself and of the world that surrounded him, among a more widespread European Christian public.[36] We can thus state that, throughout the thirteenth century, there was continuous intellectual activity in Castile based on the systematic use of the natural works of the Graeco-Arabic scientific corpus, from astronomical and astrological ones to the natural works proper. Thirdly, the contents of the above-mentioned document provide certain clues that shed light on the scientific activity of Pedro Gallego in the recently conquered Kingdom of Murcia, his love of language learning and his interest in natural questions. At the same time, it enables us to trace not only the link between Juan Gil's work and European university circles and the work of his fellow Franciscan, Bartholomew the Englishman (a link that cannot be doubted), but also a further connection with a hitherto unknown intellectual tradition characteristic of Castilian Franciscans, which had reached maturity twenty years before his probable date of birth (*ca.* 1240). The translations of medical works (it should not be forgotten that medicine, insofar as it is knowledge of all that is related to health and illness, was just one aspect of natural philosophy)[37] made by Dominican friars in late

[36] See the above-mentioned Introductory study to the edition of Juan Gil's *Historia naturalis* (note 4).

[37] 'It is the task of the natural philosopher to investigate the primary and universal principles that govern health and illness; it is the physician's task to carry out the practice of these principles... ', AQUINAS, THOMAS, *Opera omnia... Sententia libri de sensu et sensato, cuius secundus tractatus est de memoria et reminiscentia,* cura et studio Fratrum Praedicatorum, vol. XLV, 2, Rome-Paris, 1985, pp. 8-9.

thirteenth-century Murcia were not produced without precedents. In a nutshell, Pedro Gallego and Juan Gil and their works, the intellectual activity of the bishopric of Cartagena and that of the Dominican *Studium* of Murcia, were by no means isolated or chance events; neither did they come about exclusively as a consequence of intellectual activity at the Castilian court of Alfonso X in the second half of the thirteenth century, rather their roots went back to the intellectual activity of Franciscans and Dominicans in Galicia (which formed part of the lands ruled by the Castilian monarchs). This activity can be detected from the very moment at which such ideas were first introduced in this Spanish kingdom in the second decade of the thirteenth century. In fact, we should be wondering, and this is the fourth point that I would like to emphasise, whether there was any relationship between the intellectual activity of the Alfonsine court and these same Galician intellectual circles (on a variety of subjects ranging from music to the *libri naturales*).[38]

The fact that this activity was carried out by Franciscan and Dominican friars is not without significance. It should not be forgotten that after the union of the Kingdoms of León and Castile under Fernando III (1237), the Kings of Castile —Fernando III himself, Alonso X and Sancho IV— centred their policy for the Christian acculturation of the newly conquered lands of the Guadalquivir valley and the Kingdom of Murcia upon Franciscan and Dominican friaries. All three encouraged the creation of Franciscan and Dominican communities the length and breadth of a great arc surrounding the Muslim Kingdom of Granada, from Jerez de la Frontera and Seville in the west to Cartagena in the east, passing though Córdoba, Baeza, Úbeda and Alcalá de Guadaira. The large number of friars who acted as confessors to members of the royal family[39] and the fact that they carried out delicate diplomatic missions demonstrate that these orders had penetrated circles close to the king. They were also entrusted with the education of the heirs to the throne and other members of the royal circle.[40] All the thirteenth-century monarchs of Castile paid special attention to natural questions,

[38] This fourth point was suggested to me by Isabel del Val (University of Valladolid) in the discussion that followed the presentation and commentary of the Vatican document in the recently created Instituto de Historia de la Ciencia of the University of Valladolid (1995), directed by Mariano Esteban Piñeiro.

[39] For example, the *infante* D. Juan Manuel, whose confessor, Fr Ramón Masquefa, was trained in Paris and who was a lecturer in monastic centres of learning in Valencia, Gerona and Barcelona. See GALMES, L., GÓMEZ, V. T. *et al.* (note 6) p. 703.

[40] See LINEHAN, P., *The Spanish Church and the Papacy in the Thirteenth Century,* Cambridge, 1971, pp. 222 *et seq.;* (revised and updated Castilian translation published with the title of *La Iglesia española y el papado en el siglo XIII*, Salamanca, 1975 [Bibliotheca Salmanticensis V], pp. 195 *et seq.* of the Spanish edition.

especially Alfonso X and Sancho IV, in whose education Franciscans such as Pedro Gallego and Juan Gil of Zamora had played a particularly important role.[41]

The presence of these two orders in Santiago and their corresponding activity cannot be separated from the positive attention given to intellectual life and the reform of Christian life defended by the Archbishops of Santiago from the time of Gelmírez (1100-1140), who had established a cathedral school and sent his clergy to Paris and Bologna.[42] The presence at his court of a certain 'Robert, physician of Salerno'[43] is indicative of, in addition to a concern for his own health, a certain attention being paid to natural things which was characteristic of the intellectualised Salernitan physicians of this period, while such individuals also added prestige to aristocratic ecclesiastical circles.[44] This policy was maintained by bishop Pedro Muñiz (died 1224) and, in particular, by Bernardo II (1224-37), a man associated with the intellectual circles of Bologna and Paris, who was Dean of the Cathedral Chapter of Santiago from 1214. Both these prelates considered collaboration with the new mendicant orders to be an indispensable constituent of the twofold policy of reforming the clergy of their extensive diocese in both moral and intellectual terms.[45]

The Franciscans and their policy of renewing Christian intellectual life based on the attention paid to the natural things approached from both the old and the new Aristotelian traditions (Boethius, Aristotle's natural works, Avicenna and Averroes, all of which were to be found in the *Studia* of Val de Dios and

---

[41] See the above-mentioned (note 4) Introductory study to the edition of Juan Gil's *Historia naturalis*.

[42] See the book by FLETCHER, R. A., *Saint James's Catapult. The Life and Times of Diego Gelmírez of Santiago de Compostela*. Oxford, 1984, pp. 324-326. Also the articles by M. DÍAZ Y DÍAZ, 'Problemas de la cultura en los siglos XI-XII. La escuela episcopal de Santiago', *Compostellanum*, 16 (1971) 187-200, at pp. 197-198; 'La Escuela Episcopal de Santiago en los siglos XI-XIII', *Liceo Franciscano*, 2nd period, 28 (1975) 183-188, at p. 187.

[43] *Historia Compostellana*. Edidit Emma Falque, Turnholti, 1988 (*Corpus Christianorum. Continuatio Mediaevalis*, 70). Reference is here made to the Castilian translation, *Historia Compostelana*. Introducción, traducción, notas e índice de Emma Falque. Madrid, 1994, lib. II, chaps. 8 and 33, pp. 311 and 355.

[44] PARAVICINI BAGLIANI, A., *Medicina e scienze della natura alla corte dei papi nel Duecento*, Spoleto, 1991, p. 8. The archbishop of Toledo, Rodrigo Ximénez de Rada (1210-47), whose enthusiasm for the *libri naturales* was well-known, was attended by his personal physician called *Johannes* (he is not stated to be from Salerno), who was an expert on astronomy and astrology. See GONZÁLVEZ RUIZ, R., 'El traductor Maestro Juan de Toledo: una propuesta de identificación', *Toletum*, 11 (1981) 177-189, at p. 184. For the reasons for the emphasis placed on the natural philosophical dimension of medicine by mid-twelfth century Salerno physicians, see the article by LEMAY, R., 'De la scolastique à l'histoire par le truchement de la philologie: Itinéraire d'un médiéviste entre Europe et Islam', in *La diffusione delle scienze islamische nel medio evo europeo* (Convegno internazionale, Roma, 2-4 ottobre 1984), Rome, 1987, pp. 399-535.

[45] GARCÍA Y GARCÍA, A; VÁZQUEZ JANEIRO, I., 'La biblioteca del arzobispo de Santiago de Compostela, Bernardo II (+ 1240)', *Antonianum*, 61 (1986) 540-568, at pp. 558-9.

Bonaval, *items* 25-27, 6-7, 39, 42-45 in the documentary appendix below) also enjoyed the protection and respect of the powerful Benedictine order. This is suggested by the fact that the lands of Val de Dios, which lay on the banks of the River Sarela as it passed though Santiago, had been generously ceded to the Franciscans by the monks of San Martín de Pinario.[46] It is also worth noting that Pedro Gallego dedicated his compendium of astronomy (*Summa astronomiae*) —actually an abbreviated Latin translation of al-Farghani's *Elementa astronomica* (one of the works, *item* 20, handled in the *Studium* of Val de Dios in Santiago)— to Martín Gil, abbot of the Cistercian monastery of Moreruela in Zamora.[47] In fact, the first Friars Minor and Friars Preacher in Galicia were capable of making Francis of Assisi and Dominic Guzmán's new message of Christian reform and love of nature compatible with their intellectual activity, transforming the latter into a new form of love for both humankind and creatures. It is therefore not surprising that young clerics and monks, stimulated by the extremely intellectualised high-ranking clergy of Galicia and with the benevolence of the powerful monastic orders, at the same time that they were seduced by the message of Christian reform preached by the new friars and by the new intellectual currents of the new natural philosophy and the new Aristotle, should discover a new frontier which gave meaning to their twofold spiritual and intellectual concerns in these two activities.

The Bishop of Paris's condemnation of the physician David of Dinant (d. *ca.*1214), a key figure in the 'new Aristotle' movement, makes it clear that this twofold approach was neither easy nor free of risks; in 1210 this prelate ordered the notes and commentaries on the Greek scientist's works of natural philosophy that had been written by this physician and Aristotelian natural philosopher to be burnt[48]. Today the *libri Aristotelis de naturali philosophia*, as the sentence reads, used by David of Dinant are known to have included, among others, the Graeco-Latin versions of his *De animalibus* (a collection of Aristotle's three most important biological works: 'History of animals', 'Parts of animals' and 'Generation of animals', as well as the *Problemata.*[49] David is also known to have had links with the circle of Pope Innocent III (1198-1216), which paid

[46] *Ibid.*, p. 556.

[47] 'Frater P[etrus] divina miseratione cartaginensis episcopus fratri Martini egidii [*marg.*: abbati] de Morelola salutem et pacem ....', Madrid, Bibl. Nac., MS 8918, fol. 49 rb. This refers to Martín Gil, abbot of the Cistercian monastery of Moreruela (Zamora). See MARÍA I. ALFONSO ANTÓN, *La colonización cisterciense en la meseta del Duero: El ejemplo de Moreruela*, 2 vols., Madrid, 1983. I would like to thank J. A. García de Cortázar for his help in identifying this abbot.

[48] MACCAGNOLO, E., 'David of Dinant and the beginnings of Aristotelianism in Paris' in Dronke, P. (ed.), *A history of twelfth-century western philosophy* (cited in note 23), pp. 429-442.

[49] D'ALVERNY, M. T., 'Translations and translators', in Benson, R. L., Constable, G. and Lanham, G. D. (eds.), *Renaissance and renewal in the twelfth century*, Oxford, 1982, 421-462.

particular attention to the problems under consideration in this article.[50] The friars of Santiago, barely ten or fifteen years afterwards (in 1222 and 1230), under the direct protection of Archbishops Pedro Muñiz and Bernardo II, and with Benedictine approval, commented upon Aristotle's *scripta minora* (items 6-7) and the *De animalibus* (*item* 42), the latter in the recently diffused translation from Arabic into Latin by Michael Scott (1217-1220); and they continued to make use of Averroes' important commentaries on the *Metaphysics* and the *De anima* (*items* 43-44), or of the *De anima* by Avicenna (known by the name of the *Sextus liber naturalium* or *de naturalibus, item* 39), to understand Aristotle. All this occurred scarcely five years before Averroes' commentaries are first recorded in Paris (1225).[51]

As has already been mentioned, the Franciscan *Studium* was not the only centre that stimulated the intellectual life of Santiago in this period. The new Friars Preacher, with their comparable concern for the new theology and the new intellectual world of natural philosophy (in this context we should recall the names of Thomas of Cantimpré, Vincent of Beauvais and Albert the Great, who, in 1251, condensed his intellectual programme to the formula 'to make Aristotle intelligible to the Latins'),[52] must have arrived in Santiago around the same date. In fact, in the first annotation of the document under consideration (August 1222), express reference is made to two members of the order of the Friars Minor (*Petrus Oduarii* and *Martinus Fernandi*); in the fourth annotation (January 1225), the user is *Johannes Fernandi* 'de ordine predicatorum'. This would seem to be the first documentary evidence for the presence of the members of these orders in Santiago, as well as of their intellectual activity, both in the *Studium* of Val de Dios and in that of Bonaval. Both orders enjoyed the protection of the Archbishop.

The letters of Bernardo II or of his predecessor Pedro Muñiz have not been preserved, or at least they remain unknown to me. In contrast, those of their contemporary Robert Grosseteste, Bishop of Lincoln (1235-1253), are still extant. Robert was born around the year 1168; he was the first chancellor of the *Studium generale* of Oxford; he protected the first Friars Minor to reach Oxford (1224), three years after the Friars Preacher had done so, and was their first

---

[50] *Cf.* PARAVICINI BAGLIANI, A., *Medicina e scienze della natura alla corte dei papi nel Duecento* (cited in note 44), pp. 13-14.

[51] GAUTHIER, R. A., 'Le traité *De anima et de potenciis eius* d'un maître ès arts (vers 1225). Introduction et texte critique', *Rev. Sc. ph. th.*, 66 (1982), 3-55, in p. 24. De Vaux's classic study is not yet valid in this respect: 'La date limite de 1230 pour la premiѐre entrée d'Averroés chez les Latins, jadis fixée par le P. de Vaux [DE VAUX, R., 'La premiére entrée d'Averroés chez les Latins', *Rev. Sc. ph. th.*, 22 (1933), 193-245], est arbitraire', GAUTHIER, art. cit. above, p. 22.

[52] '(Libris Aristotelis) latinis intelligibles'. Comentary on the *Physica*, in *Opera Omnia*, ed. Borgnet, vol. 3,1.

master of theology.[53] These three prelates controlled extensive densely populated dioceses; the three shared the same concern for reforming the Church and the clergy. The Bishop of Lincoln (1236) painted a depressing picture of the level of clerical disintegration in his diocese,[54] a phenomenon that was fairly common in the rest of Christianity and the Spanish churches, both in the Crown of Aragon and in Castile.[55] The three bishops coincided as regards the measures undertaken to achieve the necessary degree of reform among the clergy and Christian people in general: they relied on the presence of the two new mendicant orders in the same city[56] (a method that was also noted by the people of contemporary Castile, such as the *infante* Juan Manuel)[57] and encouraged study, especially of the Scriptures.[58] It was supposed that if the clergy were intellectually prepared and respected Christian ideals, reform would trickle down to the people by means of preaching and example.[59] In 1245, Robert Grosseteste wrote the following words, which would undoubtedly have been supported by his colleagues, the

---

[53] LUARD, H. R. (ed.), *Roberti Grosseteste episcopi quondam Lincolnensis Epistolae*. London, 1861, p. xxii. For Robert Grosseteste's probable date of birth (around 1168) and, in general, his character and work, see CALLUS, D. A. (ed.), *Robert Grosseteste, Scholar and Bishop,* Oxford, 1955 (repr. 1969). On his scientific output, CROMBIE, A. C., *Robert Grosseteste and the Origins of Experimental Science*, Oxford, 1953 (3rd ed., 1971), as well as his chapter in Callus' book cited in note 22 of this article. A good and more up-to-date summary by the same scholar can be found in 'Robert Grosseteste', *DSB*, vol. 5, p. 549.

[54] *Epist.* XXII. Edition of LUARD (note 53), pp. 72-76. For a more detailed examination of the measures that he applied to improve the situation of the clergy and monks, see SRAWLEY, J. H., 'Grosseteste's Administration of the Diocese of Lincoln', in Callus, D. A. (ed.), *Robert Grosseteste, Scholar and Bishop* (note 53), pp. 146-177.

[55] See, for example, the picture painted by LINEHAN of the Spanish clergy in the first third of the thirteenth century on the basis of contemporary ecclesiastical sources: 'The Spanish clergy, as John of Abbeville found them, were incontinent, largely uneducated and total strangers to the discipline of council and synod', *The Spanish Church and the Papacy in the Thirteenth Century* (note 40) p. 29 (p. 25 of the Spanish edition). A Castilian cleric of the time, Diego García, at some date between 1214 and 1218, stated: 'Attendentes quod in partibus Hispaniae, ex defectu studiorum et litteraturae, multa et intolerabilia detrimenta animarum proveniunt', cited by Linehan, p. 30 note 7 (p. 26 note 79 of the Spanish edition).

[56] *Epist.* XX; XXIV. Edited by LUARD (note 53), pp. 71 and 120.

[57] This opinion was shared by the Infante D. JUAN MANUEL, who in 1330, at the end of his work *Libro de los Estados*, stated: 'Dos órdenes son las que al tiempo de agora aprovechan más para salvamiento de las almas... Et esto porque los destas órdenes pedrican et confiessan et an mayor fazimiento con las gentes. Et son las de los fraires pedricadores, et de los fraires menores' ('There are two orders that make most use of market time for saving souls... And this because those of these orders preach and give confession and have most contact with the people. And they are the Friars Preacher and the Friars Minor'). Edited by MACPHERSON, I. R., and TATE, R. B., Madrid, 1991, p. 374 (Clásicos Castalia, 192).

[58] *Epist.* CXXIII. Edited by LUARD (note 53), pp. 346-347.

[59] 'Cum Fratres Minores per regnum Angliae constituti sua salubri praedicatione populum efficaciter elluminant'. Edited by LUARD (note 53), p. 181.

archbishops of Santiago, to Cardinal Hugh of Saint Cher, a Dominican friar: 'The Church in England... needs men who are not only expert at both forms of law and also at theology and the Holy Scriptures, but who also live according to the contents of the latter (*sacram noverint Scripturam... et exercitio firmatam*), and this can only be found among the brethren of these orders (*latera talia, quae alibi non inveniuntur nisi in ordine fratrum utrorumque*)'.[60] To judge from their libraries,[61] the three shared a love for the study of nature and were convinced that the intellectual reform of the clergy, based on preaching, involved the harmonisation of Revelation and reasoning; this reasoning was steeped in the new Aristotelian tradition and acquired its appreciation of the natural world by means of the tools of logical and mathematical reasoning (*items* 19-21, 23, 26, 28-29, 32, 37-38)[62] or of music (*items* 25, 30), which, according to the tradition of Boethius, included the proportion and harmony not only of the sounds produced by the human voice or instruments, but also of the movements and the times of heavenly bodies, together with the harmony of the bodies that were made up by the four earthly elements (earth, water, fire and air; we should recall Francis of Assisi's *Canticle*); in brief, the harmony existing between the macrocosmos and the microcosmos. Music, therefore, restored harmony both between the body and the soul and among the various bodily elements; it also shaped human conduct and was thus a source of good health.[63]

IV

Let us consider the document in question. It is a parchment folio on which, between August 1222 and September 1230, those responsible for the episcopal library of Santiago (or for the archbishop's personal library) wrote five entries in which they noted the date, who took the books out and the works that they were

---

[60] *Epist.* CXV. Edited by LUARD (note 53), p. 336.

[61] For the Bishop of Lincoln's library, see HUNT, R. W., 'The Library of Robert Grosseteste' in Callus, D. A. (ed.), *Robert Grosseteste, Scholar and Bishop* (cited in note 53), pp. 121-145. The library was bequeathed to the Franciscan friary in Oxford. Unfortunately, it has not been preserved and it has proved possible to reconstruct only part of its contents.

[62] John Murdoch has pointed out that one of the reasons for the success of Campanus of Novara's commentaries on Euclid (1256-1259) was that they fully satisfied the intellectual requirements of the natural philosophy scholar on the basis of logical and mathematical reasoning. *Cf.* MURDOCH, J. E., 'The Medieval Euclid: salient aspects of the translations of the 'Elements' by Adelard of Bath and Campanus of Novara', *Revue de synthèse*, 49-52 (1968) 67-94; see also PARAVICINI BAGLIANI, A., 'Campano da Novara e il mundo scientifico romano duecentesco', *Novarien*, 14 (1984) 99-111 [reprinted in *Medicina e scienze della natura alla corte dei papi nel Duecento* (cited in note 44), pp. 85-115].

[63] CROMBIE, A. C., 'Robert Grosseteste', *DSB*, vol. 5, pp. 548-554.

borrowing. The total number of volumes is 39-40 with a total of 46 works being explicitly mentioned; but there were also at least a few more, the number of which it is impossible to calculate, either because they are covered by expressions such as '*cum aliis libris*', '*cum aliis scripturis*', '*cum aliis libris in eodem volumine*', '*tres caternios... in alio volumine*', or because they have been erased by the water that has damaged part of the text. Only 15 of these are works related to the Scriptures, patristics, theology, grammar or of an ecclesiastical category, such as sermons. The remaining works constitute an impressive corpus covering astronomy, astrology and natural philosophy in general. No other list with such a wide range of works on natural philosophy forming part of a library is known from the Spanish kingdoms (either from Castile or from the Crown of Aragon) at this date.[64] It is not until the closing years of the thirteenth century (an inventory of 1280) that a similar collection can be found in the library belonging to the Archbishop of Toledo, Gonzalo Pétrez (also known as García Gudiel) (d. 1299).[65]

All the signs point to the works having belonged to the episcopal (or personal) library of the Archbishops of Santiago, Pedro Muñiz (d. January 1224) and Bernardo II (d. 1240); the second of these has recently been studied by Antonio García y García and Isaac Vázquez Janeiro.[66] However, the inventory of 1236 referring to the latter archbishop's library does not include a substantial

[64] I here refer to the presence, *together*, of such a large and significant number of *libri naturales*. The names of several canons of Toledo who, in the last decade of the twelfth century and the first third of the thirteenth century, possessed important works concerning logic, geometry and astronomy, as well as of medicine, are known to us: *Stephanus* (*fl.* 1194), *Reginerius* or Reynald (*fl.* 1194) and *Johannes* (d. 1239). Similarly, the library belonging to the influential Archbishop Rodrigo Ximénez de Rada (1210-47), whose books are known to have included Avicenna's *Canon* and Ptolemy's *Almagest*, with their respective commentaries (although we do not know by whom), must have been rich in works on nature. See GONZÁLVEZ RUIZ, R., 'El traductor Maestro Juan de Toledo: una propuesta de identificación', *Toletum*, 11 (1981) 177-189 [Número *Homenaje a Rivera Recio*]; BURNETT, Ch., '*Magister Iohannes Hispanus*: Towards the identity of a Toledan translator', in *Comprendre et maitriser la nature au Moyen Age. Mélanges d'histoire des sciences offerts à Guy Beaujouan*, Geneva-Paris, 1994, pp. 425-436. See GONZÁLVEZ, R., *Hombres y libros de Toledo*, Madrid, 1998, pp. 170-3.

[65] The inventory is preserved in the Madrid Biblioteca Nacional (MS No. 13023, ff. 218r-225r). It was published by MANUEL ALONSO, P., ('Bibliotecas medievales de los arzobispos de Toledo', *Razón y Fe*, 41 (1941) 295-309) and analysed from the point of view of the history of astronomy by MILLÁS VALLICROSA, J. Mª, *Las traducciones orientales en los manuscritos de la biblioteca catedral de Toledo*, Madrid, 1942, p. 16 *et seq.* For its medical contents, see GARCÍA BALLESTER, L., 'El papel de las instituciones de consumo y difusión de ciencia médica en la Castilla del siglo XIII: el monasterio, la catedral y la Universidad', *Dynamis*, 4 (1984) 33-63, at p. 41 *et seq.* It has been studied recently by GONZÁLVEZ, R., *Hombres y libros de Toledo*, Madrid, 1998, pp. 419-549.

[66] 'La biblioteca del arzobispo de Santiago de Compostela, Bernardo II (+ 1240) ', *Antonianum*, 61 (1986) 540-568. I am unaware of the situation of the episcopal library (or that of the archbishop) during the long occupation of the see by Pedro Suárez, which started in 1173.

proportion of the works mentioned in the document housed in the Vatican Library —to be more specific, all those related to mathematics (astronomy, astrology, geometry) and the natural sciences. This absence led Manuel de Castro to put forward a hypothesis expressing the possibility that those works belonged to the recently founded Franciscan house of Val de Dios and that security reasons might have led the community of Friars Minor to deposit them, for safekeeping, in the well-controlled episcopal library until the new friary had been built. However, the brethren (*fratres*) who appear as users of the *libri naturales* belonged both to the Franciscan order (*fratres minores Vallis Dei*) and to the Dominicans (*de ordine predicatorum*). A misreading (*de ordine predictorum*, i.e. *de fratribus minoribus*, instead of *de ordine predicatorum*) led both D. de Bruyne and M. de Castro[67] to associate this important collection of manuscripts with the recently created Franciscan community alone, whose members were, according to these scholars, the only ones to be recorded in the entries referring to the works being lent. However, it is fairly logical that such an important collection of manuscripts —which included such voluminous works as Ptolemy's *Almagest*, in the Latin version translated by Gerard of Cremona (*item* 28), which in a fourteenth-century codex occupied 280 pages of folio size (33 x 23.5 cms.) with two columns per page,[68] and Aristotle's *De animalibus* (*item* 42), which similarly in a fourteenth-century codex, in the Latin version of Michael Scott, covers almost 200 pages of folio size (34 x 25.5 cms.) with two columns a page—[69] should have belonged to the episcopal library, at least in the period during which the entries referring to loans were noted down, that is, between 1222 and September 1230. It should be remembered that copies of the *Almagest* together with a commentary, and of Avicenna's *Canon*, of comparable dimensions and also to be found in Bernardo II's library,[70] were also in the possession of a canon of Toledo (*Magister Johannes*) who bequeathed them to his archbishop, Rodrigo Ximénez de Rada, in his will (August 1239).[71] The fact that there was no trace of these works in the inventory of Bernardo II's personal library, which he was to donate to the see of Santiago in 1238, only indicates that this prelate did not own them when the inventory was drawn up (1236). There are two possibilities: either 1) that Bernardo II had possessed them, but had given them to the friars prior to the date of this inventory; or 2) that they belonged to the cathedral library and, for this reason, were not included in the

[67] See the references in note 2 to this article.
[68] Cracow, Bibl. Jag. 590, ff. 3r-142v.
[69] Cracow, Bibl. Jag. 653, ff. 1v-96r.
[70] GARCÍA Y GARCÍA; VÁZQUEZ JANEIRO, 'La biblioteca del arzobispo de Santiago de Compostela, Bernardo II (+ 1240) ', (note 45), p. 568.
[71] GONZÁLVEZ RUIZ, 'El traductor Maestro Juan de Toledo: una propuesta de identificación' (note 64) pp. 177-189; BURNETT, '*Magister Iohannes Hispanus*' (note 64), p. 432.

inventory of the prelate's personal library. However, we have no documentary evidence to support either of these two conjectures. In the document there are spaces at certain points with traces of letters (were the words subsequently erased?) (*items* 1, 9, between *items* 3 and 4) after words such as '*dominus*', '*recepit a domino*' and '*de armario*'. I have completed these spaces with the words '*archiepiscopus*', '*archiepiscopo*' and '*domini archiepiscopo*' respectively, basing this conjecture on similar, but complete expressions in existence in the inventory of Archbishop Bernardo II's library (*items* 39, 51-52: '*de armario archiepiscopo*'; *items* 49-50: '*qui ... libri fuerunt domini archiepiscopi P<etri> Muñoz*'.[72]

It is evident that there must have been intense intellectual activity in the Franciscan and Dominican houses of Santiago, guided by the small community of masters who, together with their disciples, made up the respective *Studia*. The document tells us that the books were taken out by the 'brothers minor of the Val de Dios' (*fratres minores Vallis Dei)* and by a member of the Order of Preachers (*de ordine predicatorum*). Fortunately, the names of three of these brothers are also to be found alongside such expressions: *Petrus Oduarii* (Pedro de Odoario), *Johannes Fernandi (dictus Missal)* (Juan Fernández) and *Martinus Fernandi* (Martín Fernández). The first is recorded throughout the period (1222-1230) and was, together with the Dominican Juan Fernández (*fl.* 1225), the person who undertook the widest range of intellectual activity related to such subjects as natural philosophy, astronomy, geometry and mathematical calculations. Martín Fernández is only recorded in the first entry in connection with some commentaries by the Aristotelian Alexander of Aphrodisias (*item* 3), although either he did not actually taken this volume out of the library or he returned it immediately, because the entry is crossed out in the same ink.

As has already been mentioned, the books that were taken out over the period of eight years for which we have information include the subjects characteristic of a *Studium* in which the subjects comprising the *Trivium* (grammar, rhetoric and logic) and the *Quadrivium* (arithmetic, music, geometry and astronomy) were being taught and cultivated from the standpoint of the new material supplied by Arab science and the new Aristotle, together with subjects such as theology, the Scriptures, the Holy Fathers and preaching. A conscious decision was being made to opt for the new theology (Holy Fathers, Scripture and Aristotelian logic) and its new question-and-answer techniques (the *quaestio* and the *disputatio*), introduced by Peter Lombard, whose *Sententiae* and *Commentaria* on the Scriptures (*items* 1 and 18) are here mentioned in a Spanish *Studium* for the first time (1222); the document in the Vatican Library indirectly

[72] GARCÍA Y GARCÍA; VÁZQUEZ JANEIRO, 'La biblioteca del arzobispo de Santiago de Compostela, Bernardo II (+ 1240) ', (note 45), pp. 560-568.

informs of such practices at Val de Dios and Bonaval through the record of works on loan from the episcopal library. The presence of a book on practical medical therapeutics (*item* 41) in the list of manuscripts borrowed by the Franciscan Pedro de Odoario clearly indicates that the Brothers Minor may have been carrying out activities more usually associated with physicians or apothecaries.[73]

The traditional classification of the sciences into the *Trivium* and the *Quadrivium* came to be considered insufficient and gave way to a form of natural philosophy that aimed to offer a comprehensive view of creation. The fact that a significant proportion of the new scientific works dealing with knowledge of the cosmos that had been translated in Toledo in the second half of the previous century (Ptolemy, Azarquiel, al-Farghani, Alfarabi, Euclid, whether alone or accompanied by al-Nayrizi's commentaries, Albumasar's great astrological treatise, astronomical tables and the algorithmic tradition) was present, together with the great novelty of the recent and almost contemporary translations of Aristotle's works on nature (*De animalibus*) and of Averroes' commentaries on such important natural works as *Metaphysics* and *De anima*, was far from being an expression of intellectual bulimia on the part of the Franciscan and Dominican communities of Val de Dios and Bonaval; this abundance was rather the expression of an intellectual concern that was shared with the most active intellectual centres of the rest of Christian Europe, especially the Oxford school.[74] The books that were moved to and from by the Brothers Minor of Val de Dios and the brothers of the Order of Preachers at Bonaval indirectly tell us of the matters that worried, or even tormented, medieval intellectuals: the desire to find out about different astronomical theories, how to calculate the eras or land measurements, how far away the stars were, how large the cosmos was, how to calculate the movements of planetary high points and the movements of heavenly bodies, or the inclination of the ecliptic, how much precession movement there was, how much trepidation movement there was, or to find out about death, the origin and maintenance of biological life and its changes, procreation, growth and the multiplication of living beings, health and infirmity. One can imagine the conflict that arose between Holy Writ and the new Aristotle, represented by his own works and those of his commentators (eternity-creation of the world, the problem of the angels, the allegorical interpretation of Scripture etc.). The Franciscan community of Val de Dios and that of the Friars Preacher of Bonaval in Santiago de Compostela demonstrated particular interest

---

[73] This practice was known and permitted under certain conditions by the superiors of the mendicant orders themselves. See the classic book by FELDER, H., *Geschichte der wissenschaftlichen Studien im Franziskanerorden bis um die Mitte des 13. Jahrhunderts*, Frieburg i. B., 1904, pp. 390-397. See also note 98 below.

[74] See the works by CROMBIE, A. C. and CALLUS, D. A. mentioned in note 53.

in studying Holy Writ, mathematics and the natural sciences. Moreover, this interest was displayed at a particularly early date. It should not be forgotten that the document being considered records intense intellectual activity between 1222 and 1230; nor that Dominic Guzmán died in 1221 and Francis of Assisi in 1226; that the well-known Franciscan friary of Oxford was founded in 1224 nor that Robert Grosseteste taught theology, insisted on teaching Scripture in the Parisian style[75] and cultivated the natural sciences and mathematics there between 1229 and 1235, making use of the very same intellectual tools as the brothers of Val de Dios and Bonaval- works that were circulating at the schools of arts in Paris.

However, the works that the Dominican Juan Fernández used in 1225 (*items* 31-39: Azarquiel's tables, Albumasar's astrological works, al-Farghani's treatise, Avicenna's *De anima* and the *algorismus*) point towards a very different approach to the one followed by his Parisian counterparts, who suffered the consequences of the hostility of the order's Constitutions towards 'worldly sciences' in 1228.[76] The approach that can be observed among the brethren of both orders in Santiago is the same one that characterised the Oxford *Studium generale*, where Franciscan influence following the line adopted by Robert Grosseteste was predominant.[77] Unlike that of Paris, the Oxford university syllabus included the mathematical works present in Santiago,[78] while in one of his sermons in 1230 the Parisian Dominican Pierre de Bar-sur-Aube stated that 'astrology, geometry and the other worldly sciences only lead to error, draw one away from God and contribute nothing to man's salvation'.[79] On September 26th

---

[75] '*Conformitate regentium Parisius theologorum*', *Epist.* CXXIII. Edited by LUARD (note 53), p. 347. See the classic volume by SMALLEY, B., *The Study of the Bible in the Middle Ages*, 2nd edition, Oxford, 1952, and the above-mentioned work by CHENU, *La théologie au douzième siècle* (note 9) pp. 323 *et seq*.

[76] 'No estudien en los libros de los gentiles y de los filósofos, aunque los examinen algún tiempo. No aprendan las ciencias mundanas, ni tampoco aprendan las artes que llaman liberales... Tanto los jóvenes como los demás estudien solamente libros teológicos' ('They should not study the books of the gentiles or of the philosophers although they may examine them at some time. They should not learn worldly science, and neither should they learn the arts that are called liberal.... Both the young and the others should only study theological books'), *Constitutiones antiguas de la orden de predicadores*, 28, in GALMES, L., GÓMEZ, V. T. *et al.*, *Santo Domingo de Guzmán.* (cited in note 6), p. 761.

[77] CROMBIE, A. C., 'Robert Grosseteste', *DSB*, vol. 5, p. 548-554.

[78] 'Tenentur insuper omnes incepturi... juramento firmare quod sex libros Euclidis, Aritmeticam Boycii, Computum cum Algorismo, Tractatum de Spera... audierint competenter' (norm dating to earlier that 1350). GIBSON, S., *Statuta antiqua Universitatis oxoniensis*, Oxford, 1931, pp. xciii-cii.

[79] DAVY, M., *Sermons universitaires parisiens*, Paris, 1931, p. 87. Cited by BEAUJOUAN, G., 'L'enseignement de l'arithmétique élémentaire à l'Université de Paris aux XIIIe et XIVe siècles', in *Par raison de nombre. L'art du calcul et les savoirs scientifiques médiévaux,* Aldershot, Variorum, 1991, XI, pp. 93-124. A hundred years later, in the Valencia region, recently acquired for Christianity, the Catalan Franciscan, Francesc Eiximenis (*ca.* 1327-1409) expressed his opposition to

of that same year, the Franciscan Pedro de Odoario was making use of all these 'worldly sciences' just as the Dominican Juan Fernández had done five years beforehand. Nevertheless, even in Paris the true state of affairs must have been far more complex, as is indicated by the fact that, despite the Paris establishment's position, the attitude of some young students, who had been attracted by the novelty of the *libri naturales*, was very different at least to judge by Albert the Great's recollections of his time as a student at the house of Saint-Jacques in the city (1240-48), where reading the natural works of authors such as Aristotle, Avicenna, Algazel or Alfarabi and carrying out small experiments formed part and parcel of everyday life.[80] The words with which Gilson summarised the attitude of the Oxford masters could well be applied to the schools of Santiago in the first third of the thirteenth century: 'English philosophical thought put the mathematics and physics that the works of Arab scientists placed at their disposition at the service of religion'[81].

In addition to revealing these important centres of intellectual life in the north-west of the Iberian Peninsula and the names of three early participants in this intellectual achievement, the document in the Vatican Library also indicates the city's good relationship with other centres and the speed with which new works circulated among European intellectual circles. The fact that these centres were sited in Santiago de Compostela and the positive support given to intellectual activity by the above-mentioned archbishops cannot have been unrelated to the city's strategic location. 'The route to Santiago was also followed by books from the four corners of Europe'.[82]

---

the clergy and the sons of the commercial middle classes studying arithmetic, geometry and astrology, since they were not religious sciences and involved the risk of their losing their faith and becoming 'Serraïns' (Saracens) (GARCÍA BALLESTER, L., *Historia social de la medicina en la España de los siglos XIII al XVI*, Madrid, 1976, p. 53).

[80] Albert the Great's recollections are to be found in his *De mineralibus*, lib. II, tr. 2, c. 11 and lib. II, tr. 2, c. 18 (Ed. Par. V. 40 and 46), as well as in his commentaries to the books of the *Physica*, lib I, tr. 1, c. 1 (Ed. Par. III, 1). Cited by CONGAR, Y., ' 'In dulcedine societatis quaerere veritatem'. Notes sur le travail en équipe chez S. Albert et chez les Prêcheurs au XIIIe siècle', in Meyer, G. and Zimmermann, A., Hrsgbers., *Albert magnus doctor universalis, 1280/1980*, Mainz, 1980, pp. 47-57, at pp. 47-48.

[81] GILSON, E., *La philosophie au Moyen-Âge*, Paris, 1944, p. 397.

[82] GARCÍA Y GARCÍA; VÁZQUEZ JANEIRO, 'La biblioteca del arzobispo de Santiago de Compostela, Bernardo II (+ 1240) ', (cited in note 45), p. 546.

V

I should like to draw particular attention to the following details: in the first place, to the presence in 1222 of some of Aristotle's works on ethics, probably in the Latin translation from the Greek (*item* 12) and of his *scripta minora* of natural philosophy: *De plantis* (*item* 6) and *De sompno et vigilia* (*item* 7), the first of which, considered to be by Aristotle in the medieval world, had been translated from the Arabic in 1178 by Alfred of Sareshel, an Englishman working in Spain; it was derived from Nicholas of Damascus, probably via a summary by Ishaq ibn Hunayn, with corrections by Tabit ben Qurra.[83] The presence of the other work by Aristotle raises problems that remain to be solved. Secondly, one should note the presence in the library in 1230 of the *librum de animalibus* (*item* 42), likewise a work that had only recently been translated in Toledo by Michael Scott (between 1217 and 1220), before the latter's departure for the Sicilian court, where, according to the most acceptable opinion, the substantial corpus of Averroes' works on natural philosophy was to be translated from Arabic into Latin by a group of scholars, including Michael Scott himself, from 1227 onwards.[84]

Thirdly, I would like to mention that on the same date (26th September, 1230) *Petrus Oduarii* made use of the *Metafisicam Aristatelis* (sic) *cum comento* (*item* 43) and the *Librum de anima cum comento* (*item* 44), which must have been Averroes' commentaries on these works by Aristotle. This information, especially the date clearly expressed in the document, means that these important works by Averroes accompanied by Aristotle's text, were present by a year (1230) very near to the earliest possible date (between 1224 and 1227-28) for the use of these same works by the Christian intellectuals of Paris (for instance, by the anonymous natural philosopher who was the author of a work on the soul's activities: *De anima et de potenciis eius*). We have to remember that with this fact Latin scholars learned a new form of Aristotelianism, different from that offered by Avicenna.[85] It was not until 1240 and the time of Albert the Great that Aristotelian thought, via Averroes' great commentaries on the *Metaphysics* and the *De anima*, was to be clearly present.[86] Our evidence is, thus, of great interest, and should be investigated in further detail.

---

[83] MILLAS VALLICROSA, *Las traducciones orientales* (note 65), p. 60; HASKINS, *Studies in the History of Mediaeval Science* (note 21), pp. 128 *et seq.*; MINIO-PALUELLO, L., 'Aristotle: Tradition and Influence', *DSB*, vol. 1, p. 271.

[84] MINIO-PALUELLO, L., 'Michael Scot', *DSB*, vol. 9, pp. 361-365.

[85] GAUTHIER, 'Le traité *De anima et de potenciis eius* d'un maître és arts (vers 1225) ' (note 51), pp. 24-5.

[86] WEISHEIPL, J. A.: *Albert Magnus and the Sciences*, Toronto, 1980, pp. 565-577.

Fourthly, the use of the impressive corpus of astronomical and astrological works that had been brought together in Santiago should be mentioned. The following list includes some of the works taken out by Brother Pedro de Odoario and Brother Juan Fernández in January 1225: Ptolemy's *Almagest*, in the version of Gerard of Cremona, translated in Toledo in 1174-75 (*item* 28); al-Farghani's (Latin Alfraganus) *Elementa astronomiae* (*items* 20 and 36), also in Gerard of Cremona's translation, together with some astronomical tables, which, although unidentified, were usually found with these treatises; Alfarabi's *De ortu scientiarum* ('On the division of the sciences', *item* 21), which had an enormous impact on the earliest phases of scholasticism; a possible treatise on astronomy by Muhammad Yabir ibn Aflar (who lived in Seville in the later eleventh and early twelfth centuries), also translated by Gerard of Cremona (*item* 23), which was known in Christian circles as *Geber super almagesti*, in which Ptolemy's planetary theory was criticised; the *De speculis*, also translated by Gerard of Cremona (*item* 29), which was the commentary by Eutocius, a Byzantine mathematician, on Archimedes, a work that was used by such thirteenth-century writers as the Franciscan Roger Bacon on the subject of perspective; Azarquiel's *Canones in motibus celestium corporum* (*item* 33), together with the same writer's *Tabulas astronomie* (*item* 31), both translated by Gerard of Cremona, in Millás' opinion perhaps the most influentual works on later astronomers; Fadl ibn Hatim al-Nayrizi's (known as Anarazicum in Latin) commentaries on Euclid (*item* 32), likewise translated by Gerard of Cremona; the *Introductorium magnum in astrologiam* by Abu Ma'shar (known as Albumasar in the Latin world), the greatest authority on astrology in the medieval world, translated by John of Seville (*Johannes Hispalensis*) in 1133 (*item* 35); and, finally, the thirteen books of Euclid's *Elementa* of geometry, translated by Gerard of Cremona (*item* 37).[87]

Fifth, I would like to draw attention to the simultaneous presence of Boethius' arithmetical works (*item* 26) and the *algorismus* (*item* 34). The latter is characteristic of the later medieval algorithmic tradition, the first steps towards which are to be traced in John of Seville's translation of al-Khwarizmi's *Algorismi de practica aritmetica* and in Gerard of Cremona's summarised translation *Algorismus in integris*, as well as in the *Liber algorismi* by the Canon of Toledo 'Master Juan' (*Johannes Hispanus*).[88] This is effectively a *quaestio* of

[87] For details of the works referred to in this point see MILLÁS VALLICROSA, *Las traducciones orientales* (note 65), pp. 61, 148, 151, 166-170, 185, 196, 209, 212 and 220.

[88] MILLÁS VALLICROSA, *Las traducciones orientales* (note 65), p. 64. On the canon *Johannes Hispanus*, see the article by BURNETT (note 64), pp. 428 *et seq.* and the excellent book by ALLARD, A., *Muhammad Ibn Musa Al-Khwarizmi. Le calcul indien (algorismus).* Histoire des textes, édition critique, traduction et commentaire des plus anciennes versions latines remaniées du XIIe siècle, Paris-Namur, 1992.

al-Khwarizmi's *Algebra*. Moreover, according to Allard, it is the only Latin algorithmic text presented in the format of the *quaestio*, the origin of which should be sought in twelfth century Toledo. At present, there is but one extant late twelfth or early thirteenth century manuscript from Italy (Paris, BN, Lat. 15461, fols. 12v-13r).[89] The contents of the *quaestio* cover not only general aspects related to the nature of numbers but also theological aspects (for example, allusions to the oneness of God and His Trinitarian nature), rather than practical algorithmic matters proper. In this respect, it is an interesting example of how the *libri naturales* were integrated into the new theological speculations of Christian intellectuals, a subject that will be discussed below in connection with the presence of Peter Lombard's *Liber sententiarum* and commentaries on Paul's Epistles among the works loaned to our friars. Be that as it may, the presence of Boethius and the algorithm (even though this presence is characterised by the above-mentioned features) indicates the link between the Santiago schools and the modernising current within calculation, which led to the introduction of Arabic numerals (and the presence of the zero in calculations and the replacement of the abacus) and a change in the way practical arithmetic was taught, including aspects such as addition, subtraction, multiplication, division, calculation of square and cubic roots, the latter being, in addition, a totally new feature in the Latin West.[90]

Sixth, the presence in 1222 of works on theology and the Scriptures should be noted; these included Peter Lombard's *Librum sententiarum* (*item* 1) and his commentary on St. Paul's Epistles (*item* 18), which demonstrate, as has already been pointed out, that these schools expressed an interest in the new approach to

---

[89] The text of the *quaestio* begins as follows: 'Queritur cur non omnes uel plurimos numeros propriis nominibus designamus, uel cur non per adiunctionem nouorum sed post decem per repetitionem priorum semper numeramus. Ad quod dicitur. Quia non fuit possibile ut omnes numeri propria nomina haberent, idcirco quia numerorum in infinitum crescit multitudo, nominem autem in qualibet lingua infinita non potest esse inuentio. Cum enim in omni lingua certa et terminata sunt instrumenta et eorum definite naturaliter modulationes quibus uox articulata formatur, et unde litteratum figure apud omnes gentes et earum uarie scilicet diffinite sunt secundun ordinem preponendi et postponendi as representanda rerum omnium nomina compositione ...' (transcribed by A. Allard). It was M.-T. d'Alverny who demonstrated its origins to have lain in Toledo. I am indebted to André Allard for all the information referring to this *quaestio* (personal communication).

[90] See BEAUJOUAN, G., 'L'enseignement de l'arithmétique élémentaire à l'Université de Paris aux XIIIe et XIVe siècles', XI, pp. 95-98 (note 79). The opinion of THORNDIKE, L., can be found in *The Sphere of Sacrobosco and its commentators*, Chicago, 1949. The existence of the *Liber algorismi* in Toledo in the second half of the twelfth century and the reference made to it by DOMINGO GUNDISALVO, in his *De divisione philosophiae,* as the source of his learning practical arithmetic suggests that this discipline was being taught in the cathedral school of Toledo: 'Ex materia vero accidit ei [*i.e.* aritmeticae] aggregari et disgregari, multiplicari et dividi et huiusmodi, que docentur in libro algorismi'. See the edition by BAUR, L., (*Beiträge z. Gesch. d. Phil. d. Mitt.,* Münster, 1903, IV. 2-3, p. 91) (note 34 of the documentary appendix).

the teaching of theology, a feature of the most active centres —to be more precise, of Paris— and also that they were in possession of the intellectual tools that provided the new scholastic movement with its flexibility, in other words the *quaestio* and the *disputatio*, an aspect for which there is evidence in the presence and use of the *quaestio algorismi*, as was mentioned above[91].

Seventh, I would also like to draw attention to the implication of the presence of works concerning the Scriptures, science or natural philosophy (mathematics, astronomy, astrology and the natural sciences) and of Peter Lombard's *Sentences* in the same library at this date. It is evident that this small group of intellectuals, like other European communities, was confident that science (natural philosophy) was capable of providing knowledge of the true nature of the physical world and that this would supply invaluable keys for a detailed understanding and explanation of those passages of the Scriptures related to the nature of the created world and even to the very nature of God Himself (for instance, the use of the concept of infinity or eternity as applied to God). In brief, we can witness one of the most interesting phenomena of medieval intellectual life: the impact of the *libri naturales* (natural philosophy, science) on theology. In this respect, Peter Lombard's *Liber sententiarum* (*item* 1), written in about 1150, provides an interesting starting point.[92] It should be remembered that its four books deal with God, the creation, the incarnation and the sacraments respectively. The second book, devoted to the creation, gave those intellectuals familiar with the *libri naturales* an opportunity to deal with specific subjects such as the nature of light, the four elements, all the complex problem of supra-and infra-celestial waters, the order and the movement of the planets and the celestial spheres, or the day-night succession. In this way, natural philosophy shaped a new form of theology and offered new ways to interpret and comment on Holy Writ, both in the Old and the New Testament, above all because it made it possible to reconsider the question of the relationship between God and the created world and its creatures. To this was to be added, as has been pointed out, the contribution of new subjects that brought about a new approach to preaching. This line of approach (the use of the *libri naturales* in commentaries on the *Sentences*), which was started in the late twelfth and early thirteenth centuries, reached such proportions that in 1366 the University of Paris (its different attitude to such matters in comparison with Oxford has already been

---

[91] On the role of these instruments in medieval intellectual life, see CHENU, M.-D., *Introduction à l'étude de Saint Thomas d'Aquin*, Montreal-Paris, 1954. For their application to the field of medical knowledge see GARCÍA BALLESTER, L., Introduction to the edition of the *Commentum supra tractatum Galieni de malicia complexionis diverse*, Barcelona, 1985, pp. 56-137 (*Arnaldi de Villanova Opera Medica Omnia*, vol. XV).

[92] GRANT, E., 'Science and theology in the Middle Ages', in *God and Nature. Historical essays on the encounter between Christianity and science*, Berkeley, 1986, pp. 49-75.

noted) limited its use in the treatment of the *quaestiones* because the problems that were considered only dealt with physics or pure mathematics.[93]

Eighth, we must mention that the presence of a certain attitude and certain intellectual tools, recorded for the first time in an institutional context in this part of Spain, and which had no connection with the modest intellectual activity that had hitherto been the norm in the Santiago cathedral grammar school, where 'some rhetoric and logic' were taught, represented a considerable novelty.[94] As far as I know, these currents were only comparable with those circulating in intellectual circles centred upon the cathedral of Toledo and its archbishop, Rodrigo Ximénez de Rada (1210-47), a former Bishop of Osma and a contemporary of both Pedro Muñiz and Bernardo II.[95] Nevertheless, the fact that Aristotle's *libri naturales* were being used so frequently in 1222 (*items* 6, 7 and 12), and the variety and complexity of the works that were used in the years immediately afterwards (1225-1230), enable us to conjecture that there must have been a substantial change in the intellectual concerns of the circles surrounding the archbishop in the eighty years that elapsed between the death of Archbishop Diego Gelmírez (1140) and the arrival of the Franciscans and Dominicans in Santiago.[96]

---

[93] DENIFLE, H., CHATELAIN, A., *Chartularium universitatis parisiensis*, Paris, 1894, vol. 3, 144. Cited by GRANT, 'Science and theology' (note 92), p. 73, note 32.

[94] DÍAZ Y DÍAZ, 'Problemas de la cultura en los siglos XI-XII' (note 42), p. 197; *Idem* 'La escuela episcopal de Santiago en los siglos XI-XIII' (note 42), pp. 183-188. As FLETCHER states (*Saint James's Catapult*, cited in note 42, at p. 324), the main impediment to going beyond Díaz y Díaz's statement is the lack of documentation on this subject.

[95] Very little is known about scientific activity in Toledo in the first half of the thirteenth century. Burnett's article, referred to above (note 64), might be consulted as an indication of the situation. A very interesting subject which has still not been examined from the point of view here being discussed is the role played by Archbishop Rodrigo during the period of almost forty years that he held the see of Toledo, a period that was of the utmost importance in the political, religious, cultural and scientific life of Castile in the first half of the thirteenth century. It suffices to remember that Michael Scot lived and worked in Toledo during his episcopate and that he translated the highly significant corpus of Aristotle's natural philosophy works known by the name of *De animalibus* (*item* 42 in the list of books below) from Arabic to Latin in the city probably between 1217 and 1220. The original translation in his hand was preserved by Archbishop Gonzalo Pétrez (d. 1299), as is shown by the inventory he had drawn up in 1280 when he took possession of the see of Toledo ('Siete quadernos del libro de animalibus scriptos de la mano del traslador', Madrid, Biblioteca Nacional, no. 13022, fol. 185v). *Cf*. GONZÁLVEZ, R.: *Hombres y libros de Toledo*, Madrid, 1998, pp. 480-1 and 508.

[96] In fact, what happened in Santiago de Compostela, as far as the intellectual life resulting from the new attention being paid to the *libri naturales* was concerned, in the period of eighty years between the death of Diego Gelmírez (1140) and the first evidence for the presence of a large collection of scientific books, including a substantial part of the *Aristoteles latinus* (1222)? As is known, these were years of intense intellectual and translating activity, not only in Toledo, but also in the Ebro valley and in other parts of the Iberian Peninsula, particularly the nearby new Kingdom of Portugal.

Ninth, and last, I cannot leave unmentioned what is implied by the presence in the list of 1230 of the text on simple medicaments (*De simplicibus medicinis*), written by the physician of Salerno, John or Matteo Plateario (*item* 41), and more commonly known by its first two words (*Circa instans*). It is a list of varying length (with between 200 and 270 products, depending on the manuscript and date), originally drawn up in the mid-twelfth century, in which simple medicaments, mainly of plant origin, are listed in alphabetical order together with a brief description of their properties and usage. The *Circa instans* is a handbook of a practical nature, with no theoretical content, which enjoyed great popularity and which, together with the *Antidotarium magnum* and the *Antidotarium Nicolai* (both also from Salerno), provided healers (physicians, surgeons and apothecaries) with the keys to a rational approach to healing that responded to the suppositions of Galenism, an approach that had been developed in twelfth-century Salerno.[97] The Brothers Minor trained in medical attention did not hesitate to continue practising it as a practical extension of their charitable mission to their sick fellow men.[98] Did Pedro de Odoario practise medicine

---

See LEMAY, R., 'Dans l'Espagne du douzième siècle. Les traductions de l'arabe au latin', *Annales ESC*, 18 (1963), 639-665; *idem* 'De la scolastique à l'histoire par le truchement de la philologie: itinéraire d'un médiéviste entre Europe et Islam' (cited in note 21); and his article 'Gerard de Cremona', in *DSB*. Similarly, the articles by D. Pingree on 'Abu Ma'shar', 'Masha'allah', 'Al-Qabisi' and ' 'Umar ibn al-Farrukhan al-Tabari' in *DSB*.

These doubts are reinforced if it is taken into account that we are in possession of a very similar document to the one analysed in this paper (which I am studying at the moment from the point of view of the history of science), which also includes a series of loans of *libri naturales* in 1207, 1218 and 1226 between the house of Canons Regular of Santa Cruz in Coimbra and that of San Vicente in Lisbon (Oporto, Municipal Public Library, Santa Cruz cod. 34, last folio, verso. It has been reproduced by FRANCISCO DA GAMA CAEIRO, 'Fontes portuguesas da formaçao cultural do Santo (Antonio de Padua)', *Itinerarium*, 27 (1981) 130-164, at p. 156). I therefore consider that there is good reason to wonder about the origins of the Santiago library, which the earliest Franciscans and Dominicans in the city hurried to make use of.

[97] HUNT, T., 'Introduction' in *Popular medicine in Thirteenth-Century England*, Suffolk, 1990, pp. 1-63 and the bibliography referred to there.

[98] See FELDER, H., *Geschichte der wissenschaftlichen Studien im Franziskanerorden bis um die Mitte des 13. Jahrhunderts*, Frieburg i. B., 1904, pp. 390-397. The sixth General of the Franciscan Order (1244-47), Brother Crescencio (Grizzi da Jesi) was a 'medicus famosus, cuius zelum inflammavit charitas, informavit scientia, confirmavit constantia' according to Eccleston's account (*De adventu Minorum in Angliam*, ed. Mon. Franc. I, 49. *Anal. Franc.* I, 244. Cited by Felder, p. 393. There is an edition by LITTLE, A. G., (*Fratris Thomae vulgo dicti de Eccleston Tractatus De adventu Fratris Minorum in Angliam*, Manchester, 1951), which I have not been able to consult in its entirety). Robert Grosseteste's physician was a Franciscan [SRAWLEY, J. H., 'Grosseteste's Administration of the Diocese of Lincoln', in Callus, D. A., ed., *Robert Grosseteste, Scholar and Bishop* (note 53), p. 148], while the Dominican provincial chapter held in Palencia in 1249 forbade those brothers who were physicians to attend patients who did not belong to the order. 'Item, fratres phisici in nostra provincia de cetero praeter fratres nostros non recipiant infirmum aliquem in curam, nec respiciant urinas, nec dent aliquam medicinam' (DOUAIS, *Acta Capitulorum Provincialium Ord.*

himself or did he handle this brief work only because of his interest in finding out the nature of the curative materials used in the remedies prescribed by the healers of his time? The presence of a large number of prescriptions in the two works on natural history written fifty years later by the Franciscan Juan Gil (*Historia naturalis* and *Contra venena et animalia venenosa*) in his Zamora friary suggests that there were some at least among the Fransciscans who continued to pay attention to this field within the study of nature.[99]

We are, then, witnesses of the very beginnings of a tradition that, whether steadily or in fits and starts (in fact somewhat inconsistently), gradually became more prominent in the course of the thirteenth century. However, for reasons that now escape us and which have hitherto hardly been analysed, in Castile this institutionalisation of intellectual life revolving around the study of mathematics and natural matters was not maintained and even failed to be accepted in the decisive thirteenth century. Why did the Franciscan *Studium* of Oxford, which was created five years later following the same model as found in Santiago, subsequent to the initial stimulus provided by Robert Grosseteste (as from 1224-25) and, shortly afterwards, that of the Franciscan Adam Marsh (from 1237 onwards), and the Dominican centre of Saint-Jacques (Paris), despite the restrictions of the 1228 Constitutions, continue to dedicate themselves to and produce works related to the fields of theology, mathematics and the natural sciences, whereas the brilliant beginnings of the Santiago *Studia* and the intense intellectual activity of Pedro de Odoario and Juan Fernández, who initiated this same tradition in Santiago, from 1222 onwards, was not followed up in a consistent fashion? Why do we have to wait for the scientific output of Pedro Gallego between 1250 and 1267, which was admittedly interesting, but limited and hardly up-to-date for his time, or that of Juan Gil in the last third of the century, to find any continuation at all to these promising first steps? Why were the social impact of the mendicant orders in the extensive and wealthy lands ruled by Castile, or the large number of young men who flocked to join their ranks from these same kingdoms, where population numbers were relatively high by contemporary European standards, and the area's long intellectual tradition,

FF. Praed., 610, n. 7). Shortly afterwards, in Barcelona in 1299, attendance at the faculties of medicine on the part of Brothers Preacher was restricted, unless they had already studied medicine before joining the order (DOUAIS, *op.cit.*, 648, no. 14. Cited by Felder, pp. 393-394). We know the names of two Franciscans (Fr. Albert, *fl.*1295, and Fr.Arnult, *fl.*1315) of this same period, that is the late thirteenth and early fourteenth centuries, who practised medicine in royal circles in the Crown of Aragon and in the realms of Castile. See WEBSTER, JILL R., *Els Menorets. The Franciscans in the Realms of Aragon from St. Francis to the Black Death*, Toronto, 1993, pp. 188-189 and McVAUGH, M.R., *Medicine before the plague. Practitioners and their patients in the Crown of Aragon, 1285-1345*, Cambridge, 1993, pp. 72-75.

[99] See the extensive introductory study in *Johannes Aegidius Zamorensis Historia Naturalis* (note 4), vol. I, pp. 17-97.

not reflected in scientific activity of comparable significance and an associated intellectual output in the form of books and/or commentaries? What happened in the extensive realms of New Castile in the thirteenth century as regards the activities and subjects that have been discussed, especially in the three decades that elapsed between 1222 —the year when Pedro de Odoario and Juan Fernández, who were totally familiar with the 'new Aristotle' and the new mathematics (astronomy-astrology), are first recorded— and 1252, when Alfonso X started to reign and to promote the intense intellectual activity that was so much a feature of his court? The current state of research does not allow us to answer these questions; however, the discovery in the Vatican Library of this document, which reveals a hitherto unknown intellectual world by means of the books used by the Franciscan and Dominican *Studia* of Santiago de Compostela in 1222, enables us to pose questions that, until now, would have been impossible to formulate, and thereby offers an opportunity to open up a new area of research.

Appendix

[List of the manuscripts that the 'Brothers Minor' of the house of Vallis Dei (Santiago de Compostela) and the brothers of the Order of Preachers of the house of Bone Vallis (Santiago de Compostela) took out of the library of the archbishop (or archbishopric) of Santiago between 16.8.1222 and 16.9.1230].

(Vat. Lat. 659, fol. 1r)

This edition has been prepared from the photograph and the negative of the original document. It has been published on two previous occasions: in 1930 (D. de Bruyne) and in 1993 (M. de Castro). De Bruyne's edition contained serious errors as regards its date, its origin and the text itself (see note 2 of this article); that prepared by M. de Castro is more careful, but it contains a number of transcription errors, which I have endeavoured to correct. I have modified the numbers allocated by M. de Castro as it has proved possible to identify a larger number of the works it refers to.

I have inserted a (?) after all doubtful words. Whatever may be written between angular brackets < > or round brackets ( ) is not to be found in the original document. I have introduced the words 'archiepiscopus' or 'dominus archiepiscopus' in those blank spaces with traces of erased words, on the basis of the version of the text in the library of Archbishop Bernardo II of Santiago, where they figure in the original [García y García; Vázquez Janeiro (cited in note 66 of this article), *items* 39, 51-52 in Bernardo II's library].

<1>

Era m.cc.lx. et quot xvii. kalendas Septembris. (16.8.1222)

1. Habent fratres Vallis Dei a domino <archiepiscopo...> librum sentenciarum.[1]
2. Item habet ab eo frater P<etrus> Oduarii quendam librum de naturis.[2]
3. Item habet ab eo frater Martinus Fernandi quendam Alexander.[3] [*The whole item is crossed out*].
4. Item habet frater Petrus Oduarii, de ordine minorum, librum Dionisii De divinis nominibus,[4] cum aliis libris in eodem volumine.
5-7. Item habet librum De anima <et> spiritu,[5] et De plantis,[6] et <De> sopno et vigilia,[7] in eodem volumine.

---

[1] LOMBARD, PETER (*ca.* 1095/1100-1160): *Sententiae in IV libris distinctae,* ed. I. Brady, 2 vols., Grottaferrata, Rome, 1971-1981 (PL, 192, 522-963). On the presence of Peter Lombard and the Paris masters in Santiago see A. GARCÍA Y GARCÍA; I. VÁZQUEZ JANEIRO, 'La biblioteca del arzobispo de Santiago de Compostela, Bernardo II', pp. 548-552.

[2] This is probably a work by ALAN of LILLE (*ca.* 1128-1202), *De planctu naturae* or *Enchiridion de rebus naturae* (ed. by N. M. HÄRING, 'Alan of Lille, 'De Planctu naturae', *Studi Medievali*, Serie Terza, 19 (1978) 797-879; or perhaps his bestiary, *De naturis quorundam animalium* (M. MANITIUS, *Geschichte der lateinischen Literatur des Mittelalters*, 3 vols. Munich, 1911-1939, III, 804.

It cannot be excluded that it might have been ISIDORE of SEVILLE's *De natura rerum* (*Inc.*: Illustri domino et filio Sisebuto Ysidorus. Dum te prestantem ingenio facunda...) (TK 660) (PL 83, 865-1018). It is also known by the following names: *De astris caeli, De astronomia, Liber astronomicus, Rotarum liber* (published as: *Isidori Hispalensis De natura rerum liber.* Recensuit Gustavus Becker, Berlin, 1857). It brings together the cosmographical, astronomical and meteorological information scattered throughout his *Etymologies*. See DUHEM, P., *Le Système du Monde*, III, pp. 5-12.

[3] This must be the commentaries by ALEXANDER of APHRODISIAS on Aristotle (*De motu et tempore, De sensu,On matter and form, De intellectu*), which were translated by Gerard of Cremona, and by William of Moerbeke. Both translations were to be found in the library of the Archbishop of Toledo, D. Gonzalo Pétrez, according to the inventory that was drawn up when he moved from Burgos to Toledo (1280). See J. Mª MILLÁS VALLICROSA, *Las traducciones orientales en los manuscritos de la biblioteca catedral de Toledo,* Madrid, 1942, p. 18, R. GONZÁLVEZ, *Hombres y libros de Toledo*, Madrid, 1998, pp. 487 and 503.

[4] This is likely to have been the Latin version produced by JOHN THE SCOT ERIGENA (*ca.* 800 - *ca.* 877). Sancti Dionysii Aeropagitae *De divinis nominibus*, in JOANNIS SCOTI [ERIGENA], *Opera quae supersunt omnia...*, ed. H. J. Floss, Paris, 1853 (PL 122). However, we cannot reject the possibility that it may have been the version of Johannes Sarracinus (d. 1180), which formed part of the corpus on Dionysius that was brought together in Paris in the first half of the thirteenth century, with his works, letters, glosses and commentaries, a result of the entire previous Latin and Greek tradition. In fact, it is true to say that the early thirteenth century witnessed an authentic renaissance of pseudo-Dionysian studies. See H. F. DONDAINE, *Le Corpus Dionysien de l'Université de Paris au XIIIe siècle*, Rome, 1953, pp. 20-21 and 34. The 'aliis libris' that accompanied this work in the same volume are likely to have been the corpus of Dionysius' works, or part of this same corpus, as has been mentioned.

[5] From the context in which it appears, bound in the same codex with works by Aristotle or attributed to him (*items* 6 and 7), this must have been QUSTA IBN LUQA's (Costa ben Luca to the Latin West) *De differentia animae et spiritus* in John of Seville's translation. In the thirteenth and fourteenth centuries, it was often copied together with works by Aristotle, especially the *De anima*, as it was

8. Item librum De collacionibus sanctorum patrum.[8]
9. Item habet <*blank*> frater <*illegible*>.[9]
10-12. Item habent fratres minores Vallis Dei de armario <domini archiepiscopi> tres libros videlicet, Priscianum maiorem,[10] librum De Colloquio Simonis et Ihesu,[11] et librum Eciocorum Aristotilis,[12] cum aliis scripturis, in uno volumine.

---

considered to be a supplement or explanation of the same. The same association as is found in this *item* in the Santiago document (i.e. with *De plantis* and *De somno*) is to be found in MS 47-15 of Toledo Cathedral [VI in MILLÁS, *Las traducciones orientales en los manuscritos de la biblioteca de la catedral de Toledo* (cited in note 65), pp. 58-61], fol. 86rb; similarly in the Erfurt MS, Amploniana F. 32, of the second half of the thirteenth century, the contents of which are: 'Aristotelis de anima, Liber Aristotelis de memoria et reminiscencia, Liber beati Augustine de differencia spiritus et anime (*Inc.: Interrogasti me: honoret te Deus...*, TK 771, which in fact was the Latin translation of Qusta ibn Luqa's work), Libri duo Aristotelis de sensu et sensato, Libri duo A. de sompno et vigilia, Libri duo A. de vegetabilibus et plantis, Libri A. de longitudine et brevitate vite..., Liber Alphorabii de propietatibus scientiarum, (*Inc.: Cum essent plures philosophi...*, in fact Robert Kilwardby's *De divisione scientiarum*). The same association can be found in the Oxford MSS, Balliol College, 232A and 232B, Corpus Christi College CXI and Bodleian Auct. F. 5.25.

[6] This was the pseudo-Aristotelian work *De vegetabilibus* or *De plantis*. It was translated from the Arabic into Latin in 1178 by the Englishmen, Alfred of Sareshel, who worked in Spain. See Ch. H. HASKINS, *Studies in the History of Mediaeval Science*, Cambridge, 1924, p. 128. *De plantis libri duo,* ed. E. H. F. Meyer, Leipzig, 1841.

[7] Latin version translated from the Greek of Aristotle's treatise *De sompno et vigilia*, produced by an anonymous translator working in Italy in the mid-twelfth century. See L. MINIO-PALUELLO, 'Aristotle: Tradition and Influence', *DSB*, vol. 1, pp. 270-271.

[8] This was a work by JOHANNES CASSIANUS EREMITA (*ca.* 380 - *ca.* 435) entitled *Collationes patrum* (Migne, PL 49, 477-1328); he was one of the founders of western monastic life [see G. SARTON, *Introduction to the history of science*, vol. III-II, Baltimore, 1948, p. 1392 (reprinted New York, 1975)].

[9] It is impossible to identify what is written from the negative and photocopy that I have used.

[10] PRISCIANUS CAESARIENSIS (*fl. ca.* 512): *Commentariorum grammaticorum libri xviii*, above all based on Apollonius Dyscolus (first half of the second century A.D.), a fundamental work in medieval teaching. See G. SARTON, *Introduction to the history of science,* I, p. 140. This work was also to be found in Bernardo II's library (*item* 58) and was on that occasion loaned to the Brothers Preacher of *Bone Vallis* [García y García, Vázquez Janeiro (cited in note 66 to the article) p. 566]. Ed. M. Hertz, in H. KEIL, *Grammatici latini*, 2-3, Leipzig, 1855-59 (Hildesheim, 1961).

[11] M. DE CASTRO (note 2 to the article, p. 160) identified this as the work of Abbot GAUFRIDUS, a disciple of St Bernard's: *Declamationes de colloquio Simonis cum Iesu, ex s. Bernardi sermonibus collectae* (Migne, PL 184, 437-476).

[12] This was probably the Latin translation from the Greek of the *Ethica Nicomachea*, prepared at the Norman court (of which books I-III and fragments of books VII and VIII survive), earlier than the version prepared by Robert Grosseteste, who made use of these books. He carried out this task after 1230, probably around 1245-47 [D. A. CALLUS, 'Robert Grosseteste as Scholar', in D. A. Callus, ed.: *Robert Grosseteste, Scholar and Bishop,* Oxford, 1955 (repr. 1969), pp. 1-69, at pp. 62-65]. The reference to the Santiago Franciscans using Aristotle's books of *Ethics* (1222) must be one of the earliest recorded thirteenth-century examples. It should be taken into account that in his work *De Bono* (1244-46) Albert the Great stated that he still did not have all book eight of Aristotle's *Ethics* at

<2>

xviii. kalendas Decembris in Er<a> <*illegible*> (14.11.?).

13.<Item> <*illegible*> Lucam et Johannem, <in> uno volumine.[13]
14-16. Item Apocalisim,[14] Au<c>tus apostolorum,[15] Canonicas epistolas,[16] in alio volumine.
17. Item li<brum> Ezaquielis glosatum in alio volumine.[17] Et sciendum quod Epistole canonice sunt derurpate in fine ex aqua pruviali.
18. Item eadem die recepit ab eisdem fratribus duo paria epistolarum Pauli glosata.[18]

<3>

Era m.cc.lx tercia.et quot iii. idus Januarii (11.1.1225).

19. Item frater Petrus Oduarii recepit <*illegible*> fratrum minorum <*illegible*> Almagestum.[19]

---

his disposal (*De passionibus*) and he could only make use of *excerpta* (*Alberti Magni Opera Omnia. Tomus XXVIII: De Bono*. Aschendorff, 1951, tr. iii, quest. v, arts. 2 and 3, pp. 197 and 206-207). See A. PELZER: 'Les versions latines des ouvrages de morale conservés sous le nom d'Aristote, en usage au XIIIe siècle', *Rev. Neoscholastique* (1921), pp. 316-341, 378-412. In addition, *Aristoteles Latinus*, codices descripsit G. Lacombe in societatem operis adsumptis A. Birkenmajer, M. Dulong, A. Franceschini, Rome 1939, I, 67-71, and L. Minio-Paluello: 'Aristotle: tradition and influence', *DSB*, vol. I, p. 274.

[13] This work is also to be found in the inventory of Bernardo II's library (*item* 16). See GARCÍA y GARCÍA; VÁZQUEZ JANEIRO (note 66 to the article), p. 561.

[14] The same works was in Bernardo II's library (*item* 20). GARCÍA y GARCÍA; VÁZQUEZ JANEIRO, *ibidem* .

[15] Also present in Bernardo II's library (*item* 19). *Ibidem.*

[16] The same work was present in Bernardo II's library (*item* 18) although these three books of the New Testament were bound as one volume in the archbishop's library. *Ibidem.*

[17] This was probably the same work that was included in the catalogue of Bernardo II's library (*item* 8). See GARCÍA y GARCÍA; VÁZQUEZ JANEIRO, *ibid.* p. 560.

[18] This can be identified as PETER LOMBARD'S *Glossa in Epistolas beati Pauli.* Two versions are known, one prior to and the other subsequent to the *Sententiae*; there is no way of deciding which version is here referred to. Together with the *Glossa in Psalmos*, also by Peter Lombard, it is known by the name of *Glossatura Magna.* It is also recorded in the catalogue of Bernardo II's library (*item* 17); when the catalogue was drawn up, this work was on loan to the 'fratres Vallis Dei'. See GARCÍA y GARCÍA; VÁZQUEZ JANEIRO, *ibid.*, p. 561.

[19] This was the Latin version of Ptolemy's *Almagest.* The absence of the *incipit* prevents us from determining whether it alludes to the translation from the Arabic prepared by Gerard of Cremona in

20. Item recepit Alfraganum.[20]
21. Item Alfarabium.[21]
22. Item librum de cena philosophorum.[22]
23. <Item quoddam> scriptum super Almagestum.[23]
24. Item quosdam sermones Mauricii parisiensis episcopi.[24]

Toledo in 1174-75 [see Millás Vallicrosa, (cited in note 65), pp. 148-150 (MS XXXV)], or to that produced in Sicily directly from the Greek in about 1160 [Haskins, (in note 6 to the Appendix), pp. 157, 191-193], or about 1150 by Hermann of Carinthia [R. Lemay, 'De la scolastique à l'histoire par le truchement de la philologie: Itinéraire d'un médiéviste entre Europe et Islam' in *La diffusione delle scienze islamische nel medio evo europeo* (Convegno internazionale, Roma, 2-4 ottobre 1984), Rome, 1987, pp. 399-535, especially pp. 428 *et seq*.].

[20] This was almost certainly AL-FARGHANI's *Elementa astronomica*, a work which was translated into Latin twice in the twelfth century: first, by John of Seville (1135); secondly by Gerard of Cremona (before 1175). The latter's translation was more complete and therefore enjoyed greater diffusion [Millás, (work cited in note 65 to the article), pp. 141, 173-174]. The second translation is known by the name of *Liber de aggregacionibus sciencie stellarum* (see *item* 36). The absence of the *incipit* prevents us from identifying it more exactly. The ample diffusion of al-Farghani's works in European intellectual circles contributed to the popularity of Ptolemy's astronomy. This was helped by its descriptive rather than mathematical nature and the clear, educational presentation of its contents. See A. I. SABRA, 'Al-Farghani, Abu l-Abbas Ahmad ibn Muhammad ibn Kathir', *DSB*, vol. 4, pp. 541-545.

[21] It is impossible to identify this work by AL-FARABI because there is no *incipit*. It is likely to have been the *De scientiis* [42] in the translation by Gerard of Cremona. This work had been previously translated by Domingo Gundisalvo. However, it might also have been the *De Syllogismo* [3] (TK 925) (a probable commentary on Aristotle's *Prior analytics)*, or his Commentary on Aristotle's *Physics* [40], both of which were also translated by Gerard of Cremona. Domingo Gundisalvo's translation was published by M. ALONSO, *Domingo Gundisalvo. De scientiis*. Texto latino ...., Madrid-Granada, 1954; Gerard of Cremona's version was published by A. GONZÁLEZ PALENCIA, *Al-Farabi. Catálogo de las ciencias*, 2nd edition, Madrid, 1953. The translation of the commentary on the *Physics* can be found in A. BIRKENMAJER, *Aus der Geisteswelt des Mittelalters. Studien und texte Martin Grabmann zur Vollendung des 60. Lebenjahres... gewidmet*, Münster, 1935, pp. 472-475. See R. LEMAY, 'Gerard of Cremona', *DSB*, vol. 15, Supp. I, pp. 173-192 (the numbers in square brackets after the titles of Gerard of Cremona's translations refer to the list of his works as provided by Lemay).

[22] This was the *Convivium septem sapientum*. Edited by G. BUCHNER, *Die historia septem sapientum, nach der Innsbrucker Handschrift v. t. 1342*, Erlangen, 1889.

[23] This may have been the astronomical treatise by MUHAMMAD YABIR IBN AFLAH (an eleventh-twelfth century writer from Seville), which was translated into Latin by Gerard of Cremona. In the top margin of the manuscript from the cathedral of Toledo (98-16, Madrid, Bibl. Nac. 10006, XXXVI in Millás' catalogue), the following words can be read: 'Prologues Geber super almagesti. Verba Geber filii Afflay hyspalensis' [Millás (work cited in note 65 to the article), p. 151].

[24] This was MAURICE de SULLY, bishop of Paris (1160-1196). This is a further indication of the presence of the twelfth-century Parisian intellectual ecclesiastical world in Santiago de Compostela and of the city's archbishops' concern to carry out a process of ecclesiastical reform. Maurice de Sully's sermons were characterised by their 'simple approach and (their) persistent call to the Christian's moral responsibilities' (Longère, I, p. 18). See J. LONGÈRE, *Oeuvres oratories des maitres parisiens au 12 siècle. Étude historique et doctrinale*, 2 vols., Paris, 1975, vol. I, pp. 14-18,

25. Item Musicam Boetii.[25]
26. Item Arismeticam Boetii.[26]
27. Item Boetium De consolatione philosophie.[27]
28. Item quendam librum de stronomia qui incipit 'Bonum scire fuit cor sapientis'.[28]
Post istos supradictos,
29. Item quendam librum De speculis qui incipit 'Sermo de eo quod homo in speculo'.[29]

<4>

In supradicta Era. et quot iii°. idus Januarii (11.1.1225).

Frater Johannes Fernandi, dictus Missal, de ordine predicatorum, nomine conventus predicti monasterii, recepit a domino <archiepiscopo> de armario <domine archiepiscopi>,
30. Mussicam Guidonis, qui incipit 'Gignasio mussas'.[30]

88-91, 203-206, 296-300. For the sermons of Maurice de Sully, in addition to J. B. Schneyer's inventory (*Repertorium der lateinischen Sermones des Mittelalters für die Zeit von 1150-1350*, 5 vols., Münster , 1969-1974, vol. IV, 1972, pp. 170-178), one can also consult the book by J. LONGÈRE, *Les sermons latins de Maurice de Sully, éveque de Paris (+1196). Contribution à l'historie de la tradition manuscrite,* Steenbrugge-Dordrecht, 1988 (*Instrumenta Patristica,* 16).

[25] *De musica libri quinque*, by BOETHIUS (*ca.* 480-524) (Migne, PL 63, 1168-1300). Edited by G. FRIEDLEIN, *De institutione arithmetica libri II, de institutione musica libri V...*, Leipzig, 1867. See Sarton, I, 424-426.

[26] *De arithmetica libri duo* by BOETHIUS (Migne, PL 63, 1079-1168). Edited by G. Friedlein (Leipzig, 1867, see previous note).

[27] *De consolatione philosophiae libri quinque,* by BOETHIUS (Migne, PL 63, 549-862). Edited by R. PEIPER, *Philosophiae consolationis libri V* , Leipzig, 1871. See Sarton (cited in note 8 to this appendix), I, p.425.

[28] This was PTOLEMY's *Almagest* in the Latin translation by Gerard of Cremona. The *incipit* of the text is as follows: 'Bonum scire fuit quod a sapientibus non deviantibus visum est... ' (TK 180. TK = L. THORNDIKE; P. KRIBE, *A Catalogue of Incipits of Mediaeval Scientific Writings in Latin,* London, 1963). For the problems arising from the transmission of this important work see P. KUNITZSCH, *Der Almagest. Die Syntaxis mathematica des Claudius Ptolomäus in arabisch-lateinischen Überlieferung,* Wiesbaden, 1974.

[29] TIDEUS, *De speculis*. Translated from the Arabic into the Latin by Gerard of Cremona. This corresponds to Eutocius' commentary on Archimedes (*ca.* 480). The *incipit* recorded (TK 1388) is: 'Scias quod illud quod videt homo in speculo... '. See Millás (cited in note 65 to the article), 212. Published by A. A. BJÖRNBO and S. VOGL, 'Alkindi, Tideus und Pseudo-Euklid. Drei optische Werke', *Abhandlungen zur Geschichte der mathematischen Wissenschaften mit Einschluss ihrer Anwendungen*, 26, no. 3 (1912).

[30] *Micrologus de disciplina artis musicae*, by GUIDO of AREZZO (*ca.* 990 - 1050), written *ca.* 1050. The great reform in the teaching of music was based on this text: it normalised the use of lines and

31. Item tabulas astronomie qui incipiunt 'Invencio dierum(?)'.[31]
32. Item expositionem primi prologi Euclidis secundum Anarazium.[32]
33. Item canones in motibus celestium corporum qui incipiunt 'Quoniam cuiusque'.[33]
34. Item algorismus qui incipit 'Queritur cur non omnes numeros'.[34]

---

the intervals between them for musical annotation; it indicated the notes of the scales, etc. See Sarton (cited in note 8 to the Appendix), I, 720.

[31] AZARQUIEL's Toledo Tables, translated by Gerard of Cremona. See Millás (cited in note 65 to the article), p. 166.

[32] This was the Latin version of the *Commentum super X primos libros Euclidis* by FADL IBN HATIM AL-NAYRIZI (*fl. ca.* 892 - *ca.* 922) on the Arabic version of Euclid by al-Hajjaj; translated from the Arabic by Gerard of Cremona. Only the first six books and a few lines of the seventh of these commentaries survive in the original Arabic. Gerard of Cremona's translation was published by M. CURTZE, *Anaritii in decem libros priores Elementorum Euclidis commentarii... in codice Cracoviensi 569 servata*, Leipzig, 1899 [*Euclidis opera omnia. Supplementum*] [See Millás (cited in note 65), p. 209 and A. I. SABRA, 'Al-Nayrizi, Abu l-Abbas al Fadl ibn Hatim', *DSB*, vol. 10, pp. 5-7]. A new edition is in preparation, based on the Madrid manuscript (Bibl. Nac. 10010; the other manuscripts known are that in Cracow, already published, and the Vatican example, Bibl. Apost. f. Reg. Suev. 1268, derived from the Madrid manuscript) of which the first volume has been published, including books I-IV (*The Latin Translation of Anaritius' Commentary on Euclid's Elements of Geometry, Books I-IV*. Edited by P. M. J. E. Tummers, Nijmegen, 1994 (Artistarium Supplementa, 9)].

[33] AZARQUIEL, *Canones tabularum Toletanarum*, translated from the Arabic by Gerard of Cremona. These astronomical canons were of earlier date than the Toledo Tables (*item* 31). See Millás (cited in note 65), pp. 166-170 and J. Mª MILLÁS VALLICROSA, *Estudios sobre Azarquiel*, Madrid-Granada, 1943-1950.

[34] This was a gloss, whose origins are to be found in Toledo, in *quaestio* format on al-Khwarizmi's *Algebra*. Nowadays only one manuscript, of late twelfth or early thirteenth century Italian origin, is preserved (Paris, Bibl. Nat., Lat. 15461, fols. 12v - 13r). The complete text of the gloss has been transcribed by A. Allard, who expects to publish it within a algorithmic corpus (personal communication).

Neither should we forget the presence in Toledo of the *Liber Alchorismi de pratica arismetica*, a work that was written by *Magister Johannes*, a canon of Toledo, who was a younger contemporary of Domingo Gundisalvo. Developing a hypothesis of A. Allard, Charles Burnett has recently identified this figure as *Johannes Hispanus* (+ 1215), Dean of the cathedral of Toledo, and later Bishop of Segorbe and a collaborator of Domingo's. The latter, in his work *De divisione philosophiae*, alludes to it by the name of *Liber algorismi* ('ex materia - i.e. arithmetice- ..., que docentur in libro algorismi') [Ed. L. Baur, *Beiträge zur Geschichte der Philosophie des Mittelalters*, IV. 2-3, Münster, 1903, p. 91]. See A. ALLARD, ed., *Mohammed ibn Musa al-Khwarizmi. Le calcul indien*. Édition critique, traduction et commentaire des plus anciennes versions latines remaniées du XIIe siècle, Paris-Namur, 1992, pp. xiv-xx.

Be that as it may, this was a work within the medieval algorithmic tradition, and forming part of its most theoretical and speculative facets, the first steps of which are represented by the Latin translation of al-Khwarizmi's work carried out by John of Seville, Gerard of Cremona's summary translation of 'Algorismus in integris', and the work of 'Magister Johannes' (Iohannes Hispanus). See Millás (cited in note 65), p. 64, and Allard's abovementioned work.

35. Item quendam librum de astronomia qui incipit 'La<u>x Deo qui creavit celum et terram'.[35]
36. Item librum Alfragani, cum tabulis astronomie qui incipit 'Liber de agregacionibus sciencie stellarum'.[36]
37-38. Item duos libros Euclidis De geomatria, quorum uterque incipit 'Ea(?) a quibus procedit sciencia',[37] et tres caterniones de eodem in alio volumine.[38]
39. Item sextum de naturalibus.[39]

---

[35] This would appear to be John of Seville's Latin version (1133) of ALBUMASAR's (Abu Ma'shar), *Introductorium magnum in astrologiam* (TK 813). Seven years later, Hermann of Carinthia (Hermann of Dalmatia) also prepared a partly abbreviated new version in the Iberian Peninsula. The *incipit* of this translation is: 'Apud latinos artium principiis quidam ars...' (TK 116). See R. LEMAY, *Abu Ma shar and Latin Aristotelianism in the Twelfth Century*, Beirut, 1962; see also his article, 'De la scholastique à l'histoire par le truchement de la philologie... ' (cited in note 21 to this article), pp. 410-420. See also the excellent article by D. PINGREE, 'Abu Ma shar al-Balkhi, Ja Far ibn Muhammad', *DSB*, vol. 1, pp. 32-39.

[36] This was the work of AL-FARGHANI, *Liber de agregationibus sciencie stellarum*, translated from the Arabic into Latin by Gerard of Cremona (see *item* 20), accompanied by astronomical tables. This was the title by which the version of the *Elementa astronomica* by Gerard of Cremona was known and from which Dante obtained all his astronomical information. See A. I. SABRA, *DSB*, vol. 4, p. 542.

[37] EUCLID, *Elementorum libri tredecim*, translated from the Arabic into Latin by Gerard of Cremona. See the incipit in TK 479 [Millás (cited in note 65), p. 220]. This was the Latin version based on Ishaq ibn Hunayn's Arabic one, which had been checked by the mathematician Thabit ibn Qurra. See the excellent article by J. MURDOCH, 'Euclid: Transmission of the Elements', *DSB*, vol. 4, pp. 437-459.

[38] It is not possible to identify which of Euclid's works are referred to. They may have been 'quaternions' that included some of Euclid's shorter works, such as the *Liber datorum* or *Data*, the Latin translation of which by Gerard of Cremona, based on the Arabic, is now lost, but which is preserved in another Graeco-Latin version, also of twelfth century date (TK 1545), the *Optica* and *De Speculis* (TK 1313). The *Optica* was translated by Gerard of Cremona from the Arabic version of Ishaq-Thabit and the *De Speculis*, now considered to be a spurious attribution to Euclid, was also probably translated from the Arabic by Gerard of Cremona.

The 'quaternions' could also have contained the version and/or *commenta* of the 'Elements' by ADELARD of BATH, from the Arabic version of Euclid by al-Hajjaj (*fl.* 786-833). Both Adelard's translation (known as Adelard I), and his *commenta* (Adelard II and III) enjoyed widespread diffusion.

A third possibility is that these 'quaternions' could have contained the version of Euclid's "Elements" attributed to Hermann of Carinthia (*fl. ca.* 1140-50), prepared, it would seem, from the Arabic. See M. CLAGETT, 'The medieval Latin translations from the Arabic of the *Elements* of Euclid, with special emphasis on the versions of Adelard of Bath', *Isis*, 44 (1953) 16-42, and the article by J. Murdoch cited in the previous note.

[39] This was the Latin version, translated by Domingo Gundisalvo, Archdeacon of Cuéllar (Segovia), who lived in Toledo, and the Jew Avendouth (= John of Seville according to R. Lemay's hypothesis), of AVICENNA's *De anima*, also known by the name of *Liber sextus naturalium*. See S. VAN RIET: *Avicenna latinus. Liber de anima, I-II-III*, Louvain-Leiden, 1972, pp. 98*-105*. For Lemay's

<5>

Era mª.ccª.lxª.viiiª. et quot viº. kalendas Octobris. (26.9.1230).

40. Recepit <*blank*> frater Petrus Oduarii librum qui dicitur aurora.[40]
41. Item librum de medicina qui incipit 'Circa instans negocium.[41]
42. Item librum De animalibus.[42]
43-45. Item sub eadem Era, Metafisicam Aristatilis cum comento,[43] et librum De anima cum comento,[44] et Metafisicam Algazelis,[45] in uno volumine.

---

arguments, see his article, 'De la scolastique à l'histoire par le truchement de la philologie... ' (cited in note 21 to this article), pp. 410 *et seq.*

[40] M. de Castro identifies this work with one by PETRUS DE RIGA, canon of St. Dénis en Vendome (died 1209), called *Aurora* (fragments) (Migne, PL 212, 17-42), which is a verse anthology of the Bible. TK 1103 gives the *incipit* ('Primo facta dies duo celum terra leguntur...) and refers to two manuscripts, one of thirteenth century date and the other dating from the fourteenth century, which is not identical, with the text to be found in PL.

[41] This is the *De simplicibus* by the Salerno physician MATTEO PLATEARIO, known by the first two words of its *incipit*, 'Circa instans' (TK 211).

[42] This was ARISTOTLE's *De animalibus* (a collection made up by the *History of Animals, Parts of Animals* and *Generation of Animals*), translated in Toledo by Michael Scott before 1220 [Haskins, (cited in note 21 to the article), p. 277]. I would reject the possibility of it having been Avicenna's *De animalibus* (also known by the name of *Abbreviatio de animalibus*), for the translation of which from the Arabic to the Latin Michael Scott was also responsible, as he finished this second translation at the court of Frederick II in 1232 [L. MINIO-PALUELLO, 'Michael Scott', *DSB*, vol. 9, p. 362]

[43] This was probably AVERROES' commentary, which Michael Scott partially translated from the Arabic at the court of Frederick II in about the year 1230. See L. MINIO-PALUELLO, 'Aristotle: Tradition and Influence', *DSB*, vol. 1, p. 272. A Latin version of the *Metaphysics*, translated from the Greek in Italy, but without book XI, had been available since the mid-twelfth century. See L. Minio-Paluello, *DSB*, *ibidem*, pp. 270-271. See notes 51 and 85 above to the article.

[44] This was probably AVERROES' *Commentum magnum de anima*. A manuscript in Paris (Bibl. Nat. Lat. 14385) attributes the translation to Michael Scott. See the introduction to the edition prepared by F. STUART CRAWFORD, *Commentarium magnum in Aristotelis de anima libros*, Cambridge, Mass., 1953. See notes 51 and 85 above to the article.

[45] ALGAZEL (al-Ghazzali) (1058-1111), *Metaphisica* (part of the *Maqasid al-falasifa*), translated from the Arabic into the Latin by Domingo Gundisalvo in collaboration with Johannes Hispanus (+ 1215), probably a Mozarab who was Dean of Toledo cathedral and later Bishop of Segorbe [see Ch. BURNETT, '*Magister Iohannes Hispanus*: Towards the identity of a Toledan translator', in *Comprendre et maitriser la nature au Moyen Age. Mélanges d'histoire et sciences offerts à Guy Beaujouan*, Geneva-Paris, 1994, pp. 425-436]. Published by J. T. MUCKLE, *Algazel's Metaphysics. A mediaeval Translation*, Toronto, 1933 (St. Michael's Mediaeval Studies). See Millás (cited in note 65 to the article) pp. 58-59.

46-47. Item duos libros sermonum, quorum unus incipit 'Hodie fratres celebramus adventus innicium',[46] et alter 'Fili mi si spoponderis pro amico tuo'.[47]

[46] *Sancti Bernardi Sermones in adventu Domini. Sermo primus.* See the Latin text, which reproduces the critical edition of J. Leclercq, and its Spanish translation in *Obras completas de san Bernardo, III. Sermones litúrgicos (1º)*, Madrid, 1985 (BAC) (PL 183, 35-40).

[47] This would seem to be JACQUES DE VITRY (*ca.* 1165-1240), *Sermones de comuni sanctorum* (probably the third sermon, dated to between 1226 and 1228). See J. B. SCHNEYER, *Repertorium der lateinischen Sermones des Mittelalters für die Zeit von 1150-1350*, vol. III, 1971, p. 306. For his biography and the contents of his sermons, see J. LONGÈRE, *Oeuvres oratoires des maitres parisiens au 12 siècle,* 2 vols., Paris, 1975, vol. I, pp. 31-35; 168-176; 346-351. The possibility also exists that it may have been one of ST. AUGUSTINE's sermons.

III

MEDICAL LICENSING AND LEARNING IN FOURTEENTH-CENTURY VALENCIA

FOREWORD

In writing about the medieval Crown of Aragon, where both Catalan and Castilian (as well as Latin) were spoken, it is not easy to avoid arbitrariness in the spelling of proper names and foreign terms. In general, we have tried to maintain the forms particular to the linguistic region in question—thus we refer to the *corts* of Cervera but the *cortes* of Monzón—but we have not managed to do so consistently: we use the form "Lérida" rather than "Lleida," for example. We have been more consistent in employing regnal numbers, always using the Aragonese rather than the Catalan numbering (Pere IV rather than Pere III) as being perhaps more widely recognized.

The authors gratefully acknowledge the support of CICYT (L. G. B.) and the John Simon Guggenheim Memorial Foundation (M. R. M.), which made possible some of the research on which this study is based. We deeply appreciate the kindness of the staff of the Archivo de la Corona de Aragón (Barcelona), of the Archivo del Reino de Valencia, and of the Archivo Municipal de Valencia. We owe particular thanks to Dr. Francisco Gimeno, who called our attention to a number of the documents discussed below.

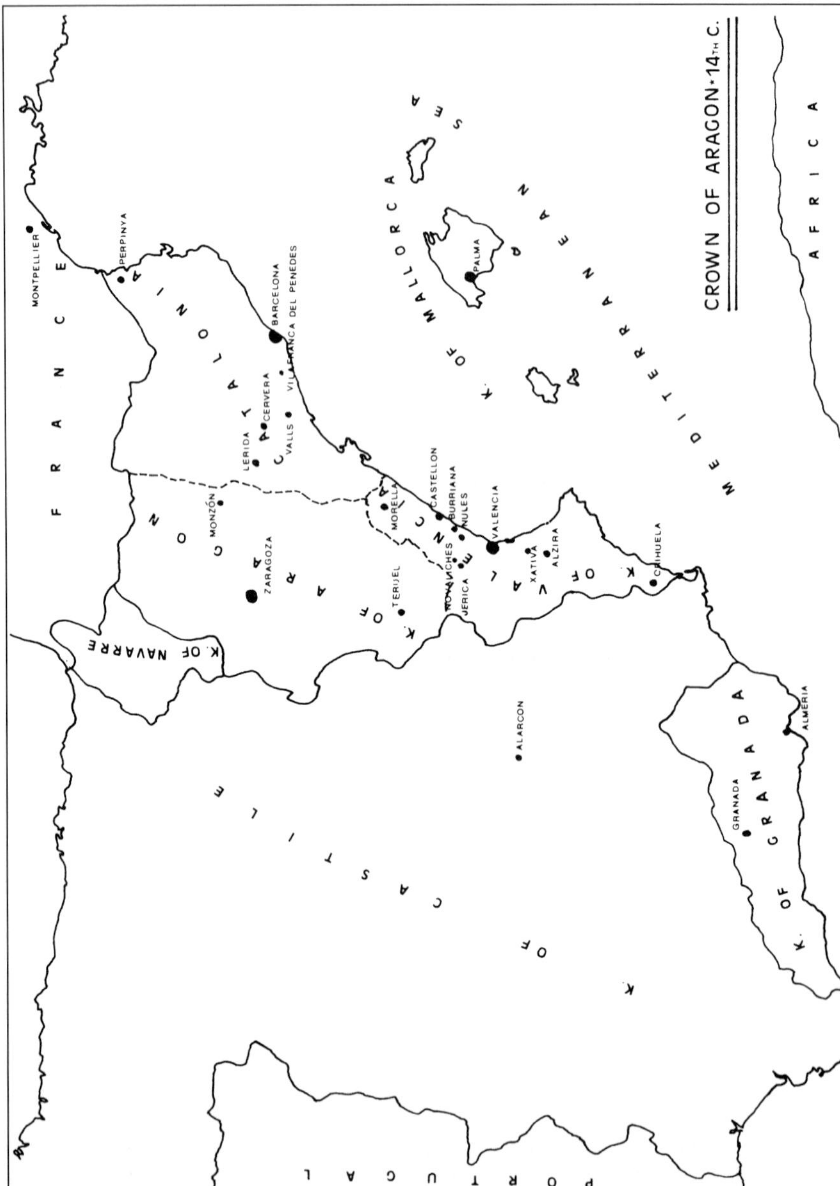
CROWN OF ARAGON · 14TH C.
FRANCE
MONTPELLIER
PERPINYA
CATALONIA
BARCELONA
VILAFRANCA DEL PENEDES
CERVERA
LERIDA
VALLS
MONZÓN
ZARAGOZA
K. OF ARAGON
TERIJEL
K. OF NAVARRE
MORELLA
CASTELLON
BURRIANA
NULES
VALENCIA
JERICA
XATIVA
ALZIRA
K. OF VALENCIA
K. OF MALLORCA
PALMA
MEDITERRANEAN SEA
AFRICA
ALARCON
K. OF CASTILE
K. OF GRANADA
GRANADA
ALMERIA
PORTUGAL

I. THE VALENCIAN *FURS* OF 1329

In the fourteenth century, the kings of Aragon in northeastern Spain governed three countries that were politically and (to a degree) linguistically distinct, and were linked only by the rule of their common monarch: the principality of Catalonia, the kingdom of Aragon, and the kingdom of Valencia—the last-named having been reconquered from Islam as recently as 1238. These realms—which we may conveniently call collectively the "Crown of Aragon," to distinguish them from the kingdom of Aragon proper (see map)—have left abundant archival materials, enabling modern historians to study their societies in particularly close detail.[1] Among the subjects that have recently received scholarly attention, the regulation, availability, and delivery of health care in these lands are proving to be of unusual historical interest. This study will focus on the development of medical regulation in the kingdom of Valencia, but in the process it will also illuminate the same topic with regard to the wider society of the Crown of Aragon and, indeed, of late-medieval Europe.

The presence of an adequate number of medical practitioners (physicians and surgeons), trained in what fourteenth-century documents call "the principles of medical science" and possessed of "verified experience" in the art of healing,[2] was a prerequisite for setting in motion mechanisms for the control of the healing professions, for such mechanisms could be established only after society had begun to institutionalize the process of acquiring medical knowledge.[3] It is not by chance that it was in the kingdom of Sicily that a specific level of training was first required of Western medical practitioners, for in that kingdom, at Salerno (near Naples), there had existed since the twelfth century a tradition of medical instruction based on a fixed corpus of medical writings. This corpus covered not only the basic theoretical aspects of medicine (anatomy, physiology, and pathology), but also the three broad divisions of medical practice or *operatio* (diet, therapeutics, and surgery), and its mastery could thus be assumed to have provided

[1] A good brief survey is T. N. Bisson, *The Medieval Crown of Aragon* (Oxford, 1986).

[2] See, for example, documents 5 ("longa e aprovada experiència") and 6 ("principis de la . . . sciència de física") in the documentary appendix (Appendix 2), below.

[3] For the relation between the institutionalized transmission of medical knowledge and the beginnings of social control of the medical profession, see Pearl Kibre, "The Faculty of Medicine at Paris, Charlatanism and Unlicensed Medical Practices in the Later Middle Ages," *Bulletin of the History of Medicine* 27 (1953), 1–20, especially p. 4.

a student with an adequate theoretical and practical background.[4] Similarly, both at Paris and at Montpellier the right to practice (*venia practicandi*) was being tied to a body of medical knowledge guaranteed by the schools of medicine existing there, schools whose syllabi centered upon the Salernitan medical corpus. The new supervision of the medical profession should not be seen merely as a pragmatic response to a political problem; it is also a social manifestation of the positive value that learning was perceived to have, and of the privileged role that medicine was coming to occupy in the thirteenth and fourteenth centuries within the *firmamentum scientiarum*.[5]

Within the Crown of Aragon, the first legislation in which we see society concerning itself with the regulation of physicians and surgeons comes from the *fueros* enacted by the *cortes* of Monzón in 1289, in which Alfons III (1285–1291) extended to physicians and surgeons a summary provision originally framed to apply to professionals in law:

> 17. Likewise we ordain and decree that no lawyer (*savi en dret*) shall take part in *inquisicions* or *advocacions* or judgments in any court unless he has been examined by the councilors (*prohòmens*) of the town together with other lawyers; and those who are examined shall swear that they will act faithfully in *advocacions* and in the other cases heard by the *veguer* or by the bailiff and the said councilors of the town.
>
> 18. Likewise we ordain and decree that the same thing be done with physicians and surgeons.[6]

---

[4] For the medical corpus used at Salerno and its European diffusion (excluding the Hispanic kingdoms), see Heinrich Schipperges, *Die Assimilation der arabischen Medizin durch das lateinische Mittelalter* (Wiesbaden, 1964). For the diffusion of Salernitan medicine in Castile, see Luis García Ballester, "El papel de las instituciones de consumo y difusión de ciencia médica en la Castilla del siglo XIII: El Monasterio, la catedral y la Universidad," *Dynamis* 4 (1984), 33–63; also idem, "La circulación de las ideas médicas en la Castilla de Alfonso X el Sabio," *Revista de Occidente* 43 (1984), 85–107. The diffusion of Salernitan medicine within the Crown of Aragon has not yet been studied, and is one of the themes we mean to pursue.

The consolidation of the Salernitan corpus or *articella* gave rise to commentaries that constituted the first medieval syllabus: see P. O. Kristeller, "Bartholomaeus, Musandinus and Maurus of Salerno and Other Early Commentators of the Articella, with a Tentative List of Texts and Manuscripts," *Italia Medioevale e Umanistica* 19 (1976), 57–87, and the literature cited there.

[5] "Quia in firmamento scientiarum inter liberales artes medicinalis scientia tanquam luminare maius noscitur prenitere, ad confovendum ipsam tanto propensius tenemur intendere, quanto per eandem salubrius humane fragilitati consulitur et egrotantibus optate sanitatis remedia conferuntur." A. Germain, *Cartulaire de l'Université de Montpellier*, I (Montpellier, 1890), p. 185; doc. 4 (15 June 1239). On the place of medicine in scholastic learning, see the chapter "The nature of medical learning" in Nancy G. Siraisi, *Taddeo Alderotti and His Pupils: Two Generations of Italian Medical Learning* (Princeton, 1981), pp. 118–146, and the literature cited there.

[6] "Capítol XVII. Item ordonam e statuïm que algun savi en dret no ús en alguna cort de inquisicions, ne de advocacions, ne de jutjaments entrò serà examinat per los prohòmens de cascum loch ensemps ab los altres savis en dret; e aquells qui seran elets, juren que se hauran feelment en advocacions e en les altres coses en poder del veguer o

With the king's approval, the *cortes* thus gave into the hands of the towns, and specifically of their councilors and physicians, the supervision of a nascent medical profession. In this way the Crown of Aragon was following a method of controlling medical practice that had been inaugurated by Roger II of Sicily in about 1140 and maintained in the Kingdom of Sicily by his successors, both the emperor Frederic II (d. 1250) and the later monarchs of the Angevin and Aragonese houses down to the fifteenth century.[7] The same tradition was in effect in Paris by about 1220,[8] and in Montpellier by 1239.[9]

As the text from the *cortes* of Monzón makes plain, it was not necessary to have studied medicine in a university in order to practice in the Crown of Aragon at the end of the thirteenth century. This does not mean that the Aragonese kings were unaware that other European societies saw this as desirable. Indeed, in 1272 Jaume I had tried to prevent the practice of medicine in Montpellier (of which he was seigneur) by men and women, whether Jews or Christians, who had not previously obtained a university degree and been certified by an examination.[10] When at Jaume's death in 1276 Montpellier passed into the hands of the kings of Mallorca, they reiterated this need for training and examination as prerequisite to practice, using his very arguments: "non solum nomen et fama eiusdem Studii denigratur, sed et multa incumbunt mortis pericula et rerum dispendia inferuntur." Both Jaume II of Mallorca (in 1281)[11] and his son Sanç (in 1316)[12] insisted on this, and their policy was explicitly endorsed by Philip VI of France in 1331.[13]

In this sense, therefore, the provision of the *cortes* of Monzón of 1289 was more than a narrowly juridical pronouncement; it was a public acknowledgment of the growing influence of medical learning. The

---

del batle e dels dits prohòmens d'aquell loch.

"Idem capítol XVIII. Item ordonam e statuim que allo mateix se fasa en los metges e cirurgians." "Usatges y constitucions de Catalunya" (Archivo de la Corona de Aragón [=ACA], Generalitat, vol. 3, fol. 40); published by J. Rubió Balaguer, in A. de la Torre y del Cerro, *Documentos para la historia de la universidad de Barcelona, I: Preliminares (1289-1451)* (Barcelona, 1971), doc. 1, p. [3].

[7] Cf. R. Calvanico, *Fonti per la storia della medicina e della chirurgia per il regno di Napoli nel periodo angiocino (a. 1273–1410)* (Naples, 1962), and Ronald Doviak, "The University of Naples and the Study and Practice of Medicine in the Thirteenth and Fourteenth Centuries" (Ph.D. dissertation, C. U. N. Y., 1974).

[8] H. Denifle, *Chartularium Universitatis Parisiensis*, II, sectio prior (1286–1350) (Paris, 1891), p. 156, n. 1; Ernest Wickersheimer, *Commentaires de la Faculté de Médecine de l'université de Paris (1395–1516)* (Paris, 1915), p. lxxii.

[9] A. Germain, *Cartulaire*, doc. 4, pp. 185–186.

[10] Ibid., doc. 14, pp. 202–203.

[11] Ibid., doc. 16, pp. 207–208 (13 April).

[12] Ibid., doc. 33, pp. 234–235 (3 February).

[13] Ibid., doc. 55, pp. 284–285 (August). Since the purchase of Montpellieret by Philip IV of France (1293) and Jaume of Mallorca's acts of homage to the same king (1307/1310), the commune of Montpellier and the studium had looked increasingly to the French monarchy for confirmation of its privileges; see Jean Baumel, *Histoire d'une seigneurie du Midi de la France* (Montpellier, 1971), II, 172–180, 203–206.

view was emerging that medical science was responsible for health, man's most precious possession, and was hence an important factor in social equilibrium and stability. With this legislation, scientific medicine began its rise to an authoritative position in the Crown of Aragon; further legislation would eventually guarantee its availability (in theory) to the entire population, and not just to a few privileged individuals around the royal court—which before the twelfth century had controlled the Aragonese (and indeed European) medical profession. Public interest in the provision was shown by its relatively rapid reenactment on the local scene: by the towns of Cervera (May 1291)[14] and Valls (August 1299), where it was applied explicitly to all the members, male or female, of the realm's three religious communities—Christian, Jewish, and Muslim; it was reiterated in the latter town in March 1319.[15]

A new and much more detailed basis for medical control was laid for the kingdom of Valencia with the promulgation of its *furs* by Alfons IV in the *corts* of 1329.[16] At the heart of this novelty was a specified level of training for the practitioner, which established a relationship between the possession of a university degree in medicine and the right to practice medicine. After the Valencian *corts* of 1329, no one (at least in theory) in that kingdom would be able to practice medicine who had not attained the level of bachelor in a faculty of medicine. The active screening of physicians desiring to practice in Valencia was based on this presumption of knowledge conveyed in a university or *studium generale*. As we will see shortly, it consisted of an examination that reflected university practice, and that attempted to determine the adequacy of the physician's theoretical knowledge and clinical experience. Those responsible for selecting physicians and authorizing their practice were still the municipal authorities, but the technical aspects of the examination and its direction would now be wholly in the hands of the Valencian physicians.

The city where this new institution was to be put into effect was, both in size and in economic and political standing, one of the most important urban centers in late medieval Iberia and indeed in all Europe. Upon its conquest from the Muslims by Jaume I in 1238, Valencia became the capital of a kingdom—the kingdom of Valencia—to which the monarch granted its own law-code (*furs*; Castilian, *fueros*) and political institutions (*corts, cortes*), incorporating it along with Aragon

---

[14] A. Duran i Sanpere, *Llibre de Cervera* (Tárrega, 1972), p. 373.

[15] F. Carreras y Candi, "Ordinacions urbanes de bon govern a Catalunya. Ordinacions de Vall (1299–1325)," *Bol. Real Academia de Buenas Letras de Barcelona* [*BRABLB*] 25 (1925), 201, 203, 286, 291.

[16] *Furs e Ordinations fetes per los gloriosos Reys de Aragó als regnícols del Regne de València* (Valencia, 1482); *furs Del Rey N'Amfós I*, rubr. xvii, I. We have consulted the facsimile edition (Valencia, 1978), pp. [209]–[210]. A corrected text has been given as doc. 1 below in Appendix 2.

and Catalonia into the federated Crown of Aragon. The newly conquered territory was repopulated with Christian immigrants from the north, primarily Catalans and Aragonese, who established themselves in the most important towns. The Muslim inhabitants were largely driven from the cities (though some Moorish enclaves, *morerias*, persisted there) into the countryside, where they continued to make up the majority of the population. Valencia itself, which at the conquest sheltered some 15,000 persons, had a small *moreria* and a somewhat larger Jewish quarter (*jueria*). The Christian majority in the city continued to swell throughout the later middle ages, and by the fourteenth century Valencia had twice the population of a hundred years before; by 1500 it had more than 40,000 inhabitants.

Agriculture was the basis for Valencia's prosperity, centered as it was on a fertile alluvial plain cut by the river Turia. The land immediately surrounding the city, the *horta*, was watered by an irrigation system dating back to Roman times but perfected under Islam; it allowed the vigorous production of grain and wine for local consumption, but also of more specialized, profitable crops, especially rice, flax, and henna, for which there was a strong export demand; the latter two were also increasingly the mainstays of a local textile industry that grew up in the city during the fourteenth century. In these years Valencia was converted into an exporter of cloth and a renowned market for all kinds of manufactured products, foods, and exotic spices. Its port, el Grau, was frequented by merchants and ships from all over the Mediterranean and became one of the routine ports of call for international commerce. In turn, the foreign activity of Valencian entrepreneurs extended from Beirut to Lisbon, from Bruges to Oran, from Seville to Cagliari.

City government depended on two institutions, the *jurats* and the *consell*. The former was an executive college, renewed annually, made up of six persons: two were members of the urban nobility and the other four *ciutadans*, that is, wealthy burgesses. The *jurats* were supervised, at least theoretically, by a sort of municipal parliament, the *consell*, whose members (also chosen every year) represented the guilds and parishes of the city. City government was thus controlled by the mercantile or artisanal class, numerically predominant, although the nobility managed after 1329 to obtain alternation with the *ciutadans* in the offices of *justícia civil* and *justícia criminal* (judges of civil and criminal cases, respectively) and of *mustaçaf* (the official charged with supervision of the market, of weights and measures, and of other matters today associated with public health). The clergy had no role in municipal affairs. The two religious minorities each had its own administrative institution, the *aljama*, which depended not on the municipal government but on a royal offical, the *batle general*. The hostility of Christian society towards them occasionally burst out in violent attacks against their enclaves, one of which, in 1391, effectively destroyed the Jewish *aljama*, whose members were forcibly baptized and made nominal Christians (*conversos*).

Within the kingdom of Valencia the capital was by far the most important center of population, and thus presented the greatest difficulties of provisioning in times of scarcity. Hence the city controlled an extensive surrounding territory capable of providing a part of the foods and materials needed by its inhabitants. Furthermore, the *furs* of Jaume I had granted it economic privileges in order to assist its development, giving it legal advantages over the rest of the towns in the kingdom. Even so, the demographic growth of late-medieval Valencia made it increasingly difficult to feed, and from the first decades of the fourteenth century its authorities extracted from successive monarchs significant new legal and economic concessions that extended and consolidated its advantageous position vis-à-vis the remainder of the kingdom. The growth of the capital thus entailed the steady increase of its power well beyond its territorial limits, and the assertion of its interests over those of the rest of the kingdom of Valencia. It was the basis of a permanent conflict, a sort of confrontation between city and country, that cropped up again and again during the last centuries of the middle ages, and it was not without its reflection in the organization of medicine and of those who practiced it.

The Valencian legislation of 1329 was not only more detailed, it was also much more comprehensive than had been the terse edict of 1289. Under the heading "De metges" it specified seven provisions.[17] Three of these have to do with concrete aspects of day-to-day professional activity: the requirement of surgeons that they provide expert testimony when asked for it by a competent authority (provision 4); the insistence that every practitioner, physician or surgeon, take an annual oath not to treat a gravely ill patient if the patient has not already confessed, and to inquire into this (provision 6); and the requirement that therapeutic instructions be made in recipes in the vernacular language, naming the different ingredients not in Latin but with their "comú e vulgar" name—that is, in Catalan—so that they may be understood by apothecaries (provision 7). But the other four provisions define the route leading through examination to practice, whether for physicians, surgeons, or barbers (provisions 1, 2, and 5), while excluding women (provision 3). The fundamental part of this legislation comes at the very beginning:

We command and ordain that the justiciar (*justícia*) and the *jurats* elect, every year, three days before Christmas, two leading physicians who shall be the

[17] For the text, see below, Appendix 2, doc. 1. See also the short note by M.-A. Belda, "Los 'metges' y 'apothecaris,' en los Furs de Valencia," in *Actas del Primer Congreso de Historia del País Valenciano* (Valencia, 1980), II, 851–854, which surveys the legislation of the thirteenth, fourteenth, and fifteenth centuries.

examiners of all the practitioners of physic who have recently come to practice in the city or in the towns of the kingdom; and those whom they find competent, and who have followed the art of medicine for at least four years in a *studium generale,* shall be admitted to practice the said art, and if not they shall not be admitted.

Those who wished to practice surgery had also to undergo examination by the medical examiners, although they were not required to have had medical studies; and this requirement of supervision via examination was extended to barbers who hoped to practice medicine or surgery: "no barber shall practice medicine or surgery if he has not been examined by the examiners of practitioners and found competent." As for the physicians who were practicing medicine or surgery at the moment when the new provisions were approved, they were required to prove their suitability before the examiners, and those who did not pass the tests were to be disqualified. Those most interested in maintaining these rules in force were naturally the physicians who already met the conditions laid down by the new *furs;* and in fact it was they who denounced all sorts of unqualified practitioners. The provisions of the *furs* stimulated the denunciation of someone who was practicing without a license by creating a system that divided his fine into thirds, destined respectively to pay the costs of the trial, to swell the treasury of the place where the denunciation was made, and to reward the accuser.[18]

In the northern lands of the Crown of Aragon, in Catalonia and Aragon proper, medical practice was still formally governed by the terse prescription of Monzón (1289), though we know of no attempts to enforce this provision during the first forty years that it was nominally in effect (the reenactments of Cervera and Valls were merely ratifications of the principle involved). In the 1330s, however, there was clearly a newly wakening sense that medical practice in Catalonia should be supervised, and that the old *constitutiones Cathalonie* provided the means to do this. It seems scarcely possible that the Valencian *fur* enacted in 1329 was not the immediate stimulus for the Catalan interest in licensing of the 1330s—particularly since one feature of the Valencian legislation that had not been enacted at Monzón, that academic medical training could substitute for qualification by examination, was by now apparently accepted in the north as well as the south. In October 1334, replying to a complaint by the "medici civitatis Barchinone" about unqualified practitioners, the infante Pere, son of Alfons IV, agreed that "by the rights and constitutions of Catalonia" no one who had not previously been examined should be allowed to practice medicine in

[18] "And anyone who practices without the said examination and licensing shall be fined 100 morabatins of gold for each infraction, of which a third shall go to the court, a third to the town, and a third to the accuser." Below, doc. 1.

Barcelona and its surroundings, except for "masters and bachelors in the art."[19] The Valencian standards were explicitly extended to the remainder of the Crown of Aragon at the *corts* of Cervera in 1359, which emphasized their innovative character in comparison with the *fueros* of Monzón that had hitherto been in effect:

Confirming the chapter from the said *cortes* of Monzón, beginning "Likewise we ordain and decree, etc.," and adding to it, we decree that no lawyer in cities, towns, or other significant places may practice law nor exercise the office of judge or assessor if he does not have all the ordinary books of civil law, or at least the ordinary books of canon law, or has not studied them for at least five years in a *studium generale,* which he must swear to have done. And we wish the same to be required of physicians in the art of medicine, except that it is enough for them to have studied for only three years in a *studium generale.*[20]

Here, for the first time outside of Valencia, a university degree was identified as the standard for medical qualification in the Crown of Aragon.[21]

As the example of the "medici Barchinone" shows, established physicians often took the lead aggressively in this new insistence that Catalan medicine be regulated, and there is certainly reason to suspect that an emergent monopolistic self-interest rather than concern for the public welfare was a principal motive. The Barcelonan physicians triumphed decisively when Pere (now King Pere IV) gave their collectivity supervisory authority over the city and a surrounding area in May 1342.[22] In rural areas, where competition was almost unknown, this

---

[19] ACA, Cancillería, reg. 571, fols. 91v-92; printed by J. Rubió Balaguer, *Documentos,* pp. [19]–[20].

[20] "Confirmants encara lo capítol en la dita cort de Muntçó fet, qui comença: Item ordonam e statuïm etc., e a aquell enadint, statuïm que negun savi en dret en les ciutats, viles, ne encara insignes altres lochs no puxe advocar, ni offici de jutge o de assessor regir si tots los libres ordinaris de dret civil no ha, o aldemenys los libres ordinaris de dret canònich. E que aquells aldemenys haja hoïts per v. anys en studi general, de la qual cosa per sagrament sie tengut fer fe. E açò mateix en los metges de art de phísica volem ésser observat, sàul que bast aquells en general studi per iii. anys tant solament haver hoÿt." "Usatges y constitucions de Catalunya" (ACA, Generalitat, vol. 3, fol. 40); published by J. Rubió Balaguer, *Documentos,* pp. [35]–[36].

[21] Of course, as in Barcelona (above, fn. 19), an academic standard had occasionally been imposed locally outside Valencia before 1359. In November 1337, the king responded to the complaint by Guido, a physician of Teruel, that persons "non experti seu docti in naturali medicinali et cirurgica scienciis" were practicing medicine in that Aragonese town, by insisting that all those in question should submit to an examination to test their proficiency; the language suggests that some sort of theoretical learning in addition to practical skill would be required of candidates. ACA, Cancillería, reg. 862, fol. 82v; published by A. López de Meneses, "Documentos culturales de Pedro el Ceremonioso," *Estudios de Edad Media de la Corona de Aragón* 5 (1952), 671–672, doc. 3.

[22] "Hanc autem ordinationem et ex ea subsequentia extendi volumus non solum ad civitatem Barchinone . . . sed etiam ad vicarium Barchinone et Vallensis et ad baiuliam . . . Barchinone ac baiulias eidem baiulie subiectas; et medici in ipsis vicariis et baiuliis habitantes ad premissa servanda existant totaliter obligati." ACA, Cancillería,

new attitude caught some practitioners by surprise. In April 1338 Ramon Roquer of Socarrats (near Castellfullit de Roca) complained to King Pere in bewilderment that "he had practiced the art of surgery for a long time, and, although he was a layman and unlettered, he owned good books and had good cures to his credit, as was well known in his district; but now some surgeons envious of him have maliciously caused royal officials to order him not to practice surgery until he has been examined *per medicos*."[23] But there was evidently public as well as professional pressure involved behind the regulatory movement in Catalonia. It was the *prohomes* of Montblanch, not its physicians, who complained in 1339 about ignorant practitioners debilitating or killing their patients, inducing King Pere to order his vicar and bailiff there to prohibit anyone from practicing medicine or surgery in Montblanch "donec examinata et approbata fuerit iuxta constituciones predictas [Cathalonie]."[24] However mixed the underlying motives, a new sensitivity to the issue of professional qualification had arisen in Catalonia by the 1330s, and this no doubt encouraged the flurry of appeals for medical certification or examination that we suddenly find there in the second half of the decade.[25]

This mixture of motives reflects the fact that the seventy years between the *cortes* of Monzón and of Cervera were a period of transition for Catalan medicine, during which the supervision and control of practitioners shifted from the towns to the medical community itself. By the *corts* of Cervera the municipal bureaucracy was in effect stripped of the responsibility, given it in 1289, of deciding whether an

---

reg. 873, fol. 154v; García Ballester, "Los orígenes," pp. 138–140, 148–149.

[23] "Raimundus Roquerii de Biania de parroquia de Soquerats nobis exposuit reverenter quod cum ipse ab antiquo uteretur et utatur officio cirurgie licet sit laycus et sine litteris tamen habeat bonos libros et fecerit et facit bonas curas et de hoc est fama in tota illa terra et nunc quidam cirurgici sibi emuli maliciose fecerit fieri sibi mandamentum per officiales nostros quod non utatur dicto officio usquequo per medicos fuerit examinatus et a dicto tempore citra vixerit pacifice et quiete sine aliqua examinacione. Et propterea supplicaverit nobis sibi super hiis de jure remedio provideri. . . . " ACA Cancillería, reg. 596, 16v (Barcelona, 10 kals. May 1338).

[24] "Petrus etc. dilectis et fidelibus suis vicario et baiulo Montisalbi presentibus et qui pro tempore fuerint salutem etc. Ne propter impericiam medicorum infirmi egentes fisicorum aut cirurgicorum auxilio confoveri incurrant irreparabilem detrimentum, in constitutionibus Cathalone provide fuit cautum ne quisque auderet medicine vel cirurgie officium exercere nisi per peritas personas in dictis artibus prius examinatus esset repertus sufficiens atque aptus. Cumque et villa et vicaria Montisalbi tam homines quam femine in dictis artibus imperiti curam infirmorum assumant et ex eorum ignorantia pluris afligant aliisque debilitent et occidant, idcirco ad humilem supplicacionem proborum hominum dicte ville vobis districte precipiendo mandamus quatenus sibi expedientibus penis vestri arbitrios apponendis ipsisque nostro erario aplicandis inhibeatis expresse voce preconia et al' ne aliqua persona uti presumat in dicta villa vel eius vicaria officio medicine vel cirurgie donec examinata et approbata fuerit iuxta constituciones predictas, vobis firmiter inungentes ut a contrafacientibus ipsas penas exhigatis adiectas et al' ipsos pro comissis taliter prehabente iustic. puniatis quod sit ceteris in exemplum. Dat. Barchinone, prid. id. Aug. (1339)." ACA Cancillería, reg. 603, 137v.

[25] For example: ACA Cancillería, reg. 863, 200v (5 kals. Apr. 1338); 863, 231v (9 kals. May 1338); 604, 103 (3 id. Nov. 1339); 873, 139 (7 kals. May 1342).

individual had the necessary knowledge to be entrusted with human health. The physicians to whom this control was turned over had not been a cohesive social group when the earlier legislation was enacted, but as we have just seen this was beginning to change by the 1330s, as physicians began to recognize and to act to further their collective interest. The Catalan towns had provided a setting in which disciplinary self-consciousness could be forged, and once that was done municipal control could no longer maintain itself against claims to professional self-regulation.

What sets the Valencian situation apart, then, is that there the municipality was able to maintain a role in the control of medical activity, by selecting the tribunal of professional examiners. A Valencian bourgeoisie had made its influence felt from the very moment of the conquest,[26] an influence evident throughout the diversity of socioeconomic and religious life within the city,[27] and medical care did not escape. Indeed, the *furs* of 1329 gave the bourgeois-dominated city government the right to control medical practice not only within the city but throughout the kingdom of Valencia,[28] a right on which it insisted throughout the fourteenth century.

---

[26] "Els primers privilegis que figuren a l'*Aureum opus* relatius al règim jurídic de la ciutat de València—i que són, és clar, posteriors a 1238—acusen ja la petjada d'aquells principis jurídics postulats per la burgesia ciutadana. El de 21 de maig de 1239 . . . ja conté una claudicació del rei. . . . Els privilegis que acabem de esmentar semblen indicar-nos clarament que la naixent burgesia ciutadana de València era qui propugnaba la constitució del nou dret valencià. . . . " *Furs de València*, ed. G. Colón i A. García, I: Introducció (Barcelona, 1970), pp. 49–50.

[27] Agustín Rubio Vela, "Una fundación burguesa en la Valencia medieval: el Hospital de En Clapers (1311)," *Dynamis* 1 (1981), 17–49; idem, "La asistencia hospitalaria infantil en la Valencia del siglo XIV: pobres, huérfanos y expósitos," *Dynamis* 2 (1982), 159–191; idem, *Pobreza, enfermedad y asistencia hospitalaria en la Valencia del siglo XIV* (Valencia, 1984).

[28] " . . . en la ciutat e en les viles del regne"; below, doc. 1.

II. THE LICENSING PROCEDURE AND ITS CONSEQUENCES

It is in 1336 that the municipal records of Valencia first give the names of the persons elected as *examinadors* for would-be medical practitioners, stating that masters Bertomeu de Casaldòria and Pere Correger had been chosen for the task. From this point on, through the rest of the century, it is possible to reconstruct the list of physicians who formally granted or refused licenses to those who wished to practice medicine and/or surgery in the city and kingdom of Valencia.[1] In spite of the *furs'* prescription that the election should take place three days before Christmas, for the first twenty years the appointment of the *examinadors* seems to have taken place on Pentecost. Until 1367 their names are inscribed in the *manuals de consell* (which recorded municipal business) along with the list of municipal *consellers* selected on that day; from that time on, however, the election of *examinadors* usually took place on 22 December, as required by the *furs*.[2]

The procedure followed in Valencia in granting licenses to practice medicine remained almost unchanged throughout this period, as can be inferred from an analysis of the texts. The candidate presented himself before the municipal authority, the civil justiciar (*justícia civil*) or his assessor, submitting a letter from the examiners that attested to the results of the examination and recommended that he be licensed to practice in the city of Valencia and the towns of the kingdom. The justiciar then administered an oath to the candidate, requiring him to swear that he would use his art or science properly and that he would observe the provisions of the chapter "De metges" of the *furs* of Alfons IV; he also had to promise to fulfill any conditions that the examiners

---

[1] The municipal records have some gaps in their listings of these names—for example in 1356–1368, 1371–1378, and 1389–1392—but these gaps can be partially filled from supplementary documentation. See Appendix 1 below for our reconstruction of the list of practitioners elected to the tribunal on a year-by-year basis during the fourteenth century.

[2] Exceptions to this choice of date occurred in 1369 and 1400, when the election was deferred for a week; Archivo Municipal de Valencia (hereafter AMV), Manuals de Consells, A-15, fol. 1r (first gathering), and A-22, fol. 49v.

In 1400 a terminological change was made, though it would not be maintained: the word *corregidors* was introduced in place of *examinadors* (though the latter term was preserved to apply to the other professions, lawyers and notaries). AMV, Manuals de Consells, A-22, fol. 49v. This usage of *corregidor* at the turn of the fifteenth century has not been mentioned by A. M. Alcover, F. de B. Moll, M. Sanchis Guarner, *Diccionari Català-Valencià-Balear* (Palma de Mallorca, 1980), III, 579.

might have imposed.[3] As he swore, he placed his right hand on the scriptures (if he were a Muslim he would also face south, towards *migjorn*, the theoretical direction of Mecca[4]). A Jew would swear by the Old Testament—"los deu manaments de la ley, los quals nostre senyor Déus donà a Moysés en lo mont de Senahí"[5]; a Muslim would swear by God and the Quran, as prescribed by Muslim religious (*zuna*) and civil (*xara*) precepts[6]; and a Christian by the Gospels, "los sants quatre Evangelis de nostre senyor Déu."[7] When this was done, the justiciar or his assessor would hand over the license in the form of a document directed to the authorities of the kingdom, certifying to them the competence of the individual in question and requesting them not to impede or hinder him in the practice of his profession.

These Valencian procedures are identical to those that eventually came into being in Barcelona. Rubió has published the text of an examination carried out in the Catalan capital in 1359[8] that conforms closely to those collected by us from Valencia in the last quarter of the century. And this practice of Barcelona and Valencia is very similar to the procedure already being followed at Montpellier in the first decade of the fourteenth century, as can be seen from a *licentia practicandi medicine* granted at Montpellier in 1307 that has fortunately been preserved. Pierre Calberte, bachelor in medicine, presented himself before the bishop's vicar—the bishop was the licensing authority for Montpellier—requesting a license to practice medicine in the city. The vicar, "conformably with the statutes and privileges of the physicians" (referring to the *collegium* or guild of physicians existing in Montpellier), summoned two masters in medicine and required them to examine the candidate in public. The two examiners chose a medical work and asked that the candidate "read" a portion of it (*ad legendum lectionem certam dicte scientie*), and his reading (*lectio*) laid the basis for an exchange of detailed questions and answers between the examiners and the candidate: *diligenter examinatus extitit in et super dicta scientia per magistros memoratos*. At the end of the exercise, the vicar asked the two masters whether they judged the candidate *sufficientem ac ydoneum* to obtain the license permitting him to practice medicine, and one spoke for both in agreeing that the bachelor was "worthy by reason of his *scientia*" to practice. Then the vicar gave "Petro Calberte, bacallario in

---

[3] In January 1338 Pere IV granted the request of the *jurats* and *prohomes* of Valencia that anyone who had taken this oath need not repeat it; apparently until then it had had to be repeated every year. ACA, Cancillería, reg. 862, 108v.

[4] Appendix 2, doc. 13.

[5] Ibid., doc. 4.

[6] Ibid., doc. 13.

[7] Ibid., doc. 5.

[8] J. Rubió Balaguer in A. de la Torre y del Cerro, *Documentos para la historia de la Universidad de Barcelona*, I (Barcelona, 1971), doc. 22, pp. [38]–[40].

medicina, practicandi et exercendi officium dicte scientie in Montepessulano et in tota Megalonensi diocesi licentiam ac potestatem plenariam," and a notary subsequently prepared the public certificate.[9]

There is every reason to suppose that in Barcelona and Valencia, as well as in Montpellier, the core of the licensing examination was a *lectio,* a technical reading of one or more of the texts that formed the basis of medieval medical education. In the Barcelonan examination reported by Rubió, a tribunal comprising four masters in medicine (three of them Valencians: Pere Ros d'Orsins, Bertomeu de Tresbens, and Arnau Germà) investigated the "aptitude and adequacy" of the candidate (Jaume de Pallars, later physician to King Pere IV) by posing him "plurima questiones, argumenta et alia." Similarly, in all the licenses so far collected from Valencia, the examiners declare whether the candidate is trained in the principles of the science of medicine. The import of "lectio" in this period of medical scholasticism could be very broad, ranging from simple explication of the meaning of words or phrases to a much more detailed analysis. Because the *lectio* possessed real flexibility, as the basis of an examination it could easily lead to a variety of *questiones et responsiones* by which a candidate's mastery of the "principles of medical science" could be explored.[10] Unfortunately, none of the licenses known from the fourteenth-century Crown of Aragon gives us information that might allow us to identify the concrete texts—Galen, Hippocrates, Johannitius, Avicenna, Haly Abbas, and so forth—on which the *lectio* was based.

Still, despite this lack of direct testimony, we can get a general sense of the content of the *lectio* and of the *questiones et responsiones* to which it gave rise from the fact that, as we have seen, the examiners tried in this part of the examination to see how familiar the candidate was with the "principles of the science of medicine." Thanks to our knowledge of the library of one of the Valencian examiners—Sanç del Miracle (c. 1290–c. 1360), who was a member of the licensing tribunal in 1351 and 1354[11]—we know the writings he was familiar with and might have viewed as constitutive of the "science of medicine." Sanç owned three encyclopedic medical works: the *Colliget* of Averroes, the *Canon* of Avicenna, and the *Pantegni* of Haly Abbas. He was familiar, too, with several treatises of Galen, most importantly *De morbo et accidenti* and *De therapeutica ad Glauconem;* with the treatise on specialized pathology by Avenzoar, the *Teisir;* and, of course, with the *Isagoge* of Johannitius, the epitome of scholastic medicine.[12] Of the two Galenic

---

[9] A. Germain, *Cartulaire de l'Université de Montpellier,* I (Montpellier, 1890), pp. 217–219; doc. 24.

[10] On the role of the *lectio* in scholastic pedagogy, see M. D. Chenu, *Introduction à l'étude de Saint Thomas d'Aquin,* second edition (Montreal and Paris, 1954), pp. 67ff.

[11] His library is included in his will, drawn up on 29 June 1351 (Archivo del Reino de Valencia [hereafter ARV], Protocolos, no. 2959, s.f.).

[12] There is no need to give a full transcription of this important library, which we have

titles, the former was that given by medieval physicians to an extensive treatise on clinical medicine and pathology (actually a conflation of four different Galenic texts: *De morborum differentiis, De morborum causis, De symptomatum differentiis,* and *De symptomatum causis*); the latter was a work on general and special therapeutics, very popular in the middle ages. Most of these had become required reading in the curriculum of the faculty of medicine at Montpellier (where Sanç del Miracle would have studied about 1310–1315) as a result of the impact of the "new Galen," the corpus of Galenic works that was introduced into Montpellier in the 1280s; many of the other texts making up the "new Galen" must also have figured in the library of our Valencian examiner.[13]

If we now examine the *Isagoge* of Johannitius or the *Pantegni*—of all those named above, perhaps the works most systematic and most balanced between what medieval physicians called theory and practice—we see that *medicina theorica* "consists of a satisfactory knowledge" of three groups of concepts: the naturals, the non-naturals, and the contra-naturals. The first are the constituents of the body (elements, complexions, humors, spirits, organs, etc.); the second, while not constitutive parts of the body, form part of its physical, biological, and social environment in interaction (normal or pathological) with it, and fall into six groups: airs, food and drink, work and rest, sleep and waking, excretions and secretions, and passions of the mind (sadness, joy, etc.); the third, the contra-naturals, include the three main areas of pathology: illness itself, the cause of illness, and the symptoms or concrete manifestations of illness. This is the skeletal system on which a theoretical understanding of medical science was built up, and we may suppose that it provided the basis for the *lectio*.

---

not yet studied fully. But certain features are of particular interest. It included ".XIX. libri qui tractant de istoriis animalium Aristotelis," which is plainly Michael Scot's Latin version (made from the Arabic c. 1217) of the biological writings of Aristotle; for some philosophically-minded physicians this work offered a biological and methodological basis for medical theory. It included many different sections of Avicenna's *Canon* with commentaries thereupon ("Item, unum alium librum apellatum primum et quartum librum Evicenne. . . . Item tertium librum Evicenne non perfectum et quintum librum Evicenne . . . unus tractatus de questionibus super primo et quarto libris Evicenne . . . et alius liber alterius voluminis . . . de questionibus super primo et quarto libris Evicenne."). And it included other classics of Arabic medicine deriving from an Iberian or Montpellier setting: "Item, alium librum cum coopertis viridis nuncupatum Gordo, cum alio libro qui est sub eodem volumine vocato Albocasim Azarahui. . . . Item, alium librum vocatum Colliet qui aliter nominatur Averrois, cum coopertis fustis. . . . Item, alium librum . . . in pergameno, vocatum Avenzuar."

[13] Sanç's will reads in part: "Item dimito Bernardo filio meo quemdam librum vocatum volumen Galieni, in quo continetur decemseptem libri, cum coopertis fustis tectis corio rubeo." On the "new Galen" at Montpellier and the reform of the curriculum of 1309, see Luis García Ballester, "Arnau de Vilanova (c.1240–1311) y la reforma de los estudios médicos en Montpellier (1309): el Hipócrates latino y la introducción del nuevo Galeno," *Dynamis* 2 (1982), 97–158. Curiously, Sanç's library contained none of the works of Arnau de Vilanova, arguably the principal figure in the introduction of the "new Galen" into Montpellier's curriculum.

The Valencian licenses we have encountered suggest, however, that there was more to the examination than a *lectio*, for it would seem that the *examinadors* were also concerned to assure themselves that those who wished to practice were familiar with routine medical activity—that is, with the diagnosis and treatment of concrete ailments. How could they arrive at an evaluation of these practical skills on the part of the candidates? There is no indication that a specific practical test was imposed (except, as we will see, when a candidate had to perform before the tribunal the particular surgical technique for which he had requested a license); but the examiners had other ways of assessing an individual's competence to practice. They could use the *lectio* to probe a candidate's familiarity with what the licenses call "malalties forts e grans" or "malalties perilloses," sometimes identified more precisely: "febres contínues, frenesis et altres malalties agudes." No one could diagnose or treat such illnesses who was not versed in the details of pathological theory, since—as one of the documents says explicitly—these are "malalties requirents sciència de física."[14]

Furthermore, the *examinadors* could complement their inquiry into the theoretical basis for practice by requiring the candidate to show the tribunal that he already possessed a certain practical experience, referred to in the licenses as "pràtica de curar les malalties" or "convinent pràtica." In the later middle ages, as now, this practice was normally acquired by attending the sick in company with other, more experienced, physicians. At the end of a certain period, the physician or physicians who had supervised the candidate in practice would provide him with a letter setting out the experience he had gained—illnesses encountered, treatments administered, successes achieved, and so forth—which would take on an official character after certification by a notary. In reporting the examination taken by Bernat Giner, the Valencian tribunal emphasized the "longua continuació que ha feyta ab metges en pràtica," testified to by "diverses metges antichs en una carta pública, la qual nós havem vista."[15] Such a letter, supplied by experienced practitioners and testifying to a candidate's clinical and therapeutic practice, may be the adaptation to new circumstances of the Arabic *ijaza*, a document originally presenting the testimony of a master physician that its bearer had read and studied certain medical books with success and was qualified himself to teach, but which with time had come to be a certification of a student's clinical training as well.[16] We have already seen that, in the *lectio*, the ritual of the examination was shaped by the Christian university culture; the incorpora-

[14] Appendix 2, doc. 8.
[15] Ibid., doc. 11.
[16] Cf. the article "Idjaza" by G. Vajda in *The Encyclopedia of Islam* (new edition; Leiden/London, 1971), III, 1020–1021.

tion into the rite of this letter may be a corresponding expression of cultural syncretism from Islam.

The tribunal did not restrict itself to granting or denying the license, did not simply declare candidates qualified or unqualified; it also granted conditional licenses to practice. In some cases, the candidate had not shown satisfactory ability in the *lectio* or theoretical portion of the examination and yet had not proved so weak as to be rejected outright. In the license granted by the *examinadors* to the Jew Hizmel Morcat in 1378 to practice medicine and surgery, they required him to attend patients accompanied by another physician who would be "suficient, abte e antich en speculativa."[17] In 1383 another candidate, this one a Christian, was required for the same reason ("havem trobat que no és tehòrich") to practice in conjunction with "metges autèntichs o de auctoritat et pus sperts"—and this in spite of a consensus that his practical skills had already been satisfactorily demonstrated: "ha covenent pràtica et antigua en física et en cirurgia . . . que ha feyta ab metges."[18]

As is perhaps understandable, however, conditional licensing more often was a response to deficiencies in practical training—when the candidate had given a satisfactory *lectio,* demonstrating the adequacy of his scientific understanding, but revealed an unsatisfactory practical background, perhaps because he had practiced for too short a time, or because he had encountered too little illness. So it was with another Jew, Içach Gabriel, of whom the examiners reported that "we have found him acquainted with the principles of the science of physic, but he has not been long involved in the practice of curing illnesses."[19] Içach was licensed provisionally, on condition that when he was called to a patient suffering from an "enfermetat fort e gran," he would ask a colleague of greater experience to collaborate with him on the case.

Restrictions like this not only affected the private realm of doctor-patient relationships, they also occasionally carried over into the public responsibilities of the physician. Not infrequently both physicians and surgeons were called to testify as expert witnesses, to provide "pronosticació o desospitació davant lo justícia criminal," in cases regarding such things as accusations of assault (where the physician would speak to the seriousness and possible consequence of wounds), certification of slaves sold with concealed illnesses, and so forth. Some newly licensed physicians were seen as incompetent to supply this expert testimony. When the Christian surgeon Sisto Fort was granted a

[17] Appendix 2, doc. 8.
[18] Ibid., doc. 11.
[19] " . . . Havem atrobat en los principis de la dita sciència de física introduhit, emperò ab la pràtica de curar les malalties no ha longament praticat ni usat." Ibid., doc. 6.

license in 1378, the examiners specified that if cases arose where he might need to give such forensic evidence, he should request the association of an expert colleague, "algun físich apte e suficient en acompanyat."[20]

It was in the practice of surgery—the dramatic and high-risk area of therapeutics—that conditions were most often imposed. Bernat Giner was granted a license to practice medicine and "minor surgery," and was expressly prohibited from having anything to do with the three great cavities—head, chest, and abdomen—or with "other dangerous wounds."[21] Similarly, in 1388 a Muslim barber from Manises, Maymó Abdochaxis, was restricted to the practice of minor surgery (which as a matter of fact was all he had asked for).[22] The Italian surgeon Tommaso de Maestre Tone, who wished to be allowed merely to operate on hernias (*potresos, potres, trencadures, ruptures*), was permitted to do so, but on condition that he fully inform everyone who chose to place himself in his hands of the risks involved: first, of the danger of death involved in the operation, and second, of the prospect of partial or total loss of the genitals.[23]

Because of the particular skills needed to carry out certain surgical operations—the cure of hernias, cutting to extract bladder stones, couching of cataracts—the *lectio* was given less importance in the examination of candidates wishing a license to perform them. Why a certification of technical competence was given more weight in such cases was made clear by the examiners (the prestigious Pere Figuerola and Guillem Ça-Fàbrega, both "maestres en artes e en medicina") who endorsed a limited license for the surgeon Johan de Sena in November 1389: "these things pertain more to experience and manual activity than to scientific understanding."[24] Two other licenses reveal that such skills might be demonstrated directly before the examiners. The first of these is from July 1389, when the *examinadors* granted a license to the surgeon Joan Gaschó to extract vesical calculi on the basis of an examination and "a demonstration carried out before us."[25] The second license is even more explicit, giving details of the patient on whom the test was performed. On 21 March 1390, the *examinadors* Bernat d'Artesa and Gabriel Dezcortell (both academically trained) examined the

---

[20] Ibid., doc. 7. The requirement that every surgeon be ready to provide a *desospitació* for a patient in his care, free of charge, is laid down by the *furs* of 1329 (though the technical term is not employed); below, Appendix 2, doc. 1 section <4>.

[21] Appendix 2, doc. 11.

[22] Ibid., doc. 13.

[23] Ibid., doc. 10.

[24] "... Com les dites coses stiguen més en speriència e hobra manual que no en theòrica de sciència." Ibid., doc. 25.

[25] Ibid., doc. 21.

surgeon Toríbio Gonçàlvez, who wished a license to operate for hernia. In their report to the justiciar they declared that, after administering the normal tests,

> since we found the said Toríbio Gonçàlvez competent to treat the said malady, and since we wished him to operate in our presence, to discharge us of responsibility, and he did treat the aforesaid malady in Minguiquo Aznar, a boy of 14 years, the son of Domingo Aznar of Novaliches in Jérica; therefore . . . we ask you . . . to grant him license to treat the aforesaid condition,[26]

and a license to practice this particular operation was duly granted.

Nevertheless, such assessments of a candidate's practical abilities might still be shaped by the examiners' familiarity with the standard texts. The license granted Andreu Martí in 1388 restricted him to treating certain kinds of hernias, and the restriction is expressed in a curious mixture of Catalan and Latin that appears to be drawn from Guy de Chauliac's *Chirurgia Magna* (1363):

> [license:]
> de ruptura dindimal, lo qual és inflació hernial, en la qual lo budell o lo cre[...] és dislogat e exit de les parts de dintre a la carn del mirach propriament *in dindimo* e *osseo seu testiculorum bursa;*[27]

> [Chauliac:]
> De ruptura dindimali: ruptura . . . est inflatio hernialis in qua intestinum aut zirbus dislocatur et egreditur ab interioribus ad carnem miracis, proprie in dindimo et ossio seu testiculorum bursa.[28]

Both Andreu's examiners were academically trained, one a master of arts and medicine, the other a bachelor of medicine, and even when judging a narrow technical skill they could not divorce themselves from the learned tradition.

---

[26] Ibid., doc. 27.
[27] Ibid., doc. 15.
[28] *Chirurgia magna*, VI.2.vii; MS Bristol, City Ref. Library 10, fol. 216va-b. The printed text in *Ars chirurgica* (Venice, 1546), fol. 73r, has minor variants.

III. THE SOCIAL IMPLICATIONS OF THE *FURS* OF 1329

The *furs* of 1329 seem immediately to have been treated as susceptible of enforcement, unlike those of 1289. In 1332 Ramon Sa Lena, an apothecary of Borriana, was accused before the justiciar of Valencia of pursuing the art or office of medicine in Borriana and other towns within the application of the *furs* in the period since they had come into effect.[1] Two years later, in December 1334, master Jacme Lama was also accused before the justiciar of Valencia of practicing medicine without a license and against the regulations established by "los furs nous . . . feyts per lo senyor rey en la ciutat de València en l'any de M. CCC. XX. IX."[2] Three years later still, in March 1338, Hamet Hatequia, a Muslim physician from Xàtiva "in arte medicine doctus et peritus," asked King Pere IV for a license to practice in the city and kingdom of Valencia; the king acknowledged in his response that "per foros novos Valentie omnes medici ad exercendo eodem officio donec examinati fuerint prohibentur."[3] These three documents of the 1330s not only show us the *furs* in effect; each also provides us with an almost paradigmatic introduction to difficulties that would arise when the new licensing procedures confronted social reality in the kingdom. Let us look at each of these cases in turn.

I

The case of the Borriana apothecary Ramon (or Raimundus) Sa Lena is interesting as our earliest proof of the application of the new *furs*, but it has other curious features as well. The apothecary was denounced before the justiciar of Valencia under the *furs* of 1329 for having practiced medicine without an examination. The justiciar absolved him, though we do not know the conditions of the judgment; we know only that Ramon subsequently came to the king to ensure that royal authority would protect him against any future accusations. Thus from the outset two authorities, king and municipality, were po-

---

[1] Archivo de la Corona de Aragón [ACA], Cancillería, reg. 485, fol. 140r.
[2] Appendix 2, doc. 2.
[3] ACA, Cancillería, reg. 863, fol. 161r.

tentially in conflict, authorities who would persist in competition for control of the Valencian medical profession throughout the fourteenth century and even beyond.

The king's response to Ramon's petition brings into evidence one major problem that had been intensified by the imposition of a qualifying examination on Valencian practitioners: a chronic shortage of medical care at every level in large sections of the kingdom, like the expanse between Borriana and Valencia. The lord of Nules had defended Ramon to the king, asserting dramatically that, in the words of the king's reply,

> in the town of Nules and in your other towns and villages there is no physician or surgeon or other skilled person from whom you and the inhabitants of these towns and villages can receive advice and assistance and medicines for sickness and other afflictions. . . . Since it would be tiresome, dangerous, and a burden for you to come to the city of Valencia or some other big city because of their distance from you for advice and treatment of these sicknesses and afflictions for you and your men, . . . to avoid these dangers we give a full license and confer power on Ramon Sa Lena, apothecary in the town of Borriana.[4]

Concerns of this sort were widespread throughout the Crown of Aragon in the 1330s, as evidenced by complaints of inadequacy of health care, on the one hand, and by signs that empirics were proliferating to supply public needs, on the other. In 1334 the physicians of Barcelona attacked the growing number of men and women who were practicing medicine in the city without the necessary qualifications.[5] This coincided with a marked scarcity of surgeons in the Catalan capital, to the point that Leon, a Greek slave "expert in surgery," was given his freedom so that he might practice the art there.[6] Again, in 1338, the inhab-

[4] ". . . asserentium quod in loco de Nules et in aliis locis et alchareis vestris non est aliquis phisicus sive cirurgicus vel alia artesana persona cum qua consilium et remedium vos et habitantes in dictis locis et alchareis possitis recipere nec ab eis res medicinales habere super infirmitatibus et aliis accidentibus. . . . Cum sint vobis tediosum periculum et onus etiam . . . recurrere ad civitatem Valentie vel alia notabilia loca propter eorum distantiam pro consilio et remedio in dictis infirmitatibus et accidentibus vobis et dictis vestris hominibus . . . et ad vitandum pericula supradicta, plenam damus licentiam et conferimus potestatem Raimundo Çalena, apothecario loci de Borriana." Ibid., reg. 485, fols. 240r–v.

[5] "Nos infans Petrus etc. quia per vos medicos civitatis Barchinone fuit nobis insinuacione humili demostratum quod in dicta civitate et vicaria eiusdem nonnulli homines atque femine, cupiditatis morbo infecti ac ignari artis et sciencie medicine, recipiunt sub eorum curis aliquos pacientes, qui eorum egritudinum causas ignorantes eis ministrare inutilia vel ven[en]osa pocula non verentur. . . . " ACA, Cancillería, reg. 571, fols. 91v–92; J. Rubió Balaguer, in A. de la Torre y del Cerro, *Documentos para la historia de la Universidad de Barcelona*, I (Barcelona, 1971), doc. 13, p. [19].

[6] "Leonus sit in arte cirurgica valde expertus et civitate Barchinone predicte multum necessarium propter cirurgicorum inopiam existere in civitate." ACA, Cancillería, reg. 571, fols. 69r–v.

itants of the Pyrenean county of Ribagorça complained to Pere IV that "in dicto committatu non sit aliquis medicus sive fisicus sufficiens."[7] In 1342 the lord of Jérica asked the king to allow a Jewish physician to move there from the city of Valencia on account of the "magna inopia fisicorum" in the town.[8] And two years later the mountain town of Morella (Valencia) complained to the king of the inadequacy of health care there, in particular its lack of surgeons.[9]

There is good evidence of this same shortage in the second half of the century. It was particularly acute during the 1350s, immediately after the Black Death—even in the cities, where the number of physicians was normally proportionally greater, as the authorities of Xàtiva made plain to Pere IV in 1352:

> By reason of the sterility of times past, as well as of the deaths which the Almighty has allowed to flourish in the world, that abundance of physicians and surgeons which used to be found in the city of Xàtiva and other large cities is now so diminished that it is scarcely possible to find a single surgeon here.[10]

The town of Castellón suffered from a lack of physicians throughout the 1370s. In 1374 the municipal *consell* acknowledged that the town needed a physician desperately;[11] in 1378 the same *consell,* confronted with a continuing need, charged the apothecary (*specier*) Pere Morades with treating the poor and with visiting the sick in hospital;[12] and the next year a delegation from Castellón was sent to Valencia to try to contract with a physician there to move permanently to Castellón.[13]

Established physicians perceived the potential problem as being one of too many unqualified practitioners, and their solution was to introduce examinations; but the local citizenry saw the problem instead as an absence of medical assistance, and viewed the requirement of an

---

[7] ACA, Cancillería, reg. 864, fol. 85r.

[8] ACA, Cancillería, reg. 874, fol. 24v (kal. Nov. 1342).

[9] ACA, Cartas reales, Pedro IV, 11 November 1344; published in A. Rubió y Lluch, *Documents per l'història de la cultura catalana mig-eval,* I (Barcelona, 1908), 131–32; doc. CXXII. The same document is enregistered in ACA, Cancillería, reg. 877, fol. 17r–v.

[10] "Attamen quia nobis constat, tam occasione temporum preteritorum sterilitatis quam racione mortalitatum que per universum orbem dudum, permittente Altissimo, viguerunt, copiam fisicorum et sirurgicorum qui in civitate Xative et aliis notabilibus locis esse solebant, in tantum fore diminutam quod vix aliquem sirurgicum invenire poterit in eadem." ACA, Cancillería, reg. 893, fol. 84r. Published by A. López de Meneses, "Documentos acerca de la Peste Negra en los dominios de la Corona de Aragón," *Estudios de Edad Media de la Corona de Aragón* 6 (1956), 411; doc. 132.

[11] A. Sánchez Gozalbo, "La sanidad en el Castellón trecentista (veterinarios, médicos y boticarios)," *Bol. Soc. Cast. Cult.* 48 (1972), 261; doc. IV.

[12] Ibid., p. 265; docs. XVI, XVII.

[13] "Item con en Bernat Cabeça, jurat, per lurs afers fos stat a València et hagués procurat si porie haver metge et hagués trobat metge quj vendrie star a la dita vila si aquell eren donats cent fflorins per pensió del any lo qual metge ere mestre Pere Castellot." Ibid., p. 267; doc. XXI (12 April 1379).

examination more as a monopolistic maneuver of the medical *collegium* or guild than as a means of improving health care. Indeed, many of those who practiced without an examination were praised by the public because "they attend the sick poor and incapacitated who lack the means to pay the salaries of physicians or to afford the price of medicines,"[14] and because they brought about "many good and useful cures."[15] Hence, in the opinion of the public, physicians who complained of violations of the Valencian *furs* often spoke "more from malice than from zeal or justice,"[16] "more from envy than from any other reason."[17] The reasons given by the monarch for granting licenses despite the provisions of the *furs*—"lack of desire for gain";[18] "practice based on the love of God and of one's neighbor"[19]—convey the impression of a similar opinion.

The physicians of Valencia seem to have been unconcerned with the general shortage of health care; in 1351 they refused even to examine an applicant who wished to practice medicine in Alzira (40 kilometers to the south) unless he first paid them 200 *sous*, despite the pleas of town officials that Alzira had no doctor whatsoever, "no one to cure the ill and take care of their needs."[20] This was a problem unfortunately common to all Europe. Talbot reminds us that, at the end of the thirteenth century, the reason why one cleric taught another medicine was so that the poor might receive medical care without charge, since they had been "abandoned by physicians and surgeons."[21]

II

The complaint brought by the notary Miquel de Roures in 1334, against Jacme Lama "who calls himself a physician," alleged that "Jacme Lama presented himself for examination but was not approved by the examiners nor given a license by them to practice medicine in the city, nor was he determined to have studied four years in a *studium generale*; he gave back nonsense and inanities to the questions put to

---

[14] ". . . quamque aliquibus pauperibus et egenis pacientibus, qui non habent unde medicis salaria inde valeant ministrare. . . . " ACA, Cancillería, reg. 683, fols. 99v–100r; published by López de Meneses, "Documentos culturales," p. 695; doc. 31.

[15] Rubió y Lluch, *Documents*, I, 132; doc. CXXII.

[16] ACA, Cancillería, reg. 1909, fol. 150v; cited by R. Jordi González and J. L. Gómez Caamaño, "Mujeres y varones médicos por decisión real en el reinado de Juan I de Aragón," *Boletín Soc. Esp. Hist. Farmacia* 19 (1968), 150.

[17] "Plus inductus invidia quam alia ratione"; Rubió y Lluch, I, 132; doc. CXXII.

[18] ACA, Cancillería, reg. 1893, fol. 174r.

[19] López de Meneses, "Documentos culturales," p. 695; doc. 31.

[20] ". . . quod non est aliquis qui in eorum infirmitatibus et necessitatibus curet eosdem." ACA, Cancillería, reg. 894, fol. 29v; published by López de Meneses, "Documentos culturales," p. 690; doc. 25.

[21] C. H. Talbot, *Medicine in Medieval England* (London, 1967), p. 96.

him by the examiners, and was held to be incompetent."[22] This complaint is worth studying for a number of reasons. It is the only document yet found from fourteenth-century Valencia—indeed, from the Crown of Aragon—containing details of the accusation and of the proceedings in such a case. It is also the one case so far found in which the complaint includes not only practicing without an examination but also those other activities prohibited by the first and seventh provisions of the *fur* of 1329: paying fees to apothecaries as well as to physicians, and prescribing medicines in Latin. Moreover, it is our only proof that the municipal system of *examinadors* was already functioning between 1331 (when Jacme Lama arrived in Valencia) and December 1334 (when the suit was brought before the justiciar of Valencia), since the municipal documentation has recorded the election of examiners of physicians and surgeons only after 1336.

Another feature of this case allows us to assess certain concrete aspects of physicians' daily practice that are otherwise difficult to measure. Because by the terms of the *furs* an accuser had a financial interest in the denunciation, it was necessary for Miquel de Roures to estimate the number of calls made by Jacme Lama, as well as the number of prescriptions he had had drawn up without proper municipal authorization. He claimed that they averaged some ten consultations daily—"ha usat de medicina o físicha deu vegades per cascun jorn poch més o menys en la dita ciutat"—and about one hundred Latin prescriptions during the three years that Jacme had practiced in the city. These details allowed Miquel to calculate the fine that Jacme Lama should pay, in this case the respectable sum of 185,000 pounds, with over 60,000 pounds thus going each to accuser, court, and municipality. Obviously economic issues were not irrelevant to the operation of this system of control over medical practice, and they were a serious threat to the unlicensed practitioner; that is, even though the system did not function particularly rapidly, even though the pressure from established physicians cannot have been particularly strong (since three years had passed before the accusation was made), the advantages of illegal professional activity had to make up for the risk of high fines.

But perhaps the most important aspect of this case to emphasize is the fact that the accused was a tonsured cleric. Jacme Lama insisted upon this before the justiciar, for it permitted him to claim the *privilegium fori*, one of the most important of the clerical privileges laid down by Innocent III at the beginning of the thirteenth century, by virtue of which clerics enjoyed immunity in any affair governed by civil law and falling under the jurisdiction of civil judges. Moreover, no cleric could be brought before such judges by a layman, and al-

---

[22] Appendix 2, doc. 2.

ready in the fourteenth century laymen were prohibited from hearing cases in which clerics were involved.[23] All these points were raised by Jacme Lama in his response to the charge:

> And the said master Jacme Lama says . . . that he is not required to reply to the accusation nor to pursue it before you, lord justiciar, for the following reasons:
>
> First, because the said master Jacme is a tonsured cleric . . . he is not required to submit to your authority, lord justiciar, since he is not in your jurisdiction, nor can you, lord justiciar, proceed against him or his goods on the strength of the said unjust demand, since possessions fall under the law of their possessor.
>
> Likewise, because by inspection of the said complaint it is manifest to you, lord justiciar, that the said Miquel has no right to bring it since it does not pertain to him either directly or indirectly.
>
> The said justiciar, having studied the complaint . . . and the replies proposed to it could not imprison him in accordance with the said complaint.[24]

Probably because the calculated fine was so large, the justiciar ordered as a precaution that a written inventory be made of the cleric's goods in case the accusation should be carried further, so that in this way "the lord king's right in the said goods might be preserved." The suit continued, but thenceforth it centered exclusively upon Lama's clerical status rather than upon his medical activities, and the remainder of the arguments heard by the tribunal, like the family quarrel that apparently underlay the complaint,[25] have no interest for us.

Between 1163 and 1298 the church had laid down a series of restrictions meant to regulate the situation of monks, friars, and clerics who wished to leave their residence to study medicine. As Amundsen has pointed out,[26] none of these ecclesiastical regulations prohibited clerics from practicing medicine. We have few evidences of medical practice by clerics or monks in the Crown of Aragon in the fourteenth century—that is, of a general practice rather than one carried on within the heart of an ecclesiastical community—and those that we do have come from the first third of the century.[27] In Jacme Lama's case his

[23] The *privilegium fori* goes back to the time of Constantine and was one of the most important privileges enjoyed by clerics; see Pearl Kibre, *Scholarly Privileges in the Middle Ages* (Cambridge, Mass., 1962), pp. 7ff. and references there.

[24] Appendix 2, doc. 2.

[25] As it proves, the notary Miquel de Roures was related to Jacme Lama by marriage, and his denunciation was apparently the continuation of a family quarrel. The accusation does not appear to have been successful: Jacme Lama was still called "metge" in 1340 and was evidently alive as late as 1347, when he was tried for having sworn an oath to the *Unió* in opposition to royal authority (below, ch. 5, n. 61).

[26] D. W. Amundsen, "Medieval Canon Law on Medical and Surgical Practice by the Clergy," *Bull. Hist. Med.* 52 (1978), 22–44.

[27] For example, on 22 August 1326 the *consellers* of Barcelona "wrote to the superior of a religious order whose name is illegible in the document to ask that brother Bartomeu

clerical status seems only to have been nominal, perhaps that of minor orders; clerical status was regularly adopted in fourteenth-century Valencia as a device for escaping civil jurisdiction.[28] The "maestre Lama" practicing in Valencia 1279–1304 was probably his father, and medicine the occupation to which Jacme had been brought up.[29] Thus his case focuses attention on an inherent tension between ecclesiastical authority and a secular occupation moving towards professional status in this period. The tension was heightened by the oft-made contrast between healers of the soul and physicians of the body.[30] The interests of these two could sometimes conflict, as indeed is suggested by the fourth provision of "De metges," which required physicians and surgeons to provide a confessor before treating a gravely ill patient.

III

The case of Hamet Hatequia, the Moor of Xàtiva who asked Pere IV to grant him a license to practice in the city and kingdom of Valencia, introduces us to the difficult situation in which the Jewish and Muslim minorities found themselves after the promulgation of the *furs* of 1329. Members of these minorities did not have access to university studies,[31] and hence could scarcely comply with the requirement of

---

de Podiolo (Dez-Pujol?), who had already attended various patients successfully in Barcelona, be sent to the convent of that city." Rubió Balaguer, *Documentos*, p. [14]. Archivo Histórico de la Ciudad de Barcelona, Llibre del Consell, IX (1325–1326), 47.

[28] The tonsure was a subterfuge for avoiding ordinary justice, since everyone tonsured—and hence every cleric—fell under ecclesiastical jurisdiction. In the wrangles that disturbed the city's life the use of this recourse by persons attached to the bishop's party (or that of some other important ecclesiastic) was so common that the *jurats* finally wrote (in a letter to the king of 18 July 1399) that to bear the tonsure had become the sign of a scoundrel; "car són molts de cascuns bandos, axí conjugats com no conjugats, axí de paratge com d'altres, portants e al.legants corona e opposants declinatòria que no són del for seglar, mas de la Ecclésia, per la qual són emparats e defeses de fet ab excomunicació dels officials reyals, no contrastant que aquells aytals no sien en sacres órdens, (ne) servesquen a la Ecclésia, mas tenguen sola corona, la qual, axí com era e ésser deuria senyal de simpla onestat, ara és penó de malendrinea." A. Rubio Vela, *Epistolari de la València medieval* (Valencia, 1985), p. 306.

[29] In November 1279 Pere III gave "magistro Lame phisico nostro et domine Regine" the right to transport into the city of Valencia all the salt produced at the coastal saltworks; he subsequently served Jaume II as physician as well (ACA, Cancillería, reg. 44, fol. 166r; 105, 148v). Lama was alive in December 1304 but dead by March 1307 (ACA, Cancillería, reg. 134, fol. 189v; reg. 296, fol. 35v).

[30] This has been closely studied by J. Agrimi and C. Crisciani, *Medicina del corpo e medicina dell'anima* (Milano, 1978), and C. Crisciani, "Valeurs éthiques et savoir médical entre le XIIe siècle," *History and Philosophy of the Life Sciences* 5 (1983), 33–52, esp. 38–39.

[31] To understand the evolution of this problem, as regards the Muslim (later Morisco) minority until its expulsion at the beginning of the seventeenth century, see Luis García Ballester, *Historia social de la medicina en la España de los siglos XII al XVI*, I (Madrid, 1976); idem, *Los moriscos y la medicina* (Barcelona, 1984); idem, "Academicism versus Empiricism in Practical Medicine in Sixteenth-Century Spain with Regard to Morisco Practition-

following medicine for four years in a *studium generale*.

Despite the demographic importance of the Muslim population in the kingdom of Valencia—in many parts of the kingdom it was not just the dominant but the only community—we have been able to find only two Muslim requests for a medical license in all the fourteenth century: one in 1338, made directly to the king to be allowed to practice medicine,[32] and one just fifty years later, made in 1388 to the justiciar of Valencia (as the *furs* required) for permission to practice surgery.[33] Obviously this number of licenses bears no relation to the actual number of practitioners in the Muslim community. It is extremely difficult, of course, to know what kind of health care was available to the great numbers of Muslims in the kingdom of Valencia, or who attended them; yet in spite of a lack of documentation offering concrete details, everything seems to indicate that they were treated by healers from their own community who, with rare exceptions, did not practice among Christians or Jews.

Because these healers could not acquire the training in theory demanded by the examiners, they had virtually no means of penetration into Christian society, which was governed by its own model for professional health care.[34] Muslim healers, whether physicians or surgeons, appear in our records only when that socioreligious boundary was crossed: sometimes legally, when a member of the Muslim community accepted the professional model of the Christian society and requested an examination, but more often illegally. In these latter instances, our few data reveal "subprofessionals," in effect *curanderos* or *curanderas*, and show us how deeply medicine was affected by the broad cultural disintegration that afflicted the Valencian Muslims living under Christian rule. In the years after the conquest of Valencia (1238), most of the Muslim intellectual minority—including learned physicians—left for Muslim realms (especially the kingdom of Granada), and the situation of the Muslims who remained in the new Christian kingdom did not encourage the survival of a scientifically sophisticated medical elite. Both King Jaume II (1292–1327) and his son Alfons IV (1327–1336) held learned Arabic medicine in high esteem, but when they sought expressly to be attended by Jewish and Muslim physicians, the best representative they could find of the latter group

---

ers," in A. Wear, R. K. French, and I. Lonie, eds., *The Medical Renaissance of the Sixteenth Century* (Cambridge, 1985), pp. 246–270, 338–342.

32 ACA, Cancillería, reg. 863, fol. 161r.

33 Appendix 2, doc. 13.

34 In studying and comparing charters granted and renewed to Muslim communities in Castellón during the thirteenth and fourteenth centuries, María del Carmen Barceló Torres has found something common to all: "el reconocimiento (por parte del grupo cristiano dominante) de una sociedad *distinta* que se seguirá rigiendo según los preceptos islámicos." "L'Alfondeguilla y Castro. La situación de los mudéjares castellonenses en el siglo XIII," *Bol. Soc. Cast. Cult.* 56 (1980), 126–139 (our emphasis).

in the entire kingdom of Valencia was a woman, a "metgessa mora."[35]

The Jewish minority was in a somewhat less difficult situation during most of the fourteenth century, both socio-economically and culturally, and was more successful in obtaining entrance into the medical occupations. What was at issue, of course, was the possibility of practicing within the Christian community, since (as with Muslims) the authorities were not concerned to regulate Jews who limited themselves to caring for members of their own faith: in 1342 King Pere agreed with Astruga, wife of master Astruch of Barcelona, that because she practiced surgery only on other Jews she was not subject to the requirement that all practitioners undergo examination.[36] In spite of the fact that the *furs* required a medical degree, which made it legally impossible for either minority to practice medicine, it seems likely that some Jews were enabled to practice under another provision of the *furs*, one designed to verify the qualifications of those who were practicing medicine or surgery at the moment when the laws came into effect:

> practitioners who are now practicing medicine or surgery shall be examined, and those who are found competent may remain in practice, but not the others, under a fine of 100 gold morabatins. . . .[37]

Potentially, at least, this allowed for the continuation in practice of Jewish (and Muslim) physicians, even though they could not have acquired their training in a medical faculty.

As time went on, Jews continued to be allowed to practice medicine by meeting the requirement of an examination; nothing was usually said about academic studies. It is not clear whether in these cases a Jew was expected routinely to sit on the examining tribunal, but certainly this did sometimes happen. In May 1346 Pere IV granted the Jew Jaffudà Abenvives a license to practice medicine in the city and kingdom of Valencia, having had verification of his professional qualifications from an examination carried out by two of the royal physicians—Pere Ros d'Orsins, a Christian, and Alatzar Avinardut, a Jew.[38] Pere, although a Valencian, was not one of that year's municipal examiners, but the king commanded the examiners to accept his assessment of Jaffudà and ordered royal authorities throughout the kingdom to accept Jaffudà's qualifications and to offer no obstacles to his practice. Abenvives had to swear to fulfill not only all the medical provisions of

---

[35] Michael R. McVaugh, "Islamic Medicine in the Kingdom of Aragon in the Early Fourteenth Century," in Proceedings of the Third International Conference on Islamic Medicine; *Bulletin of Islamic Medicine* 3 (1984).

[36] ACA, Cancillería, reg. 873, fol. 160v (kals. Jul. 1342).

[37] Appendix 2, doc. 1.

[38] ACA, Cancillería, reg. 880, fol. 186v; published by López de Meneses, "Documentos culturales," pp. 682–684; doc. 16.

the 1329 *furs*, but also their requirement of academic study—"quod audiverat per spatium quatuor annorum vel ultra arte seu scientia medicine"[39]—though the place and manner of such study was perhaps deliberately left vague.

Whether the form of Abenvives' examination—that is, by both a Christian and a Jewish physician—was routine in the 1340s,[40] by twenty years later it had become formally established throughout the Crown of Aragon. The *cortes* of Monzón of 1363 paid little attention to the problem of medical licensing except to ratify a particular method of professional examination for Jewish and Muslim physicians:

> Jewish and Saracen physicians should be examined by physicians of their law or sect, if there are any, although one Christian physician should assist in their examination; and if there are no physicians of their law or sect, they should be examined by two Christian physicians; and once the examination is carried out, if they are found qualified, they must swear to practice well and loyally before they are admitted to practice. [41]

The provision may simply have been designed to legitimate a system that had gradually come into being, and it certainly did not ensure that all Jews practicing medicine after 1363 underwent examination.[42]

What was legislated for Aragon or Catalonia did not necessarily affect the kingdom of Valencia, and despite the precedent of Abenvives' examination in 1346, despite the ruling of the *cortes* of Monzón, the municipality of Valencia does not seem to have included Jewish physicians on tribunals called to license other Jews to practice medicine. At

---

[39] Ibid., p. 683.

[40] We have earlier testimony to the examination of Jewish physicians, in Barcelona as well as in Valencia, but they are always examined by Christian physicians. In Catalonia such examinations were routinely given by master Pere Gavet, "in artibus licentiatum et in scientia medicine professorem." He examined David Abrahe of Cervera in 1334 (ACA, Cancillería, reg. 576, fol. 62r; published by J. Rius Serra, "Més documents sobre la cultura catalana medieval," *Estudis Universitaris Catalans* 13 [1928], 135–170; doc. 10, p. 140); Salomon Caravida of Copons in 1338 (ACA, Cancillería, reg. 863, fol. 231v); Rouen Caravida of sa Reyal in 1339 (ACA, Cancillería, reg. 604, fol. 103); and Mahir Caravida Çaporta of Barcelona in 1342 (ACA, Cancillería, reg. 873, fol. 139; published by Rubió y Lluch, *Documents*, I, pp. 123–124; doc. CXXI)—declaring the last-named qualified to practice *surgery*. In 1343 the *examinadors* of Valencia examined a Jewish physician whose name is not recorded: "Encara en la examinació de . j. metge de fehica (*sic*) juheu, fo acompanyat al dit maestre Bernat Ferrer, maestre Bertomeu de Casaldòria, metge de fehica (*sic*)" (AMV, Manuals de Consells, A-4, fol. 196r).

[41] "Usatges y constitucions de Catalunya" (ACA, Generalitat, ms. 3, fol. 40); published by Rubió Balaguer, *Documentos*, pp. [45–46]; doc. 25.

[42] For example, the infante Joan, finding himself in Vic on 1 August 1385, commanded an official of the court at Lérida that he should punish those Jews who were practicing medicine without having been examined: "infans Johannes etc. fideli nostro Petro Minoris, curie Ilerde . . . , quod de omnibus et singulis criminibus, et specialiter de delictis . . . medicorum judeorum non examinatorum . . . , diligentissime inquiratis et . . . extingatis. . . . " ACA, Cancillería, reg. 1732, fol. 78v; Rubió Balaguer, *Documentos*, p. [73].

any rate, no member of that community figures in any of the licenses we have found granted to Jewish physicians or surgeons of the city. In Barcelona, on the other hand, a license of 1368 identifies the Jewish member of an examining tribunal convoked by Pere IV (the Valencian Humer Tauell), and adds that "other Jewish physicians were present."[43] Perhaps it should be emphasized that in both these cases where a Jewish physician was allowed to sit as an examiner (1346 and 1368) the license was authorized by royal rather than municipal authority. Does this imply a different attitude on the part of the king and of the Valencian municipality towards admitting Jews to practice medicine in the Christian community?

IV

The three cases we have just considered show us that the regulations of the *furs* of 1329 had very real social consequences. Curiously, however, another provision of the *furs* seems to have had no effect at all, the explicit statement that

> no woman may practice medicine or give potions, under penalty of being whipped through the town; but they may care for little children, and women—to whom, however, they may give no potion. [44]

The prohibition would seem to reflect what has been called "the supposedly natural subordination or inferiority, generally recognized both in canon law and scholastic theology, [that] women experienced in the legal system of James I"; a situation that manifested itself in "limitations or restrictions on their power in civil life."[45] Prior to the *furs* of 1329, in fact, there is very little direct testimony to the practice of medicine by women in the Crown of Aragon (except as unofficial *curanderas*). Yet what regulation there was seems to have envisaged sanctioning their practice as at least an abstract possibility; the ordinances of the town of Valls (1299 and 1319), like those of Jaume I for Montpellier (1272), exclude from practice anyone "who has not learned the science of medicine, be they man or woman, Christian, Jew, or

[43] " . . . presentibus aliis medicis judeis." ACA, Cancillería, reg. 946, fols. 195v–196v; published by Rubió Balaguer, *Documentos*, pp. [73], [75]; doc. 46. A. Cardoner Planas, "El médico judío Selomó Caravida y algunos aspectos de la medicina de su época," *Sefarad* 3 (1943), 377–392.

[44] "Alcuna fembra no ús de medicina, ne de dar bouratges, sotz pena de córrer la vila açotan, mas puxen pensar de infans pochs e de fembres, a les quals, emperò, no donen alcun bouratge." Appendix 2, doc. 1.

[45] P. López Elum and M. Rodrigo Lizondo, "La mujer en el código de Jaime I de los *Furs* de Valencia," in *Las mujeres medievales y su ámbito jurídico* (Madrid, 1983), p. 128.

Saracen."[46] This may have been a mere formalism, but it makes the much more general prohibition of 1329 seem unexpectedly severe.

The prohibition seems all the stranger when we discover that in the period *after* the *furs* there is much better evidence available of the practice of medicine by women in the Crown of Aragon. In 1334 the physicians of Barcelona defended a policy of forbidding anyone "of whatsoever law, status, sex, or condition . . . to practice the office of medicine" who had not passed an examination or received an academic training, and in the process they indicated that "many men *and women* in this city and its surroundings are taking patients under their care."[47] Four years later Pere IV noted the rumor that an unnamed woman was practicing surgery in Barcelona and was harming her patients by her incompetence; rather than forbid her practice outright, he ordered that she should be examined by "expert surgeons" who could test her skill.[48] In the kingdom of Valencia itself the evidence is even more concrete. Here the practice of women included activity in virtually all aspects of medicine: as midwives; as specialists in, for example, eye ailments; and as practitioners of general medicine and surgery, treating men as well as women. We have continuing documentation of this practice in Valencia from 1332, when a woman named Çahud is found practicing surgery in the royal household, until 1436, when the king granted a license to Peregrina, wife of Martí Navarro of Morella. The presence in the kingdom of Valencia for over a hundred years of *metgesses*—that is, women (almost all of whom were Muslim) practicing medicine as a more or less normal occupation, often without bothering to seek formal exemption from the *fur*—would seem to indicate that the prohibition of 1329 was essentially a dead letter.[49]

How are we to interpret this contradiction between the *furs* and the medical reality? It may perhaps be useful to reformulate this as two associated problems: 1) what was the motive behind the enactment of the *fur,* and 2) why was it not enforced? Monica Green has recently suggested that the medical licensing introduced generally in the later Middle Ages was partially aimed at restricting or prohibiting the prac-

---

[46] "Encara an stablit et ordenat, que no sia null hom ni nuylla fembra, crestià o cristiana, jueu o juhya, sarray o sarraÿna, de qualque condició sia, qui no aja appresa scièntia de medicina, qui gos donar a persona malauta metzina. . . . " F. Carreras y Candi, "Ordinacions urbanes de bon govern a Catalunya. Ordinacions de Vall (1299–1325)," *BRALB* 25 (1925), 201.

[47] "In dicta civitate et vicaria eiusdem nonnulli homines atque femine . . . recipiunt sub eorum curis aliquos patientes." Rubió Balaguer, *Documentos,* doc. 13, p. [19].

[48] ACA, Cancillería, reg. 594, fol. 23 (5 id. Jan. 1337/8). The woman was probably a Christian, for she was living *in platea Sancte Anne,* which lay well outside the Jewish quarter.

[49] A. López de Meneses, "Cinco catalanas licenciadas en medicina por Pedro el Ceremonioso (1374–1382)," *Correo Erudito* 5 (1957), 252–254; A. Cardoner Planas, "Seis mujeres hebreas practicando la medicina en el reino de Aragón," *Sefarad* 9 (1949), 441–445; idem, *Història de la Medicina a la Corona d'Aragó (1162–1479)* (Barcelona, 1973), pp. 103–104; Luis García Ballester, *Historia social de la medicina,* pp. 42–44.

tice of medicine by women.[50] But if this was the motive behind the ordinance of 1329, why are there no known attempts to implement it? Why do we continue to find women practicing with impunity in Valencia? And why was the activity of female practitioners in Barcelona, noted above, not met by a similar prohibition in Catalonia?

A possible answer emerges from the pattern observable in the few licenses known to have been awarded to Valencian *metgesses* in the fourteenth century. First, none received her license from local Valencian *examinadors* and the municipal *consell*; in every case it was granted by the king. We see again that, as his sympathetic policy towards Jewish physicians has already suggested, the monarch found it in his interest to interfere in the monopoly over medical control that the *furs* had nominally given to the municipal authorities. Second, most of the women seeking to practice were Muslims rather than Christians (or Jews). Together, these facts suggest that the prohibition of 1329 may have been a response to a regional phenomenon that was perceived as a cultural and religious threat rather than a professional one: the practice of medicine—perhaps particularly gynecology and obstetrics—by Muslim *metgesses,* within an expanding Christian society. For Muslim *metgesses* enjoyed real prestige, and their ability to penetrate into Christian families and practice generally within the Christian population (which was still very much in the minority in the kingdom of Valencia as a whole) was clearly a cause of concern to some in local authority. The hidden purpose of the *furs* may have been made explicit in 1338 when the *batle general* of Valencia, Arnau Çamorera, specifically forbade "any Saracen woman who acts as *metgessa* to women to bring a Christian woman into her house for treatment."[51]

If this is the case, and the ordinance of 1329 was really aimed not so much at women in general as at Muslim women wishing to practice medicine, we can understand why it would not have been strictly enforced against Christians or Jews; but why were Muslims also allowed to practice, with or without a license? For practice medicine they certainly did, without any noticeable restrictions enforced by local government. In 1379 the *jurats* of Valencia, called to the house of Francesc Monyoç (an important figure in the city), found him attended by a Muslim *metgessa* who was treating his ailing hand and foot, as they mentioned in passing—casually, and perfectly naturally—in the letter they wrote to the governor of the kingdom.[52] Again, in 1391 the mu-

---

[50] Monica Green, "Women's Medical Practice and Health Care in Medieval Europe," *Signs: Journal of Women in Culture and Society* 14 (1989), esp. 446–452.

[51] "Que serrahina alcuna ques faça metgesa als dones no gos acollir en casa sua christiana alcuna a metgar." García Ballester, *Historia social de la medicina,* p. 42, n. 87.

[52] The letter was sent to Olfo de Pròxida, governor of the kingdom of Valencia, on 5 September 1379: "E anam a.N Francesch Monyoç que anàs a vós per ço que vós poguéssets venir ací per usar de vostra e nostra comissió, e trobam aquell ab la mà e ab lo peu malalts, e la mora metjessa qui.l curava." AMV, Lletres Missives, g3–4, fol. 110r-v; pub-

nicipality of Castellón agreed to request the presence of a Muslim *metgessa* specializing in the care of eye ailments, noting

> that she had been only a short time in the town and had brought about marvelous cures of the eyes. . . . The *consell* said that if she came it would be thankful because of the good she would do.[53]

There is no hint in such passages that the activity of such *metgesses* was anything but normal and unremarkable, the *furs* notwithstanding.

The simplest answer is probably the obvious one, that women—Muslims, Jews, or Christians—recognized as medically proficient were too valuable to exclude from practice. Those whom we find continuing to practice after the enactment of the *furs* were obviously not just midwives, with an exclusively gynecological clientele; indeed, significantly, they rarely appear in the treatment of women's ailments. Nor does it seem appropriate, socially, to view them as mere empiric healers or *curanderas*, for their occupational niche was acknowledged and supervised by those who controlled medical activity, the Valencian municipality and the king.[54] Whatever its original inspiration, the law of 1329 was unlikely to be enforced as long as competent women practitioners could be identified in a society where there were so few men qualified to practice medicine (or surgery) as to leave much of the public without the health care it wanted. If we now turn to look closely at the actual level of the practitioner population in fourteenth-century Valencia, we will see that it was indeed perceived as dangerously low.

---

lished by J. Sanchis Sivera, "La enseñanza en Valencia en la época foral," *Boletín Acad. Hist.* 108 (1937), 171.

[53] "Qui era ja estada poch temps havje en la dita vjla e havja fetes de grans cures de hulls . . . lo consell dix que sich venje que li fos fet plaer que fer li pusque per la bona obra que y fa." AMC, 4 July 1391; published by A. Sánchez Gozalbo, "La sanidad en el Castellón trecentista," *Bol. Soc. Cast. Cult.* 48 (1972), 246–274.

[54] We have testimony that in 1374 Floreta, a Jewish woman, received royal licence to practice *in arte medicina* throughout the territories of the Crown of Aragon: "Nos Petrus . . . quoniam fidedigna relatione percipimus quod tu, Floreta, uxor Jucefi Ça Noga, judei, quondam, habitantis in villa Santa Columba de Queralto, in arte medicina apta et suficiens es et propter tuam industriam et longam practicam in arte medicine uti per quevis loca regnorum et terrarum nostrarum . . . tibi plenam huius serie concedimus facultatem." A. López de Meneses, "Florilegio documental del reinado de Pedro IV de Aragón," *Cuadernos de Historia de España* 17 (1952), 171. Cf. the licence granted in 1394 to Francisca, widow of Berenguer Sa Torra, cited by Teresa Maria Vinyoles, *Les barcelonines a les darreries de l'Edat Mitjana (1370–1410)* (Barcelona, 1976), pp. 45–48, 174–75.

IV. THE DEMOGRAPHIC CONSEQUENCES OF THE *FURS*

It may be possible to understand some further implications of the Valencian licenses we have identified if we introduce here some additional demographic information about the kingdom of Valencia, in particular about the number and distribution of medical practitioners active there in the fourteenth century. What the proportion of practitioners was to the population as a whole is almost impossible to say, for—except at certain instants of time, and then only for the capital and a few other towns—we have no figures that will allow us to determine the population of the kingdom of Valencia during the fourteenth century. It is even more hazardous to make quantitative judgments about the distribution of this population among Christians, Muslims, and Jews. Tentatively, however, we can estimate that the city had 30,000 inhabitants and the kingdom 200,000 or so, at least two-thirds of whom were Muslims and 5–10% Jews.[1]

Fortunately we can provide somewhat more concrete information about the number of practitioners in the kingdom, based on several years' work in the Valencian and Aragonese archives and a thorough search of the secondary literature. Table I presents the numbers of individual physicians and surgeons whom we have so far identified as practicing in the kingdom in each quarter of the fourteenth century (subdividing the practitioners into Christians, Moors, and Jews); these

[1] The present state of research does not permit us to offer any more precise figures. According to the calculations of J. C. Russell ("The Medieval Monedatge of Aragon and Valencia," *Proceedings of the American Philosophical Society* 106 [1962], 502), the city's precincts held some 25,895 inhabitants in the period 1359–61. J. Hinojosa Montalvo estimates that the *jueria* of Valencia in the second half of the fourteenth century held 2,500 to 3,000 inhabitants, which would imply 10% of the total of the urban population. (Cf. "La comunidad hebrea de Valencia: del esplendor a la nada [1377–1391]," *Saitabi* 31 [1981], 66.) J. R. Magdalena Nom de Déu has found that the *jueria* of Castellón in 1371 had 27 inhabitants and has estimated that the Jewish population was "6 percent of the total of the town" ("Población, propiedades e impuestos de los judíos de Castellón de la Plana durante la Baja Edad Media," *Sefarad* 34 [1974], 274 and n. 8). As regards the fifteenth century, everything suggests that the Muslim population of the town of Castellón was almost double that of the Jews (idem, "Estructura socioeconómica de las aljamas castellonenses a finales del siglo XV," *Sefarad* 32 [1972], 341–370). The first trustworthy information for the city of Valencia is from 1489, when 8,840 hearths or homes were counted, without regard to their inhabitants: see A. Rubio Vela, "Sobre la población de Valencia en el Cuatrocientos. Nota demográfica," *Bol. Soc. Cast. Cult.* 56 (1980), 158–170.

TABLE I

PHYSICIANS AND SURGEONS ACTIVE IN VALENCIA, 1300–1400

	physicians			surgeons		
	C	J	M	C	J	M
1300–1325	21	5	0	18	1	0
1326–1350	35	8	1	16	0	2
1351–1375	37	4	0	12	2	0
1376–1400	48	8	3	37	0	1

numbers, therefore, are minima. The great majority of these practitioners were associated with the great urban nucleus of Valencia and its surroundings.

Finding evidence of so many physicians and surgeons actually practicing in Valencia makes it something of a surprise to have discovered so few municipal (as distinct from royal) licenses in the fourteenth-century Valencian documentation. This small number of licenses that have surfaced from the first seventy years after the promulgation of the *furs* seems to indicate that licensing was not a necessary prerequisite to practice, as a professional diploma or degree is today. The formal license may have been issued under circumstances that are impossible to understand with the information presently available to us. It may have been a hurdle that was invoked in a variety of circumstances—by municipal or royal authority, by physicians, or by individuals—but that was not automatically required in order to practice; otherwise the threat of examination would not have been such a useful weapon for personal enemies or professional competitors.[2] Indeed, in practically all the licenses we have collected, whether those issued by the municipality in conformity with the *furs* or those granted directly by the king, it is more or less expressly indicated that those who had submitted to questioning by the *examinadors* had already been practicing before presenting themselves for examination. This suggests that perhaps those who submitted to the provision of the *furs* were in some way forced to do so, which could help explain the striking differences between Tables I and II. The data in Table I are also consistent with our earlier conclusion that whatever healers practiced within the Valencian Muslim majority must have done so outside normal channels;

[2] For invocation by personal enemies, see the case of Jacme Lama, above, p. 24 n. 25. For invocation by professional competitors, consider the case of Ramon Bonet, a surgeon who was lured from Tarrega (in Catalonia) to Morella (in Valencia) by the *universitas* of the latter town in 1344. He began a successful practice there that cut into the livelihood of another Morellan surgeon, Guillem Ça Selva, who thereupon, "plus inducta invidia quam alia ratione, acusavit dictum Raimundum . . . dicendo ipsum in nonnullas penas incidisse eo quia sine examinatione usus fuerit arte predicta." The document is cited above, p. 21, n. 9.

TABLE II

LICENSES GRANTED TO VALENCIAN PHYSICIANS AND SURGEONS, 1375–1400

physicians			surgeons		
C	J	M	C	J	M
2	6	0	18	1	1

their practice was simply ignored by the machinery of control. Only in isolated cases—arising from the confrontation of cultures (as when, for example, Muslim healers were formally accused of conjuration in offering prognoses),[3] or from the fame of a particularly successful individual summoned to care for the court, a town,[4] or a hospital[5]—do such practitioners make an appearance in the archival materials.

It is not easy to reconcile this apparently inconsistent application of the *furs* with the vigorous terms in which the Valencian authorities regularly denounced unlicensed practice in the city and kingdom.[6] The subject was sensitive enough that despite the liberal policy that (as we have seen) the Aragonese monarchs generally followed in this regard, the king himself occasionally refused to grant licenses to practice, recognizing explicitly "that according to the new *furs* of Valencia all physicians are prohibited from practicing that craft in the city and kingdom of Valencia before they have been examined."[7] If the city really did care about licensing physicians, why have not more licenses survived? There are many other questions, too, to which we would like to have answers. What happened to those who sought a license and were rejected for having failed one requirement or another of the

---

[3] The same accusation was prominent in the inquisitorial investigation of the Muslim healers of Valencia in the sixteenth century: Luis García Ballester, *Los moriscos y la medicina* (Barcelona, 1984).

[4] On this subject see Luis García Ballester, *Historia social de la medicina*, pp. 42–45 (and references there).

[5] Cf. the admiring tone of the writer who recorded the payment to a Muslim *metgessa* for her successful care: "Item foren dats a Iª. mora que la guarí de la melsa, que tenia en lo vent gros, que lo metge de l'espital no la podia guarir, e la mora guarí-lla: III sous." Agustín Rubio Vela, *Pobreza, enfermedad y asistencia hospitalaria en la Valencia del siglo XIV* (Valencia, 1984), p. 125. In the sixteenth century Christian institutions (and individuals) continued to apply to Moorish healers when their own physicians failed them; cf. Luis García Ballester, *Los moriscos y la medicina*, pp. 108ff.

[6] For example, in the denunciation of a Muslim physician dated 13 March 1342: " . . . tam in civitate Valencie quam in . . . locis aliis regni Valencie arte medicine quamvis examinatus non fuerit in dicta arte, ut fieri debet iuxta forum." ACA, Cancillería, reg. 619, fol. 10r; reprinted by A. Rubió y Lluch, *Documents per l'història de la cultura catalana mig-eval*, II, 67; #67.

[7] ". . . Attendentes quod per foros novos Valentie omnes medici ab exercendo (in civitate et regno Valentie) eodem officio donec examinati fuerint prohibentur." ACA, Cancillería, reg. 863, fol. 161r.

examination? Was it possible to apply for a license repeatedly until successful? Did those who had been denied a license continue to practice illegally until another complaint was made against them, or did they shift their practice to a new locale in which they were unknown? None of these problems can yet be resolved on the basis of the existing documentation.

The additional demographic information available from archival sources can also help us to understand the otherwise unexpected pattern by which municipal supervision of medical care was extended to the lesser health occupations during the fourteenth century. The Valencian *furs* of 1329 had already extended the requirement of examination beyond physicians and surgeons to one of these lesser occupations: "a barber may not practice medicine or surgery if he has not been examined by the medical examiners and found adequate."[8] This requirement was peculiar to the kingdom of Valencia and was maintained throughout the fourteenth century;[9] it was undoubtedly one of the elements in the social dynamic responsible for the professional conflict between the barbers and surgeons of Valencia that became especially acute during the fifteenth century.[10] In contrast, in none of the laws applying to the Crown of Aragon as a whole are barbers mentioned, neither in the *cortes* of Monzón of 1289 nor in the later *corts* of Cervera (1359) or Monzón (1363). Indeed, not even surgeons are referred to explicitly in the *furs* after the Cerveran *corts*. Pere IV noted this in 1384, while rebuking his son, the infante Joan, for his excessive zeal in punishing Arnau and Bernat Oliva, two barbers of Perpinyà, for having practiced surgery without having passed a professional examination: he remarked in passing that in Catalonia it was not the custom to examine barbers who practiced surgery: "for the provision stating that physicians who practice must be examined does not mention surgeons, or at least in Catalonia it is not the custom that barbers who routinely practice surgery be examined."[11] The reason why barbers were included in Valencian legislation that purported to control the practice of medicine and surgery can only be that in the 1320s barbers were there perceived as performing the tasks of physicians and

---

[8] Below, Appendix 2, doc. 1.

[9] There is however no documentary evidence of the examination of a barber wishing to practice surgery in Valencia until 1388; Appendix 2, doc. 13.

[10] M. Gallent Marco, "Profesionalización y control del personal médico en el siglo XV," *Saitabi* 23 (1983), 97–103. The process discussed by this author really belongs to the fourteenth rather than the fifteenth century.

[11] "Car la constitució que parle que.ls metges hajan ésser examinats ans que usen de lur art, no comprèn cirurgians, o almenys no és acostumat en Cathalunya los barbers qui comunament usen de cirugia ésser examinats." ACA, Cancillería, reg. 1288, ff. 19v–20; reprinted by J. Rubió Balaguer, *Documentos*, p. [73]. Surgeons are also found excluded from provisions for professional control in Montpellier in 1239: "ut nullus de cetero praticari [medicina] presumat, nisi prius examinatus fuerit a duobus magistris . . . exceptis cirurgicis, quos huic nolumus examini subjacere." A. Germain, *Cartulaire de l'Université de Montpellier*, I, 186; doc. 4.

TABLE III

HEALTH PRACTITIONERS IN BARCELONA AND VALENCIA, 1325–1334

	physicians		surgeons		apoth's		barbers		total	
	B	V	B	V	B	V	B	V	B	V
1325	3	13	14	12	30	17	7	18	54	60
1326	6	12	11	13	30	17	7	17	54	59
1327	5	12	12	12	27	17	10	17	54	58
1328	8	11	11	11	26	16	9	17	54	55
1329	6	12	11	10	25	18	10	16	52	56
1330	7	12	12	9	24	16	10	16	53	53
1331	7	12	10	10	22	19	10	17	50	58
1332	6	12	9	11	23	18	10	19	47	60
1333	9	11	10	12	23	24	11	19	53	66
1334	8	11	7	9	23	18	11	16	49	54

surgeons, and hence as providing health care to a significant portion of the population.

The Catalan and Valencian archives allow us to assess the number of health professionals on a year-by-year basis in the two great cities, Barcelona and Valencia, during the period 1325–1334 that encompassed the promulgation of the *furs*, data presented in Table III. If we consider the barbers, the first thing to strike the attention is how many more there were in Valencia, both proportionately and absolutely: they made up almost a third of the practitioners, being far more numerous than the surgeons and roughly equal to the physicians or apothecaries. Leaving aside the latter (because although apothecaries could also carry out medical tasks, they were not yet covered by the *furs*), barbers amounted to almost half of the health practitioners legally recognized as performing a medical role in the city of Valencia. And the almost equal numbers of physicians and barbers in 1325–1334 would tip in favor of the barbers by 1347, a year before the Black Death, when there were but 12 physicians practicing as against 31 barbers, so that the legislation does not seem to have limited the growth of the barber population in Valencia.

The relative importance of the barbers within the practitioner populations of Valencia and Barcelona shows that at the moment when the *furs* went into effect barbers played a much larger role in Valencia than in Barcelona and were perceived as requiring examination or control. On the other hand, the city of Barcelona may have grown stricter in its supervision of barbers practicing surgery, at least by the end of the fourteenth century. In April 1386 Pere IV granted a license to practice surgery to Bernat Bertomeu, a barber of Barcelona, but added that he would have to undergo an examination "if the city councilors required it."[12] It may be that the demographic features we have already discussed influenced the attitude of the *consell*. Certainly by the end of the century the distribution of health professionals had changed in Barcelona as it had in Valencia, and so had the social role of the barber.[13]

By 1350 apothecaries as well as barbers were being publicly perceived as having an important role as health providers. In the aftermath of the Black Death of 1348 there was a growth of irregular practice in Valencia, and the municipal *consell* reacted firmly against what appeared to them to be a consequent lowering of standards. The councilors expressed their alarm in their session of 5 November 1350: "since some physicians and apothecaries have recently appeared in the city and are practicing their craft without being examined as the *furs* require, they should be so examined."[14] It was important to bring this irregularity to an end "because it is dangerous for them to practice without such an examination, and furthermore apothecaries may sometimes give one herb or one substance [by mistake] instead of another because they do not know or understand the said herbs or medicinal substances."[15] The municipal government resolved "that the said physicians active in the city be examined, as is ordained and established by the *furs*,"[16] and also provided for "two apothecaries who will examine the said [new] apothecaries as best they can"[17] under the supervision of the *examinadors*: "The *consell* also ordains that apothecaries be examined by the *examinadors* of physicians, joined by two apothecaries knowledgeable in the art."[18] Their motive was the public

[12] ". . . Hoc tamen proviso quod si consiliarii civitatis Barchinone, aut alii nomine ipsorum, requisiverint seu instanciam fecerint pro predictis, quod vos iuxta mentem dictarum constitucionem huiusmodi examen subeatis, quodque id facere et complere teneamini infra duos menses postquam inde fueritis requisitus." ACA, Cancillería, reg. 947, fol. 32v–33; reprinted by J. Rubió Balaguer, *Documentos*, p. [77]; doc. 47.

[13] Our treatment here of the precocious development of the Valencian barbers has been given greater amplification in Luis García Ballester and Michael R. McVaugh, "Nota sobre el control de la actividad médica y quirúrgica de los barberos (*barbers, barbitonsores*) en los *furs* de Valencia de 1329," *Homenatge al Doctor Sebastià García Martínez* (Valencia, 1988), I, 73–88.

[14] ". . . Com alcuns metges e speciés novellament sien en la ciutat e pratiquen de lurs arts sens que no són examinats, segons qu.és fur los dits metges deuen ésser examinats." Appendix 2, doc. 3; cf. A. Rubio Vela, *Peste negra, crisis . . .* , p. 74.

[15] "Com sie cosa perillosa aquells usar o pratichar sens la dita examinació, e semblantment los dits speciés s'entrameten a les vegades donar .I. erba per altra, o una cosa per altra, per tal com no són sabents ni conexents les dites erbes o les coses medecinals." Ibid.

[16] ". . . Que.ls dits metges ussants en la dita ciutat fossen examinats, segons que per fur és ordenat e stablit." Ibid.

[17] "Et axí meteix .II. speciayres qui examinassen los dits speciés segons que mills puxen." Ibid.

[18] "Encara ordenà e volch lo dit consell que los speciés fossen examinats per los dits examinadors de metges ensemps ab .II. speciés sabents bé de l'art." Ibid. The *consell* named as examiners for the year masters Miró de Corçà and Bernat Minguet, together with En Jacme Metge; it also decreed that together with the two knowledgeable *speciers*

health—"a pprofit e utilitat de la cosa pública"—for the Black Death seems widely to have reinforced the sense that health was a definite responsibility of municipal authorities. Evidently the upheaval produced by the plague of 1348 set in motion a broadening of medical supervision to include all the health occupations, completing a process foreshadowed by the *furs* of 1329.

This broader control of the medical occupations was soon felt throughout the kingdom: in 1355 Pere IV had to intervene to protect the Valencian apothecary Guillem Caner, accused of practicing medicine illegally in that he had not fulfilled the four years of study required by the *furs.*[19] Another apparent consequence of the upheaval of the 1350s was the appearance of demands by the examiners for a fee from candidates for a license, a practice complained of as early as 1351.[20] In the Valencian *furs* of 1403 King Martí I confirmed the municipal control of the apothecaries, and took action to prevent the imposition of fees by the *examinadors.*[21] When in 1441 the apothecaries established themselves as a guild they accepted their supervision by physicians, with the assurance that the two apothecaries on the tribunal would be elected annually by their own body rather than by the *consell.*[22]

Evidently the 1350s and the aftermath of the Black Death mark a moment of medical disintegration in Valencia. We have noted the reaction of municipal authorities to this disintegration, but there was also a response from the physicians and surgeons who were already qualified *secundum formam fori Valentie*. There is reason to think that, from this moment on, the Valencian physicians began to develop a professional cohesion and to assume a directing role in the scrutiny of would-be practitioners—a role that in the 1330s had been solely held

they should examine the apothecaries, and that two *jurats* should be present at the examinations in order "to determine those who are unqualified" so as to prevent them from practicing the craft in the city or kingdom.

[19] A. López de Meneses, "Documentos culturales," pp. 694–696; docs. 30–31.

[20] The complaint, by a Jewish physician of Alzira, is published by López de Meneses, "Documentos culturales," p. 690; doc. 25. However, it may be that this abuse was an inveterate one, dating back almost to the moment when the examination system went into effect. A surgeon of Mallorca, Samuel Içach, complained to the king in 1339 that "ipse intendat habitare in regno Valencie et uti officio cirurgie et propterea requisiverit ut asserit deputatos ad examinandum cirurgicos ut iuxta forum Valencie per examinationem accipiant ab eodem, hocque dicti deputati facere contradicant," and that this had happened three or four times. The king's (favorable) response to the complaint does not specify the reason for the examiners' refusal, but it is plausible that (as in the Alzira case) they had demanded a fee that the candidate was unwilling to pay. ACA, Cancillería, reg. 598, fol. 227r–v (8 kals. Feb. 1338/9).

[21] "Los examinadors dels metges, elets segons forma de fur, no reeben alcun salari, do ne servey per examinar alcuns metges de física o de sirurgia o barbers ne de examinatió de speciers. E si lo contrari faran, sien encorreguts en pena de deu morabatins per quantes vegades contrafaran." *Furs e Ordinations . . . del Regne de Valencia* (facsimile ed., Valencia, 1978), p. [380].

[22] F. Barberà, *Códice del antiguo colegio de boticarios de Valencia* (Valencia, 1905), p. 8.

by the municipal bourgeoisie. We may remember that in 1334 in Barcelona, in a similar situation—that is, in response to an intrusion of unqualified "healers"—, physicians had taken the lead in protesting such an invasion. Now in 1356 the physicians of Valencia also arrogated to themselves alone the title of "medicus" and denounced its usurpation by those who practiced medicine without abiding by the *furs*, reiterating their content: no one shall practice in the city or kingdom "nisi prius per quatuor annos audiverit in studio generali et postmodum examinatus fuerit et repertus sufficiens per examinatores ordinatos in civitate predicta."[23] In Valencia, as earlier in Barcelona, physicians were addressing the king as a cohesive social group and asking for action against the unauthorized practice. The original leadership of the city government in this protest is undeniable, but it is important too to recognize that the Valencian physicians were beginning to show signs of acknowledging their collective identity and self-interest by the second half of the fourteenth century.

---

[23] ACA, Cancillería, reg. 690, fols. 69v–70; published by A. López de Meneses, "Documentos culturales . . . ," pp. 700–701; doc. 37. We will look more closely at this document later, for it is of particular importance for an understanding of the tensions between king and town over control of the medical occupations.

V. THE PRESSURES FOR MEDICAL SUPERVISION IN VALENCIA

I

How are we to explain the promulgation of a specific licensing code for Valencia in 1329, and the extent to which it was implemented there? We may conveniently begin by considering the role of educational and ecclesiastical institutions in shaping the activity of its physicians. The absence of controls over the practice of medicine in thirteenth-century Valencia was perhaps rooted in the Muslim model for the transmission of knowledge,[1] in which anyone could give instruction; but it had been formally established by the original Valencian *furs* of Jaume I (1238), which affirmed explicitly that "any cleric or other man may freely and without service or tribute teach medicine anywhere in the city."[2] The change in attitude was initiated by the founding in 1300 of the University of Lérida, by which Jaume II introduced into his realms the educational revolution associated with the medieval universities.[3] This gave Lérida the monopoly on higher education (including medicine) in the Crown of Aragon,[4] explicitly applying the university model adopted in Sicily in 1224 by the emperor Frederic II.[5] There were thus two kinds of medical practitioners in the Crown of Aragon (and hence in Valencia) in the early fourteenth century: those who had acquired their medical knowledge more or less informally, and those who had been trained in a faculty of medicine and might possess a university degree (bachelor, licenciate, or master). It was quite natural to proceed to demand a university degree for the practice of medicine,[6] eliminat-

---

[1] Cf. Luis García Ballester, *Historia social de la medicina*, p. 24.

[2] "Tot clergue o altre hom pusque francament e sens tot serví e tribut tener studi . . . de física . . . en tot loch per tota la ciutat." *Furs e Ordinations . . . del Regne de Valencia* (facsimile ed., Valencia, 1978), p. [189].

[3] H. Rashdall, F. M. Powicke, A. B. Emden, *The Universities of Europe in the Middle Ages* (Oxford, 1936), II, 93.

[4] "Nulla persona cuiuscumque preheminencie, dignitatibus, condicionis, statibus aut legis existat tam audax reperiatur quod in aliquo loco terre et dominationis nostre . . . libros medicine . . . audeat vel presumat aliquibus scolaribus legere vel docere. . . . " A. Rubió y Lluch, *Documents per l'història de la cultura catalana mig-eval*, I (Barcelona, 1908), p. 15, doc. xv.

[5] Rashdall, *Universities*, II, 93.

[6] "Thus one of the purposes of the university was to initiate the professional into a set of attitudes and controls, to give him a professional conscience, and to develop a feeling of group solidarity." V. L. Bullough, "Achievement, Professionalization, and the Univer-

ing this two-fold route into practice, and this step was taken by the new *furs* of Jaume's son Alfons IV.

The founding of the new university at Lérida was in effect a "Christianizing" act, for it gave special recognition to Christians, who alone were entitled to pursue studies there and to receive its degrees. By the same token, it tended to weaken the importance of the freedom of teaching traditional within the Muslim and Jewish communities.[7] The *furs* of 1329 merely consolidated this cleavage between the religions: it was "Jews, Saracens, and apostates" who were attacked with such contempt in 1356 by Valencian physicians and surgeons licensed *secundum formam fori Valentie*.[8] The new *furs* may thus be interpreted in part as an attempt to make medicine an essentially Christian activity, and to weaken the socio-cultural importance hitherto enjoyed by Jews and Muslims, who made up the overwhelming majority of the kingdom's population.

The *furs* further provided for the "Christianization" of medicine by insisting that physicians and surgeons summon a confessor before treating the gravely ill, or at least warn the patient of his need for confession. In this respect the condition was one long required by the church, for (as Tentler has emphasized)[9] the sacrament of confession could be an effective instrument of social control. The *furs* drew specifically from canon 22 (*Cum infirmitas*) of the Fourth Lateran Council (1215), which declared that physicians should advise and persuade—"moneant et inducant"—their patients to confess.[10] The conflict between the interest of the physician for the health of the body and that of the priest for the health of the soul was of concern to the church

---

sity," in J. Ijsewijn and J. Paquet, eds., *The Universities in the Later Middle Ages* (Louvain, 1978), p. 508.

[7] Cf. L. Barthélémy, *Les médecins à Marseille avant et pendant le Moyen-Age* (Marseille, 1883), pp. 13–14 and pièces no. 1 (28 August 1326) and 2 (19 September 1443), pp. 31–32.

[8] A. López de Meneses, "Documentos culturales," p. 701, doc. 37.

[9] T. N. Tentler, *Sin and Confession on the Eve of the Reformation* (Princeton, 1977), p. xv.

[10] "XXII. Quod infirmi prius provideant anima quam corpori. Cum infirmitas corporalis nonnunquam ex peccato proveniat, dicente Domino languido quem sanaverat: 'Vade et amplius noli peccare, ne deterius aliquid tibi contingat': decreto presenti statuimus, et districte praecipimus medicis corporum, ut cum eos ad infirmos vocari contigerit, ipsos ante omnia moneant et inducant, quod medicos advocent animarum: ut postquam infirmis fuerit de spirituali salute provisum, ad corporalis medicinae remedium salubrius procedatur, cum causa cessante cesset effectus. . . . Si quis autem medicorum, hujus nostrae constitutionis, postquam per praelatos locorum fuerit publicata, transgressor extiterit, tamdiu ab ingressu ecclesiae arceatur, donec pro transgressione hujusmodi satisfecerit competenter.

"Caeterum cum anima sit multo pretiosior corpore, sub interminatione anathematis prohibemus, ne quis medicorum pro corporali salute aliquid aegroto suadeat, quod in periculum animae convertatur." J. D. Mansi, *Sacrorum conciliorum nova amplissima collectio* (repr. Graz, 1960–62), v. 22, cols. 1010–11. The position of canon law is expressed in the *Decretales* of Gregory IX (lib. V, tit. 38, cap. 13) in the following terms: "Medici, vocati ad infirmos, debent ante omnia inducere infirmum ad confessionem, nec quicquam persuadere pro salute corporis, tendens in animarum periculum [idem in eodem (concilio generali)]." E. Friedberg, ed., *Corpus Juris Canonici* (repr. Graz, 1959), II, col. 888.

generally,[11] but it had particular relevance to the predominantly Muslim society of Valencia, where originally there were virtually no Christian physicians available; no doubt for this reason, the confessional injunction of canon law had already been firmly insisted upon by the original Valencian *furs* of 1238.[12] The reiteration of this injunction in the "new *furs*" ninety years later shows that this tension had not disappeared with time; so does the warning of the Valencian St. Vicent Ferrer (1350–1419), at the end of the fourteenth century:

> Morally, when a physician takes a man under his care, he must first get him to confess; he is required to do this by the decretal "Mandamus etc.," and sins mortally if he does not do so.[13]

In one final respect the impact of institutional Christianity upon the shaping of the practitioner needs to be emphasized. As we have just seen, the thirteenth-century formulation of canon law stressed the need for physicians to require their patients to confess. More broadly, in such collections as the *Decretales* of Gregory IX (1234), it established the norm of annual confession under penalty of excommunication, and encouraged confessors to investigate the circumstances and characteristics of the sinner and his sin. This and other recommendations gave rise in following years to a religious literature that was practical in nature, intended to train confessors and help them in the various problems presented to them by an increasingly complex and changing society. These guides or manuals, *Summae confessorum,*[14] insisted that confession should examine every aspect of daily life. Nothing was to fall outside the scope of confession, from the most intimate details of domestic life to those of economic and social activity—including that of physicians.

One such guide was the *Summa de casibus conscientiae* (c. 1317), usually cited as *Astesana,*[15] which expressly emphasized the sinfulness of the physician "who claims to practice his profession without a knowledge of medical science (*cum sit idiota*),"[16] and described such ignorance as a *culpa ante factum.* The *Astesana* went on to develop a

---

[11] Cf. D. W. Amundsen, "Casuistry and Professional Obligations: The Regulation of Physicians by the Court of Conscience in the Late Middle Ages," *Trans. and Stud. Coll. Phys. Philadelphia* 3 (1981), 22–39, 93–112, and bibliography in n. 73.

[12] "Negun metge no reeba alcú o alcuna que sie greument malalt o malalta en cura, si donchs primerament lo malalt no haurà presa penitèntia." *Furs e Ordinations,* loc. cit.

[13] " . . . Moralment, que quan lo metge deu pendre en cura hun hom, *primo* lo deu confessar; e són-o tenguts fer, car axí.u diu la decretal *Mandamus,* etc., e per ço pecque mortalment si fa lo contrari." Sant Vicent Ferrer, *Sermons,* ed. J. Sanchis Sivera, I (Barcelona, 1932), 209.

[14] Amundsen, "Casuistry," pp. 28ff.

[15] Astesanus de Asti, *Summa de casibus conscientiae* (Venice, 1478); cited by Amundsen, p. 25.

[16] *Astesana,* 6.14, following Amundsen, p. 29 n. 27.

distinction that reinforced still further the need for an adequate apprenticeship for the professional physician (a training that, given the terminology used, could only take place in the new university contexts): a distinction between the *culpa in facto,* "when the physician does not follow the established practices of the *ars* and attempts risky procedures," and the *culpa post factum* when, properly trained and having acted responsibly, "he does not follow up the patient's case diligently."[17] The *culpa ante factum* would be evoked later in the century by the Franciscan Eiximenis (a Catalan living in Valencia) in his condemnation of those who practice medicine without adequate knowledge, whom he views as murderers if their practice leads to a patient's death:

> Fourth, it is homicide if someone kills another, for example someone who stupidly throws a stone from a high place, or who attaches the clapper of a bell insecurely which, falling, kills someone; or who declares himself to be a physician and, without knowing the art, gives medicines or advice which cause the patient to die.[18]

The church was thus portraying a full and systematic education as not merely practically desirable but morally imperative for the physician, and in this way it implicitly supported the demands of civil authorities (municipalities or king) for specialized training of would-be practitioners.

II

The royal family was by no means indifferent to the nature and availability of medical care in the Crown of Aragon. In particular, Jaume II—who died in November 1327, only two years before the Valencian *furs* were issued—had been a visible patron of medicine, especially of learned medicine, during his long reign of thirty-six years.[19] This patronage manifested itself at a number of different levels of royal activity, certainly within the court but also more widely within the kingdom, and may very well have contributed to the atmosphere of belief and expectation that underlay the new legislation.

---

[17] *Astesana,* 6.16 and 6.14; Amundsen, p. 30.

[18] Francesc Eiximenis, *Lo libre de les dones,* ed. F. Naccarato (Barcelona, 1981), II, 306.

[19] "La vertadera passió de tota sa vida fou la medicina"; Rubió y Lluch, *Documents,* II (Barcelona, 1921), p. xxxi. At the moment, the best discussion of the king's concern for medicine is that of J. Ernesto Martínez Ferrando, *Jaime II de Aragón: Su vida familiar* (Barcelona, 1948), I, 54–63 and elsewhere; one of us is preparing a fuller study of this subject.

For one thing, from the moment Jaume succeeded to the throne he displayed a preoccupation with his health and with keeping medical care continually available to him—and, in lesser degree, to his family. He kept at least one and usually two physicians in ordinary throughout his reign, and if in his travels through his realms he felt ill he would supplement their care with physicians from the immediate region in which he found himself.[20] The supply of physicians was so scant, however, and the rewards available to entice them to stay with him so slim, that he was not able to achieve a permanent medical staff until 1306; from that time on he was served by the same two physicians, Joan Amell and Martí de Calça Roja.[21] This medical staff was expanded, as time went on, to include physicians responsible for his family's care; as his children grew up, he appointed physicians to serve each of them, as Guillem de Carcassonne served Jaume's daughter Constança from 1307 to 1315, or as Pere Cellerer served four of the children between 1316 and 1334.[22] Such physicians were typically "on call"; they lived and practiced in Valencia (like Guillem) or Daroca (like Pere), but they enjoyed a supplement to their income in the form of a retainer from the king, and in turn they were expected to come attend the infantes whenever necessary. In this way the royal concern for family health both directly and indirectly ensured a certain growth in the level of health manpower in the kingdom, and in order to ensure a larger pool of practitioners to fill this role, the king routinely did his best to entice foreign physicians and surgeons to move into his lands—not necessarily to enter into his own employment, but to settle and practice among his subjects.

The king was not, however, unconcerned about the type of medicine that such practitioners carried on; he was in particular a patron of learned academic medicine rather than of mere empirical skill. As a young man, Jaume had had first-hand experience of a system requiring the qualification of physicians on the island of Sicily, first as his father's lieutenant and then as ruler there (1283–1291); it is difficult not to believe that his continuing associations with southern Italy (in 1295 he married the daughter of Charles II of Anjou, king of Naples) helped

---

[20] When the king fell ill in Jaca in June–July 1302, for example, he called no fewer than nine physicians to attend him, from Huesca, Zaragoza, Lérida, and Pamplona: Eduardo González Hurtebise, *Libros de Tesorería de la Casa Real de Aragón*, I (Barcelona, 1911), 56–57, 61–62.

[21] The appointment of Martí goes back to the end of 1304 (ACA, Cancillería, reg. 235, fol. 144); that of Joan is published by Martínez Ferrando, *Jaime II de Aragón*, II, 22 (doc. 36).

[22] The letter of Guillem's appointment is published by Martínez Ferrando, II, 30 (doc. 50); see also pp. 115–116 (doc. 170). Pere cared for the infante Jaume in 1316, Maria in 1320, Joan in 1321–1334, and Constança in 1326. On Pere's relation to Arnau, see the information provided by John F. Benton, "The birthplace of Arnau de Vilanova," *Viator* 13 (1982), 245–57. A full study of the archival material pertaining to Pere is in preparation.

shape his policy of support for academic medicine. Jaume's creation of a university at Lérida was expressly designed to make his new realm self-sufficient in medical and legal training.[23] He saw to it thereafter that his household physicians were supplied with copies of scholastic medical texts as needed, and he subsidized the translations of still others from Latin into Catalan (for example, the *Tasrif* of Abulcasis[24]).

For a variety of reasons, Jaume found Arnau de Vilanova the embodiment of what learned medicine could offer. Arnau was Valencian by culture, academically trained, the translator of medical works from the Arabic, and the author of a vast range of knowledgeable medical treatises; his skill was acknowledged by his colleagues, who would even refuse to treat a case before Arnau had arrived to give advice. Unable to persuade Arnau to return permanently to the Crown of Aragon, Jaume settled for repeated short visits and for consultation, as it were, at a distance, via medical writings. About 1307 Arnau composed for the king a *Regimen sanitatis*, largely traditional in form but personalized to the extent of adding a final chapter on hemorrhoids that responded to the king's own concerns; at the queen's request, the surgeon Berenguer ça Riera translated Arnau's work into Catalan.[25] The next year Jaume wrote to Arnau asking for a copy of his chef d'oeuvre, the *Speculum medicine*, promising him to show it to no one "nisi eum cui volueritis."[26] And the year after that, Arnau visited Jaume at the siege of Almería and presented him with a unique little treatise on military hygiene for the army's use—trying (unsuccessfully, as it proved) to ingratiate himself with the monarch against the day when Jaume would learn of Arnau's recent tales to the pope of the king's religious beliefs.[27] Jaume was enraged at Arnau when he did learn of these, the next year, and Arnau never returned to Aragon, dying in 1311.

It is characteristic of Jaume's commitment to scholastic medicine that shortly before Arnau's death he should have sought out Arnau's disciple, Pere Cellerer, and begun to make use of him in caring for the royal family[28]—Arnau's learning was too valuable to neglect, even in his disgrace. We should certainly understand the king's personal involvement during these years in the establishment and direction of the medical faculty at his new university of Lérida in the light of this same

---

[23] See the text published by Jaime Villanueva, *Viage literario a las iglesias de España*, XVI (Madrid, 1851), 196.

[24] Rubió y Lluch, *Documents*, II, 22 (doc. 29); A. Cardoner Planas, "Nuevos datos acerca de Jafuda Bonsenyor," *Sefarad* 4 (1944), 287–93.

[25] Ana Trías Teixidor is preparing an edition of the Latin text for vol. VII of the *Arnaldi de Villanova Opera Medica Omnia*.

[26] Heinrich Finke, *Acta Aragonensia* (Berlin, 1908), II, 876–878 (docs. 554–555).

[27] An edition of this text, known in sixteenth-century editions as the *Tractatus de regimine castra sequentium*, will be included in vol. VII of the Arnaldian *Opera Medica Omnia*.

[28] ACA, Real Patrimonio, reg. 273, fol. 56v.

commitment; and we should probably acknowledge that his obviously high valuation of medical learning, communicated to his son and heir Alfons IV, helped to form a climate of expectation that his subjects had come to share by the time of his death in 1327.

III

There were political as well as personal reasons for the fourteenth-century kings of Aragon to have taken a direct interest in the supervision of medical care in their realms, as evidenced by the continuing struggle between the king and the municipality of Valencia over the power to license physicians. Although the *furs* of 1329 had made it explicit that control of the medical profession lay in the hands of the municipal *consell,* the monarchs tried increasingly to assert their own authority in this area. At the beginning of Pere IV's reign he seemed ready to acknowledge the city's prerogative. We have already remarked upon his response in 1338 to Hamet Hatequia, who had appealed directly to him for permission to practice medicine in the city and kingdom of Valencia: Pere had refused to grant such permission, explaining that the new *furs* gave this power to the municipal *examinadors.* Yet six months later Pere showed that he was fully prepared to override the new *furs* when he responded quite differently to a comparable request. Thomas Gallesii assured the king in August 1338 that he had practiced surgery successfully in Zaragoza and Lérida for more than twenty-five years and now wanted to continue his practice in Valencia; Pere thereupon granted Thomas the right "to exercise the art of surgery in the city and kingdom of Valencia freely and without any sort of examination or obstacle, notwithstanding the *fur* of Valencia which says that practitioners (*medici*) must be examined before they begin to practice any sort of medicine."[29] Again, as we have already seen in another context, Pere granted a license to practice medicine in the kingdom of Valencia in 1346 to the Jew Jaffudà Abenvives, whose qualifications he had had verified by two royal physicians who had given Jaffudà an examination.[30] Was the royal intervention in this case owing to the fact that, as a Jew, Abenvives could present no documentation of having followed medicine in a university and hence had anticipated difficulties with the municipality? We do not know; but, as we have already pointed out, the *furs* of 1329 made it difficult for the

---

[29] " . . . Quod vos, foro Valencie dicente quod examinentur medici antequam arte uti incipiant medicine modo aliquo non obstante, in dicta civitate et regno Valencie uti dicta arte cirurgie libere et absque examinatione et alio quocumque obstaculo valeatis." ACA, Cancillería, reg. 864, fol. 94v (13 kals. Sep. 1338).

[30] ACA, Cancillería, reg. 880, fol. 186v; publ. by A. López de Meneses, "Documentos culturales," pp. 682–684; doc. 16.

members of the Jewish and Muslim minorities by requiring an academic training. Whatever the reason, it is evident that there were in fact *two* license-granting authorities in fourteenth-century Valencia: one, established by the *furs*, was the municipal government of the city of Valencia; the other was the Crown.

The royal assertion of the right to license, first observed in the late 1330s, can be better understood against the broader background of events, for a decade of acute political tension between city and king was beginning. These years culminated in the establishment of the *Unió*, a movement of rebellion whose formation "was owed essentially to the authoritarian characteristics that the royal government was taking on."[31] It was in fact in May 1347 that the *consell* of Valencia summoned the country in order to constitute the *Unió*, claiming "that the juridical structure that ruled the life of the kingdom was being violated by the king, royal officials, and judges delegated by the Crown—who (what is worse) justified their violation by claiming the authoritarian principle, derived from Roman law, that the royal power was above all laws and rights of the land."[32] The royal intervention in the control of a nascent medical profession was only one aspect of a wider assertion of authority feared by the king's Valencian subjects.

Nor, apparently, did the episode of the *Unió* bring such medical interventionism to an end, and in 1356 this provoked a serious protest to the king from those physicians and surgeons who were practicing legally. In April, led by the (Valencian) royal physician Pere Ros d'Orsins, they merely asked the king to confirm that anyone who wished to practice in Valencia had to be examined *iuxta forum*.[33] In October, however, still dissatisfied, they pointed out to the king that it was he who was violating the *furs*;[34] that the procedure of getting royal authorization for medical practice in the kingdom had given rise to a dangerous intrusion into the profession "of ignorant men who are not worthy of the name of physician, from which follows no little harm and consequent danger for patients."[35] They asked the king that "he not overstep by granting a license against the *furs*," and they charged him with issuing licenses above all to "apothecarii, tintorerii, judei, sarraceni et apostate."[36] The monarch's reply was conciliatory: he promised to annul all authorizations granted by him contrary to the

[31] M. Rodrigo Lizondo, "La Unión valenciana y sus protagonistas," *Ligarzas* 7 (1975), 135.

[32] "Com lo senyor rey e sos officials e jutges letrats hajen fet e usat contra furs e privilegis, bons uses e libertats de la ciuitat [sic], al.legants que lo senyor rey és en possessió de no servar furs e privilegis, bons uses e libertats. . . . " Ibid., pp. 137–138.

[33] ACA, Cancillería, reg. 898, fol. 253.

[34] A. López de Meneses, "Documentos culturales," pp. 700–701; doc. 37.

[35] " . . . Cuius rei occasione sequitur dampnum non modicum et per consequens pericula personarum, cum sint ignari hominis [*sic*] et non vocari debeant medici sed verius si tales sunt in sciencie eis ignote"; ibid., p. 701.

[36] " . . . Aliquam cartam contra dictos foros concessisse excedere debuisse"; ibid.

furs, ordering all authorities in the kingdom to apply the law strictly in all matters pertaining to medical supervision, whatever circumstances might seem to permit its evasion—the latter perhaps an allusion to particular circumstances (e.g., lack of professionals, unavailability of medical care to the poor) that had encouraged the king to intervene. The monarch's deference to the *furs* thus appeared to concede the hegemony of the Valencian *consell* and indicates the growing strength of the group formed by those "approved in medicine and surgery."[37]

This concession does not mean that after 1356 conflicts of authority did not still arise over this subject between municipality and Crown. There are no signs of them in the remainder of Pere's reign, but it is clear that Pere's son and successor, Joan I (1387–1396), repeatedly violated his father's promises of 1356. The licenses granted by Joan, without any examination and in open defiance of all provisions for regulation, are fairly numerous, both to men and to women, in various parts of the Crown of Aragon. The grant of such licenses was sometimes justified by reference to a lack of medical assistance for a local population, whether because examined and "qualified" physicians were lacking or because, although present, they charged more than their patients could pay. Such is the explanation for the license granted in 1387 to Francesc Martí, an apothecary of Vilafranca del Penedès, "for the rest of his life, even though he has not taken the required examination."[38] Again, in May 1393 the king granted a license to practice in the city of Valencia "and all our lands" to Joan Forner, even though he had not been examined, "since you are competent and satisfactory in the art of medicine by virtue of having learned from experience."[39] A few months later, in December 1394, he granted another license, this time to a woman—Bevenguda, wife of Joan Mariner of Valencia—"since it is clear that by licit rather than prohibited means . . . you are vigilant in treating and curing many men and children of both sexes of serious conditions and illnesses." The license explicitly provides that "contrary *furs*, privileges, uses and other practices of the kingdom of Valencia shall in no way interfere";[40] indeed, the document suggests a certain animosity towards the body of "qualified" physicians when it refers to the group that had originated the attacks on Bevenguda's medical practice as "those who call themselves expert in medicine." Once more we must recognize the possibility that

---

[37] "Nullus cuiuscumque conditionis existat, audeat vel presumat uti medicinali sciencia vel cirurgia in civitate et regno predictis, nisi prius per quatuor annos audiverit in Studio generali et postmodum examinatus fuerit et repertus sufficiens per examinatores ordinatos in civitate predicta." Ibid.

[38] "Et . . . concedimus vobis dicto Francisco et licentiam elargimur quod possitis licite et impune uti de cetero quamdiu vixeritis dicta arte fisice non obstante quod examinatus non fueritis." ACA, Cancillería, reg. 1893, fol. 174r.

[39] " . . . In arte fisice suficientem et ydoneum experientia edocente." ACA, Cancillería, reg. 1905, fol. 55r.

[40] ACA, Cancillería, reg. 1909, fol. 150v.

the motives behind professional attacks on empiric healers may have been economic, as well as based on a concern for public health—the license repeats Bevenguda's complaint that the attacks made on her by physicians arose "more from malice or envy than from a desire for justice."[41]

It may be that this string of royal licenses is a manifestation of a political conflict between the municipality of Valencia and King Joan I, as had been the case in his father's reign; or it may be that the Crown had economic motives, that in these licenses it hoped for a source of income. We have already indicated that still other motives, which might be termed sociomedical (e.g., lack of medical care in certain communities), are hinted at in the texts. But whatever the motivations for royal policy, they were ones to which the educational qualifications set up by the *furs* of 1329 were irrelevant, for the king recognized quite well that his licensees were merely empirics, whose "manner of curing [does not] extend to the art of medicine, since that consists not only in practice but in science."[42]

IV

To a certain degree, the origin of the Valencian *furs* was shaped by the peculiarities of local circumstances. At the beginning of the fourteenth century Valencia enjoyed a particular reputation for the excellence of its medicine. Contemporaries associated its name with the other Mediterranean centers of medical renown. The Castilian Archpriest of Hita, after listing a wide range of medicinal products used in contemporary therapy in his *Libro de Buen Amor* (1330–1343), linked Valencia with Montpellier in the Christian West and Alexandria in the Muslim East as places equally famous for the variety of spices and electuaries they marketed.[43]

---

[41] Ibid. Used by R. Jordi González and J. L. Gómez Caamaño, "Mujeres y varones médicos por decisión real en el reinado de Juan I de Aragón," *Boletín Soc. Esp. Hist. Farmacia* 19 (1968), 150.

[42] ACA, Cancillería, reg. 1908, fol. 143r.

[43] "Muchos letüarios dan a ellos: a las de vezes / dïacitrón, codoñate e letüario de nuezes, / ë otros de más quantía -de çahanorias, rehezes, / embían unas a otras, cada díä, a revezes-;/

"cominada alixándria, con el buen diagargante, / el diacitronabatis, con fino jingibrate, / mielrosado, diacímino, diantosio, vadela[n]te, / la rosata novela, que devía dezir ante;/

"adragea e alfenique, con el estomaticón, / e la garïofilata, con dïamargaritón, / trïasándalis muy fino, con dïasaturïón, / quë est para doñear preciadö e nobre don. /

"Sabet que todo açucar allí anda bal.lonado: / polvo, terrón e candi, e mucho del rosado, / açucar de confites e açucar vïolado, / e de otras muchas guisas que ya hë olvidado. /

"Monpesler, Alixandría e la nombrada Valencia / non tienen de letüarios tantos ni

Moreover, Valencia prided itself on the superiority of its physicians. In January 1315 the Valencian physician Guillem Barberà, sent by Jaume II to attend his daughter Constança (who was married to don Juan Manuel), reported disturbing news back to the monarch about the condition of his daughter, who was then in Alarcón. Immediately upon receiving the news, Jaume II wrote to Constança's Castilian husband, proposing that she be moved to Valencia:

> here she will have the benefit of the air in which she was born and grew up, and will have pleasure and comfort with [her sister-in-law] the infanta doña Leonor, and with the infanta doña Violante, her sister, and we will send some of her brothers there specifically to give her comfort; and she will have abundance of physicians and of all sorts of medicinal things, which are better there than in [Alarcón].[44]

Medical learning was by no means absent from the kingdom before 1329. Valencia had already produced one famous figure in the academic medical world, Arnau de Vilanova, whose thought exerted a strong effect on its powerful mercantile bourgeoisie.[45] The period when the new *furs* were being drawn up coincides with the activity of Berenguer Eymerich (c. 1300-c. 1365), who had studied medicine at Montpellier about 1320 and is one of the most interesting physicians of the fourteenth century. To affirm, as we have done, the municipal leadership in matters of public health in the 1330s does not mean that learned physicians were lacking in Valencia or indifferent to the new policies of the *furs*; after all, they too formed a part of the directing bourgeoisie.[46]

Although Valencia thus seemed particularly well suited to introduce qualifying standards, there were other features of civic life there which in time tended to weaken the application of the first provision of the *furs*, the one requiring four years' training in a *studium generale* for any would-be practitioner. There was, to begin with, some continuing sup-

tanta ëspecia." J. Ruiz, *Libro de Buen Amor*; ed. J. Corominas (Madrid, 1967), pp. 507–509. Corominas' notes on the materia medica listed here are extremely interesting (cf. pp. 500, 502, 504). Many of the products and materials named by Juan Ruiz figure in the list of drugs bought by the Valencian hospital of En Clapers in the years after 1374: Agustín Rubio Vela, *Pobreza, enfermedad y asistencia hospitalaria*, Appendix II and Index, pp. 197–246.

[44] Cited by Martínez Ferrando, *Jaime II de Aragón*, I, 136–37.

[45] Agustín Rubio Vela, "Una fundación burguesa en la Valencia medieval: el Hospital de En Clapers," *Dynamis* 1 (1981), 17–49; idem, "Un hospital medieval según su fundador: el testamento de Bernat dez Clapers (Valencia, 1311)," *Dynamis* 3 (1983), 373–387; M. Rodrigo Lizondo, "La protesta de Valencia de 1318 y otros documentos inéditos referentes a Arnau de Vilanova," *Dynamis* 1 (1981), 241–273.

[46] The most important academically trained physicians in Valencia in the first generation after the promulgation of the *furs* were Miró de Corçà (d. c. 1368), Pere Ros d'Orsins (d. c. 1367), and Sanç del Miracle (d. c. 1360), on whom see Luis García Ballester, *Historia social de la medicina*, p. 25, and references there. On Pere Ros d'Orsins, see also Rubió Balaguer, *Documentos*, pp. [38]–[41] and [75].

port in Valencia for opening the teaching of medicine to more than just those who had been trained by a *studium*. This was encouraged by intellectual developments that distinguished the capital, particularly the growth of Lullist philosophy. In 1369 Pere IV granted Berenguer Fluvià the privilege of teaching the Lullist doctrine, both in medicine and surgery and in philosophy and astronomy, and of conferring the mastership on whomever he found qualified;[47] and on 12 October 1392 Joan I conceded a similar privilege to the Valencian physician-surgeon Francesc Surià.[48]

Ramon Llull's peculiar philosophy, an all-encompassing vision of man and his relations with his surroundings (carrying with it a particular system of medicine and surgery), found special strength and penetration in Valencian society in the second half of the fourteenth century. It enjoyed great prestige among physicians of the city.[49] Indeed, Pere Geronés, *examinador de metges* in various years between 1380 and 1393,[50] was one of the leaders of Valencian Lullism;[51] Pere Figuerola (also an *examinador*, and associated with Pere Geronés in this capacity in 1393) was another prominent Lullist.[52] Both had an active role in the events that took place between the city of Valencia and the inquisitor Eimeric in the latter's attempt to condemn the Lullist vision as heretical. The medical aspects of this philosophy have been inadequately studied, and sources for their development in Valencia or the Crown of Aragon in the last thirty years of the fourteenth century are extremely hard to locate. It is clear, nevertheless, that Lullist medicine offered a popular alternative to the medicine of the orthodox faculties, and that its attraction for the Valencian bourgeoisie would have weakened the faculties' claim to a monopoly on medical education and qualification.[53]

If a *studium generale* had been set up in Valencia itself, its claims to supervise all medical training would no doubt have been considered,

---

[47] ACA, Cancillería, reg., 917, fol. 213v; published by Rubió y Lluch, *Documents*, I, 222 (doc. 230).

[48] Luis Comenge, "La medicina en el reino de Aragón. Siglo XIV," *El Siglo Médico* 44 (1897), p. 468.

[49] J. de Puig i Oliver, "El procés dels lul.listes valencians contra Nicolau Eimeric en el marc del Cisma d'Occident," *Boletín de la Soc. Cast. de Cultura* 56 (1980), 319–463.

[50] See Appendix 1, below.

[51] J. de Puig i Oliver, "El procés," pp. 339 n. 21, 352–356.

[52] Ibid., pp. 356–360. Pere Figuerola was likewise prosecuted by Eimeric (ibid., p. 359).

[53] We know that Pere Figuerola was trained c. 1370 at Montpellier; he wrote a brief but interesting *Regimen sanitatis* to his sons in 1415 (ed. by L. Thorndike, "Advice from a Physician to his Sons," *Speculum* 6 [1931], 110–114; Thorndike's date for the work is mistaken) and a commentary on the surgery of Guy de Chauliac that is unfortunately lost. We know of the commentary by the reference to it in the library of Martín de Overna, of which the inventory was drawn up in 1416: "Item, Catappell de mestre Guido ab suplements de maestre Pere Figuerola, scrit en pergamí, cubert de fust, ab camisa de aluda blancha." A. Ivars, "Inventario de los libros de don Martín de Overna. Año 1416," *Archivo Iberoamericano*, 1913, p. 449.

but no such *studium* was created before the late sixteenth century—and then it was one whose principal emphasis lay in the teaching of Greek and Latin. Indeed, even though physicians in the city displayed enough corporate self-consciousness to address the king as a body in 1356, at no time during the century did they receive recognition as a *collegium* (as Barcelona's physicians did in 1342 from Pere IV); certainly they did not display that common identity that a shared academic formation would have instilled, and probably relatively few had been so schooled. For without a *studium* near at hand, Valencian society was unable to find enough university graduates to provide even a minimally adequate level of care.

In 1373 the Valencian *consell* did actually resolve to establish a *studium generale* in the city, and it charged the physician Pere Figuerola with drawing up plans for the project. The bishop of Valencia, however, protested, pointing to papal and conciliar privileges in favor of the church's right to control such education. In the following year, after a sharp debate, the municipality abandoned its plans and chose in retaliation to endorse the freedom to teach originally established by the *furs* (c. 1238). A similar situation arose again in 1399 and 1400, and again the *jurats* agreed to return to the *furs* of Jaume I,

> allowing every master, under the last provision of the said *fur* entitled 'De metges,' that he may hold a school with or without another master in association, in whatever place that he wishes and can find within the city, without hindrance or opposition from other masters.[54]

This clear restatement by the *consell* of a general freedom to offer medical instruction would appear at first glance to be an outright repudiation of the first provision of the *furs* of 1329.

Signs of a similar resistance are to be found in Catalonia, in the reaction by the Barcelonan physicians to the creation in 1401 by Martí I of a "*studium generale de medicina*" in Barcelona; in the charter of foundation, the king affirmed that "no one in the city of Barcelona may practice unless he be distinguished by the title of 'magister.'"[55] Neither

---

[54] "Los dits honrats jurats, vista lur disceptació, attés que.ls capítols que.s dien formats sobre tal unitat són exhorbitans a fur . . . , revocaren e hagueren per revocats de fet e per nul.les, e no servadors, los dits affermats capítols, sots qualsevol concepció de paraules sien concebuts, donants facultats e leer a cascun maestre per observança del dit fur, posat sots rúbrica 'De metges,' lo capítol últim, que puxa tenir escola ab altre companyó maestre e sens aquell, en aquell loch de la ciutat que.s volrà e trobar porà, sens embarch e oppòsit d'altre maestre." AMV, Manuals de Consells, A-22, fol. 21v; published by V. Vives Liern, *Las casas de los estudios de Valencia* (Valencia, 1902), pp. 97–98; doc. 3. On these problems, see L. García Ballester, *Historia social de la medicina*, pp. 26–27.

[55] ACA, reg. 2196, fols. 2v–3v; published by Rubió Balaguer, *Documentos*, p. [104], doc. 67. On these themes, see Luis García Ballester, *Historia social*, pp. 23–29; and idem, *Los orígenes de la profesión médica en Cataluña*, pp. 144ff.

the government nor the medical guild of Barcelona accepted this royal imposition of an educational monopoly over professional medical activity, which gave rise to a series of tensions.[56]

How are we to interpret this apparent contradiction between Valencia's refusal to restrict the teaching of medicine, on the one hand, and its continuing enforcement of the *furs*, on the other? We would suggest that by the end of the fourteenth century the requirement of graduation from a *studium generale* was not being strictly enforced, and perhaps never had been. In our view, the *examinadors* regarded an academic education more as a prospective ideal than as a minimal criterion for qualification. They still acted to punish certain individuals who for whatever reason could not or would not satisfy their requirements, as we know from the cases of the Jew Blanqua (fined 100 *sous* in 1384 for practicing medicine without accepting the *furs*)[57] and of Gento Morcat (fined 22 *sous* in 1390 for practicing surgery without having been examined).[58] But of the 28 candidates we have found licensed by the city of Valencia between 1378 and 1396 to practice medicine, only one—the Italian Tommaso de Maestre Tone, licensed in 1380—actually had a university degree.[59]

At the end of the fourteenth century, the number of physicians and surgeons per 10,000 inhabitants in Valencia was only 6–7, and this figure falls to about 5 if physicians alone are counted.[60] This level is only slightly higher than that of 1347, just before the Black Death, when it varied between 3 and 4 Christian physicians (we do not know the number of surgeons) per 10,000 inhabitants.[61] So low a figure—comparable to what we find today in the most underdeveloped pockets of Southeast Asia or in certain African or Latin-American countries—helps to explain why empirics and other healers continued to prosper,

---

[56] C. Carrère, "Refus d'une création universitaire et niveaux de culture à Barcelone: hypothèses d'explication," *Le Moyen Age* 34 (1979), 245–273; García Ballester, *Los orígenes*, pp. 143ff.

[57] J. Hinojosa Montalvo, "La comunidad hebrea en Valencia: del esplendor a la nada (1377–1391)," *Saitabi* 31 (1981), 66.

[58] ARV, *Maestre Racional*, 6441, fol. 14v; cited by Hinojosa, loc. cit.

[59] Appendix 2, doc. 10.

[60] On 15 November 1400 there were 19 physicians in the city of Valencia (7 *maestres en medicina* and 12 *licenciats en medicina*) and eight surgeons; AMV, Lletres missives, g3–7, s.f., published by A. Rubio Vela, *Peste Negra, crisis y comportamientos sociales en la España del siglo XIV. La ciudad de Valencia, 1348–1401* (Granada, 1979), pp. 130–31 (doc. xxiv). The population of the city at this time has been estimated as 35–40,000 inhabitants.

[61] On 6 June 1347 the city had 11–12 physicians: En Francesc Çabruguera, maestre Jacme [Lam]a(?), maestre Bertomeu de Vernet, Pere de Vernet, En Guillem Tortosa, En Pere Correger, maestre Bernat Ferrer, Folquet Colom, Guillem Galceran, Arnau Pastor, maestre Berenguer Eymerich, and Pere Roís (probably also a physician); ACA, Real Audiencia histórica, Procesos, leg. 120, cuaderno 13a, fol. 4r and cuaderno 10, fol. 32v. The city also had 31 barbers; ibid., leg. 120, cuaderno 12, fol. 50r. These data come from the oaths sworn to the *Unió* of Valencia by the inhabitants of the city and various parts of the kingdom; these signers were all from the city. (We thank Mateo Rodrigo Lizondo for furnishing this information.) There were 10,625 signatories from the city, which has given us a demographic basis (of ca. 20–25,000 inhabitants) for our estimate here.

despite the attempt of the *furs* to eliminate their activity. The system of unrestricted instruction in medicine that the Valencian *consell* finally endorsed at the end of the fourteenth century led to an even greater proliferation of practitioners who, although "they should not be called physicians,"[62] nevertheless acted as such. In the end, therefore, the activities of the *examinadors* had to focus on the worst of this sort of medical practice. The system of medical examination that had evolved in Valencia by the end of the century maintained a balance between a perceived need for medical standards, on the one hand, and an objective need for enough practitioners to satisfy the health care demands of the inhabitants of the kingdom, on the other.

---

[62] "Et non vocari debeant medici"; A. López de Meneses, "Documentos culturales," p. 701, doc. 37.

APPENDIX 1

MUNICIPAL EXAMINERS OF PHYSICIANS AND SURGEONS IN VALENCIA, 1336–1400*

1336:	Bertomeu de Casaldòria
	Pere Correger
1337:	Francesc Ça-Bruguera
	Berenguer Eymerich
1338:	Bertomeu de Casaldòria
	Jacme d'Avinyó
1339:	Berenguer Eymerich
	Pere Correger
1340:	Pere de Lambilles
	Ramon Pere
1341:	Berenguer Eymerich
	Jacme d'Avinyó
1342:	Pere Correger
	Miquel del Miracle
1343:	Bernat Ferrer
	[Miquel del Miracle]
	[Bertomeu de Casaldòria]
1344:	Miró de Corçà
	Pere Lambilles
1345:	Miró de Corçà
	Pere Lambilles
1346:	Bernat Ferrer
	Francesc Ça-Bruguera
1347–1348:	*missing*
1349:	Berenguer Eymerich
	Bernat Minguet
1350:	Miró de Corçà
	Bernat Minguet
	Jacme Metge
1351:	Andreu Ponç
	Sanç del Miracle

* The names have been drawn from the lists in the Manuals del Consell, AMV, except for those placed in square brackets, which have been supplied from other documentation of the period.

1352: *missing*
1353: Berenguer Eymerich
Nicolau Barceló
1354: Sanç del Miracle
Jacme d'Avinyó
1355–1357: *missing*
1358: [Sanç del Miracle]
[Andreu Ponç]
1359–1368: *missing*
1369: Romeu Bruschà
Arnau Guillem, *alias* Metge
1370: Andreu Ponç
Nicolau Barcelò
1371: *missing*
1372: [Gabriel Dezcortell]
[Jacme d'Avinyó]
1373–1377: *missing*
1378: [Jacme Maderes]
[Francesc Cambres]
1379: Pere Soler
Gabriel Dezcortell
1380: [Jacme Maderes]
[Vicent Serra]
1381: Jacme Maderes
Pere Geronés
1382: Pere Figuerola
Pere Soler
1383: Jacme Maderes
Pere Geronés
1384: [Pere Geronés]
1385: Guillem Ça-Fàbrega
Jacme d'Avinyó
1386: Jacme Maderes
Pere Geronés
1387: [Pere Figuerola]
[Bernat d'Artesa]
1388: Bernat Minguet (replaced by Jacme Maderes)
Jacme d'Avinyó
1389: [Guillem Ça-Fàbrega]
[Pere Figuerola]
1390: [Bernat d'Artesa]
[Gabriel Dezcortell]
1391–1392: *missing*
1393: Pere Figuerola
Pere Geronés
1394: *missing*

1395: Jacme d'Avinyó
Jacme Rotg (*sic*)
1396: Pere Figuerola
Vicent Serra
1397: Pere Soler
Bernat d'Artesa
1398: Pere Urgellers
Lluís d'Ordis
1399: Pere Soler
Guillem Piquó
1400: Jacme Maderes
Bernat Oliver

APPENDIX 2

DOCUMENTS CONCERNING THE EXAMINATION AND SUPERVISION OF MEDICAL PRACTITIONERS

(Editorial emendations or comments have been put within parentheses; letters supplied where the manuscript is defective have been put within square brackets. Each document is followed immediately by its English translation. We are deeply grateful to Germà Colón for furnishing us with the transcription of document 1.)

1

Valencia, 1329.

King Alfons IV el Benigne establishes provisions in the Cortes of Valencia governing the examination and supervision of those wishing to practice medicine in the kingdom (AMV, Furs de València, ms B of Boronat Péra, fols. 119v–120r).

De metges.

<1> Manam e establim que.l justícia e els // jurats cascun any lo terçer jorn ans de Nadal eligen .II. físichs de actoritat, los quals sien examinadors de tots los metges de físicha qui novellament vinguen per praticar en la ciutat e en les viles del regne, e aquell que trobaran suffitient, e que almenys haja oÿda art de física o medicina per .IIII. anys en estudi general, sia reebut a praticar la dita art, e en altra manera no y sia reebut. E si sens la dita examinatió e licèntia usarà, sia caygut en pena per cascuna vegada de .C. morabatins d'or, dels quals la terça part sia de la cort, e la terça de la universitat del loch, e la terça de l'acusador. E sots la dita pena partidora segons que dessús, alcun físich no particip en los salaris dels apotecharis, e que açò juren cascun any l'endemà de Ninou, per lo qual sagrament prometen e sien tenguts de tatxar tempradament lo salari dels apotecharis quantesque vegades ne serà qüestió. E si alcun físich caurà en la dita pena e pagar no la porà, sia gitat del loch a tots temps.
<2> Los metges qui ara usen de física o de cirurgia sien examinats, e aquells qui seran trobats suffitiens romanguen en l'offici, e los altres no usen, sots pena de .C. morabatins d'or, partidors segons que dessús.

<3> Alcuna fembra no ús de medicina, ne de dar bouratges, sotz (*sic*) pena de córrer la vila açotan, mas puxen pensar de infans pochs e de fembres, a les quals, emperò, no donen alcun bouratge.
<4> Tot cirurgià qui tinga alcun nafrat en poder sia tengut de dir, ab sagrament, sens alcun salari, quantesque vegades request ne serà, si.l nafrat és fora de sospita o no.
<5> Barber no ús de medicina o de cirurgia, si donchs no serà examinat per los examinadors dels metges e donat per suffitient. E si sens lur examinatió e licèntia ne usarà, pac per pena cascuna vegada que contrafarà .L. morabatins d'or, dels quals haja la terça part la cort, la terça la universitat del loch, e la terça l'acusador.
<6> Cascun metge axí de físicha con (*sic*) de cirurgia jur cascun any en poder del justítia, en lo començament de la aministratió d'aquell, que no reeba en cura alcun o alcuna qui sia greument malalt o nafrat si donchs primerament lo malalt o nafrat no haurà confessat, sinó en tal cas de perill de mort que la triga fos perillosa, e ladonchs no sia feta la segona visitatió tro lo patient haja confessat.
<7> Metges axí físichs com cirurgians les receptes que dictaran hajen dictar en romanç, declaran los noms de les erbes e de les altres coses medicinals en lur nom comú e vulgar. E axí meteix hajen a declarar los noms del pes o mesura de les dites coses en manera que.s puxa clarament entendre per la gent popular. E qual qui contra açò farà, pach per pena cascuna vegada .X. morabatins d'or, dels quals haja la cort la terça part, e la terça la universitat del loch, e la terça l'acusador.

* * *

Concerning [medical] practitioners.

1. We command and ordain that the justiciar and the *jurats* elect, every year, three days before Christmas, two leading physicians who shall be the examiners of all the practitioners of physic who have recently come to practice in the city or in the towns of the kingdom; and those whom they find competent, and who have followed the art of medicine for at least four years in a *studium generale*, shall be admitted to practice the said art, and if not they shall not be admitted. And if they practice without the said examination and license, they shall be liable to a fine of 100 gold morabatins for each occasion, of which a third part shall go to the court, a third to the town, and a third to the accuser. And under the same penalty, allotted as above, no physician shall share in the fees of apothecaries, and each year they shall swear an oath the day after New Year's promising to set apothecaries' fees moderately, as often as necessary. And if any physician shall be assessed the said fine and not be able to pay, let him be expelled from the town forever.

2. Practitioners who are now practicing physic or surgery shall be examined, and those who are found competent may remain in practice but not the others, under a fine of 100 gold morabatins allotted as above.
3. No woman shall practice medicine or give potions, under penalty of being whipped through the town; but they may care for little children, and women—to whom, however, they may give no potion.
4. Every surgeon who has a wounded patient in his care shall be required to state on oath, for no fee and as often as he shall be asked, whether the patient is out of danger or not.
5. No barber shall practice medicine or surgery if he has not been examined by the examiners of practitioners and found competent. And if he should practice without their examination and license, he shall pay a fine of 50 gold morabatins every time he transgresses, of which the court shall receive a third, the town a third, and the accuser a third.
6. Every practitioner, whether of physic or of surgery, shall swear each year before the justiciar at the beginning of his term that he will not treat anyone who is seriously ill or wounded, man or woman, if the patient has not first made confession—except in a potentially fatal case where a delay would be dangerous, and then he will not make a second visit until the patient has confessed.
7. Practitioners, both physicians and surgeons, shall give prescriptions for medicines in the vulgar tongue, naming herbs and other medicinal things by their common or popular names. Likewise they shall give weights and measures of the said things in a manner that can be readily understood by the ordinary people. And whosoever shall disobey shall pay each time a fine of 10 gold morabatins, of which the court shall receive a third, the town a third, and the accuser a third.

2

Valencia, 9 December 1334.

Miquel de Roures, notary of Valencia, accuses master Jacme Lama to the justiciar of Valencia of having practiced medicine without having been approved by the examiners, as required by the furs *of 1329* (ARV, Justícia Civil, 42, s. f.).

Anno Domini millesimo .CCC°. tricentesimo tricesimo (sic) quarto, die veneris intitulata quinto idus decembris. Comparech denant l'onrat En Bernat Çanou, justícia de València en lo civil, En Michel de Roures de una part, et maestre Jacme Lama de l'altra. Et lo dit En Michel de Roures, per escrit, posà ço que.s segueix:

Davant vós, sènyer En Bernat Çanou, justícia de la ciutat de València en lo civil, claman, proposa En Michel de Roures, notari, contra En

Jacme Lama, qui.s diu metge, dién e afferman en juhii contra aquell que.l dit En Jacme Lama, sens que no és estat examinat e provat ne atrobat sufficient per los físichs los quals són elets per cascun any per lo justícia e per los jurats segons la forma del fur nou, e sens que per los dits físichs no és estada a aquell donada o atorgada licència de praticar de físicha, ne ha hoÿt en estudi general .IIIIe. anys, ha cessat (*sic*) e praticat de física e de medecina en la dita ciutat de .III. anys a ençà contínuament .X. vegades per cada dia e pus, que munta per cascun any .CLXXX. míl.lia *libras* poch més o menys. Et no-res-menys, per lo dit temps ha participat lo salari o salaris ab apotechari o apotecharis .C. vegades poch més o menys, e ha ordenades receptes en latí .C. vegades poch més o menys. On, com segons lo dit fur nou alcun metge o físich lo qual vengués aprés de la confecció d'aquells per praticar en la ciutat no deja usar o praticar de física o medicina en la dita ciutat ni en les viles del regne si donchs no serà examinat e atrobat suficient e donada licència a aquell de pratichar e usar de físicha o medicina, et que haja hoÿt .IIII. anys en estudi general, e.n altra manera sia encorregut e caygut en pena de .C. morabatins per cascuna vegada que usarà; et si participa los salaris ab los apotecharis, sia caygut en semblant pena, et si darà receptes en latí als apotecharis, sia caygut en pena de .X. morabatins per cascuna vegada, et lo dit En Jacma (*sic*) Lama, aprés la confecció dels dits furs nous, sia vengut en la dita ciutat per praticar e usar de físicha o medicina, per tal, lo dit En Michel de Roures demane e requer que per vós, sènyer dit justícia, lo dit En Jacme Lama sia condempnat a.quelles penes en lo dit fur posades, enaxí que al dit En Miquel de Roures sia feit compliment de dret e de justícia en tot ço que de fur e de rahó sia faedor, et per tot dret que li pertanga o pertànyer-lo.s puscha [o].s deça. Et açò demane ab les messions del pleyt feytes e a ffer, salvu dret de créxer e minvar, *etc.*

Et com tot demanat deja dar fermança de dret, per tal, lo dit En Michel de // Roures requer que per vós, sènyer dit justícia, lo dit En Jacma Lama encontinent sia forçat e destret de donar fermança de dret e de pagar la cosa jutjada; et si aquella donar no porà o no volrrà, que sia retengut a presó, com axí sia faedor segons fur. En altra manera, si contrafahíets, ço que no creu, o lo dit En Jacme Lama s'asentava, com sia hom vagabunt, proteste lo dit En Michel de Roures que sia imputat a vós, sènyer dit justícia, e a vostres béns e de vostre assessor. Et no-res-menys requer que tots los béns d'aquell sien encontinent escrits e emparats, per tal que aquells no sien abcegats e que.l dret del senyor rey no sia perdut.

Et enaprés, addén e milloran, fa e posa les declaracions infrasegüents:

Primerament diu e declara que los furs nous foren feyts per lo senyor rey en la ciutat de València en l'any de .M.CCC.XX.IX., .V. anys ha poch més o menys.

Item diu e declara que .III. anys ha poch més o menys que.l dit En Jacme Lama vingué en la dita ciutat per usar e praticar de física o medicina.

Item diu e declara que.l dit En Jacme Lama, dels dits .III. anys ençà, ha usat de medicina en la dita ciutat comunament e sens que no fo examinat per aquells per qui devia ésser examinat.

Item diu e declara que sí.l dit En Jacme Lama vengué a examinació, que aquell no fo aprovat per los examinadors ni li fon donada licència per aquell de praticar, usar de medicina o físicha en la dita ciutat, ne fo atrobat que agués hoÿt .IIIIe. anys en estudi general, ans dehia e responia peguots e fatuïtats a les interrogacions que li fahien los examinadors, e fon donat per insuficient.

Item declara que.l dit En Jacma Lama, per los dits .III. anys, ha usat de medicina o físicha deu vegades per cascun jorn poch més o menys en la dita ciutat.

Item declara que.l dit En Jacme Lama ha praticat lo salari ab apotechari o apotecharis [.C.] vegades poch més o menys.

Item diu [e] declara que.l dit En Jacme Lama ha ordenades (o) dictades receptes en latí .C. vegades poch més o menys.

Item declara que de les dites coses és fama. //

A les quals demanda e declaracions demanà ésser respost per la dita part adversa, atorgan o negan, car si negades seran o fer-se provador, proteste, emperò, que no.s requer *nomen* (?) a provar totes les dites coses, mas tan solament aquelles que poran e a la sua intenció a fundar bastaran.

Fo interrogat per sagrament lo proposant qui havia dictada la present demanda, e dix que En Domingo Eymerich e En Domingo de Monçó, savis en dret de València.

E en aquell instant mateix, lo dit maestre Jacme per escrit posà ço que.s segueix:

E lo dit maestre Jacme Lama diu, excipién, que no és tengut de respondre a la dita demanda, ne enantar ne proceyr en aquella denant vós, sènyer dit justícia, per les rahons següents:

Primerament per ço com lo dit maestre Jacme és clergue e tonsurat, e ab tonsura e hàbit clerical atrobat e ja tengut per clergue per vós, sènyer dit justícia, per què no és tengut de fer dret en poder de vós, sènyer dit justícia, com no sia de vostra juredicció, ne vós, sènyer dit justícia, per vigor de la dita injusta demanda, no podets ni devets enantar contra ell ni sos béns, com lo for de la persona seguesque.n lurs béns.

Item per ço car per inspecció de la dita demanda és clar e manifest a vós, sènyer dit justícia, que.l dit En Michel no ha loch de proposar aquella, com no pertanga a ell principalment ne accessòria.

Item per ço com lo dit En Michel és demanat de crim de fur(t) denant lo justícia criminal, del qual crim de furt no és encara purgat; et axí no pot estar en juhii tro s[ens] que.l dit crim sia purgat e per d'altres rahons; per què requer que vós, sènyer dit justícia, cessets de enantar o proceyr contra lo dit maestre Jacme e sos béns com fer-o dejats. En altra manera protesta de tot son dret.

Et lo dit justícia, vista la demanda per lo dit En Michel de Roures proposada e les rahons e excepcions per lo dit maestre Jacme Lama contra aquella proposades e al.legades, de continent féu venir lo dit maestre Jacme Lama denant si, lo qual trobà ab tonsura e hàbit clerical e, per consegüent, la persona de aquell lo dit justícia no podia fer retenir a presó per rahó de la dita demanda. Emperò, quant als béns de aquell, lo dit justícia tramés En Bernat d'Auriach, escrivà de la cort, per scriure // aquells, per ço que si loch per alcun temps la dita demanda pot ésser vista haver, que dels dits béns, per la rahó damunt dita, al senyor rey pusca ésser feta conservació de dret en los dits béns per la rahó damunt dita, si alcun li és pertanyent. Et nores-menys, assigne dia a les parts damunt dites a comparer denant ell per enantar el dit feyt degudament diluns següent de matí, ans de cort partida.

* * *

In the year of our Lord 1334, Friday the fifth day of the ides of December, there appeared before the honorable En Bernat Çanou, civil justiciar of Valencia, Miquel de Roures on the one hand and master Jacme Lama on the other. And the said Miquel de Roures set out the following, in writing:

Before you, Bernat Çanou, civil justiciar of the city of Valencia, Miquel de Roures, notary, complains against Jacme Lama, calling himself a physician, and publicly affirms against him that the said Jacme Lama, without having been examined and found competent by the physicians who are elected each year by the justiciar and by the *jurats* according to the form of the new *fur,* and without having been given a license to practice physic, or attending a *studium generale* for four years, has practiced physic and medicine in the said city continuously for three years, ten times a day or more, which comes to 180,000 pounds more or less per year. Moreover, during the said period he has shared fees with apothecaries 100 times more or less, and has drawn up prescriptions in Latin 100 times more or less. Wherefore, since according to the said new *fur* no practitioner or physician who arrives to practice in the city after the promulgation of [the *fur*] may not practice physic or medicine in the said city nor in the towns of the kingdom if he has not been examined and found competent and given a licence to practice physic or medicine or attended a *studium generale* for four years, and otherwise shall be fined 100 morabatins for each time he has practiced; and if he shares fees with apothecaries shall suffer a like penalty, and if he writes prescriptions in Latin to the apothecaries shall be fined ten morabatins for each offence; and since the said Jacme Lama arrived in the said city after the promulgation of the new *furs* to practice medicine, therefore, the said Miquel de Roures demands the said Jacme Lama be condemned by you, lord justiciar, to the penalties prescribed by the said *fur*, so that the said Miquel de Roures shall receive his full rights in law according to the *fur*. And he asks as well all the costs of this suit, past and present, reserving to himself the right to increase or decrease them.

And as every complainant asks that the law be fulfilled, therefore the said Miquel de Roures asks, lord justiciar, that you force the said Jacme Lama immediately to observe the law and to pay the fine assessed; and if he cannot or will not, let him be imprisoned, so as to comply with the *fur*. And if you will not do this (which he does not believe), or if the said Jacme Lama disappears [from the city] (for he is a vagabond), the said Miquel de Roures protests that you will be to blame, lord justiciar, and will be held responsible with your possessions. And moreover he demands that all his goods be immediately inventoried and frozen so that they may not be concealed and so that the rights of the lord king may not be lost.

Subsequently, enlarging on this, he makes the following statements:

First he declares that the new *furs* were promulgated by the lord king in the city of Valencia in the year 1329, five years ago more or less.

Likewise he declares that three years ago more or less the said Jacme Lame came to the said city to practice medicine.

Likewise he declares that the said Jacme Lama has routinely practiced medicine generally for those three years without being examined by those by whom he ought to be examined.

Likewise he declares that in fact the said Jacme Lama has presented himself at examination, but he has not been approved by the examiners nor given a licence by them to practice medicine in the said city, nor has he been determined to have studied four years in a *studium generale*, but he gave back nonsense and inanities to the questions put to him by the examiners, and was held to be incompetent.

Likewise he declares that the said Jacme Lama has practiced medicine in the said city ten times every day more or less for the said three years.

Likewise he declares that the said Jacme Lama has shared fees with apothecaries 100 times more or less.

Likewise he declares that the said Jacme Lama has prescribed recipes in Latin 100 times more or less.

Likewise he declares that these things are common knowledge.

To which complaints he demands that the defendant reply, with admission or denial; if he denies them, he [Miquel] will prove them, but he insists that he should not have to prove all the said things, only those which will be sufficient to justify his assertion.

The plaintiff was asked on oath who had drawn up this complaint, and he named Domingo Eymerich and Domingo de Monçó, jurists of Valencia.

And at that very moment, the said master Jacme replied in writing as follows:

And the said master Jacme Lama says in response that he is not required to reply to the said complaint nor to pursue it before you, lord justiciar, for the following reasons:

First, because the said master Jacme is a tonsured cleric and has already been acknowledged by you, lord justiciar, in tonsure and clerical habit as a cleric, lord justiciar, wherefore he is not required to submit to your authority, lord justiciar, since he is not in your jurisdiction, nor can you, lord justiciar, proceed against him or his goods on the strength of the said unjust demand, since possessions fall under the law of their possessor.

Likewise because by inspection of the said complaint it is manifest to you, lord justiciar, that the said Miquel has no right to bring it since it does not pertain to him either directly or indirectly.

Likewise because the said Miquel is accused of the crime of theft before the criminal justiciar and is not yet absolved of the theft, and hence cannot take part in a case until the said charge is resolved, and for other reasons; wherefore he demands that you, lord justiciar, cease to proceed against the said master Jacme and his goods as you wish to. He protests his rights to the contrary.

And the said justiciar, having studied the complaint by the said Miquel de Roures and the replies proposed to it by the said master Jacme Lama, straightway caused the said master Jacme Lama to come before him, and found him with tonsure and clerical dress and consequently the said justiciar could not place him in prison in accordance with the said complaint. However, as to his goods, the said justiciar sent Bernat Auriach, scribe of the court, to inventory them, in order to assure that if at some point the said complaint were accepted, for the abovementioned reason the lord king's right in the said goods might be preserved, if any should pertain to him. And furthermore he named the day for the abovementioned parties to appear before him to hear the said case properly, next Monday morning before the court rises.

3

Valencia, 5 November 1350.

The consell *of the city of Valencia commands the examination of all physicians and apothecaries who have recently arrived in the city, in accord with the provisions of the* furs (AMV, Manuals de Consells, A-9, fols. 122v–123r).

En lo qual consell fon proposat per los dits honrats jurats que, com alcuns metges e speciés novellament sien en la ciutat e pratiquen de lurs arts sens que no són examinats, segons qu.és fur los dits metges deuen ésser examinats, enaxí com sie cosa perillosa aquells usar o pratichar sens la dita examinació, e semblantment los dits speciés s'entrameten a les vegades donar .I. erba per altra, o una cosa per altra, per tal com no són sabents ni conexents les dites erbes o les coses medecinals; per ço, que seria bo que en los dits metges fos tenguda la forma del dit fur, e que hi fossen assignats, per examinadors de aquells, metges qui tots aquells examinassen, e a.çò que fossen talls persones o metges sabents del dit art assignats que fessen examinació de aquells. Et axí meteix .II. speciayres qui examinassen los dits speciés segons que mills puxen, a pprofit e utilitat de la cosa pública. Per què lo consell, concordantment, ordenà e tench per bé que.ls dits metges ussants en la dita ciutat fossen examinats, segons que per fur és ordenat e stablit, e per examinadors d'aquells que y ordenaven maestre Miró // de Cur[ç]à, maestre Bernat Mi(n)guet e.N Jacme Metge, los quals dejen aquells examinar.

Encara ordenà e volch lo dit consell que los speciés fossen examinats per los dits examinadors de metges ensemps ab .II. speciés sabents bé de l'art. Et de present ordenà y En Antoni Pautrer e En Guillem Caner, los quals, ensemps ab los dits metges, regoneguen e vegen e.xaminen aquells e les coses medecinals que en lurs obradors o cases tenen; e si n'hi trobaran de incovinents, que aquells puxen cremar e vessar tantes quantes vegades n'ich trobaran. Emperò, que a les dites examinacions sien .II. dels jurats per certifficar-se dels que no seran sofficients, axí dels dits metges examinadors com dels dits speciés, per tal que puxe ésser provehit ab lo dit consell o justícia a fer a aquells inhibicions o altres forces per les quals no puxen mal.lament de lurs arts ussar. Et que cascun any d'ací enant los dits jurats hajen poder de assignar los dits examinadors de metges e de speciés.

* * *

In which council session it was proposed by the said honorable *jurats* that since some practitioners and apothecaries are newly come to the city and are practicing their arts without having been examined, as such practitioners ought to be examined under the terms of the *fur*, since it is a dangerous thing for them to practice without such an examination, and likewise the said apothecaries at times engage in giving an herb for this or an herb for that without being acquainted with the said herbs or medical things; and because it would be good that the form of the *fur* be observed for the said practitioners, and that there be appointed examiners of such practitioners who would examine all such, and that such persons be appointed as are knowledgeable in the said art, that they may carry out examinations on them—likewise two apothecaries who would examine the said apothecaries as best they can—for the good of the public. Wherefore the council, agreeing, commanded that the said practitioners practicing in the said city be examined, as is ordained by the *fur,* and appointed master Miró de Curçà, master Bernat Minguet, and Jacme Metge as examiners of such.

The council also commanded that apothecaries be examined by the said examiners of practitioners together with two apothecaries knowledgeable in the art. And they appointed Antoni Pautrer and Guillem Caner, who, together with the said physicians, shall inspect and examine them and the medicines that they have in their shops or houses; and whenever they discover anything incorrect, they may destroy it. Furthermore, let there be two *jurats* present at the said examinations to certify those who are incompetent, together with the said examiner-practitioners and the said apothecaries, so that the said council and justiciar may be able to provide means whereby such may not misuse their arts. And that henceforth every year the said *jurats* shall have the power to appoint the said examiners of practitioners and of apothecaries.

4

Valencia, 11 October 1378.

Grant of a license to practice "the art of physic" in Valencia and its kingdom to the Valencian Jew Içach Çaroxel.la (ARV, Justícia Civil [Lletres], 391, s. fol.)

[Anno a nativitate Domini] millesimo .CCC°.LXX°. octavo, die lune hora tertiarum que [fuit] .XI^a. mensis octobris. Comparech davant l'onrat En Martí Fuster, justícia de la ciutat de València en lo civil, Içach Çaroxel.la, juheu de la dita ciutat, e presentà a aquell una letra certifficatòria dels honrats e discrets maestre Jacme Maderes, maestre en arts e en medicina, e En Francesch Cambres, maestre en arts e licenciat en medicina, metges de la dita ciutat, examinadors deputats e assignats per los honrats jurats de la dita ciutat, en paper scrita, uberta, e dins aquella ab dos sagells dels dits examinadors en cera vermella sagellada, la qual és de la tenor següent:

A l'honrat e discret lo justícia civil de la ciutat de València, o a son lochtinent. De nós, En Jacme Maderes, mestre en arts e en medicina, e En Francesch Cambres, mestre en arts e licenciat en medicina, metges de la dita ciutat, examinadors deputats e assignats per los honrats justícia e jurats de la dita ciutat de tots los metges de físiqua e de cirurgia vinents novellament per praticar en la dita ciutat e vil.les del regne de València. Salut e honor. A la discreció de vós per tenor de les presents certifficam ésser comparegut denant nós Yçach Çarrochel.la, juheu de la dita ciutat, lo qual, volent usar de art de físicha dins les ciutat, viles e lochs del dit regne, és estat per nós examinat segons forma de fur e havem aquell atrobat abte e sufficient per longa e aprovada experiència de usar e pratichar de la dita art de físicha, per què, instant e requirent lo dessús dit Yçach Çarrochel.la de la sua sufficiència, per les presents [cer]tifficam per ço que sens alcun dubte donets e atorguets licència e plen poder a aquell de usar e praticar de la dita art de físicha. *Data Valentie tricesima et ultima die mensis septembris anno a nativitate Domini millesimo .CCC°. LXX°.octavo.*

Et presentada la damunt dita letra, lo dit Iach Çarrochel.la requerí lo dit honrat j[ustícia] que li donàs licència de usar e pratichar en la dita c[iutat], vil.l[es] e lochs del r[eg]ne de València de la dita art // de físicha, e no-res-menys que li manàs ésser feyta letra [a uni]verses e sengles officials e loch de senyoria tinents dins lo dit regne de València constituïts, que d'açí avant hajen per metge de físicha lo dit Iach Çarrochel.la e de la dita art lo lexen usar e pratichar sens alcun contrast o embarch e sens alcuna pena.

Et lo dit honrat justícia, vista e regoneguda la damunt dita letra e coses per lo dit Içach proposades e requestes, de consell de son assessor, rehebut primerament e abans sagrament de aquell sobre los deu manaments de la ley, los quals nostre senyor Déus donà a Moysés en lo mont de Senahí, de fer e ser[var] les coses contengudes e expressades en lo fur nou del rey N'Amfós, en rúbrica "De metges," los capítols .VI. e .VII., les quals li foren lests de mot a mot e donats a entendre, donà e atorgà licència al dit Içach Çarrochel.la de usar e praticar de la dita art de medicina en les ciutats, viles e lochs del regne de València sens temor de alcuna pena. Et no-res-menys lo dit honrat justícia, a instància e requisició del dit Içach Çarrochel.la, manà ésser feyta a aquell la letra dejús següent:

Als honrats universes e sengles officials e loch de senyoria tinents dins lo regne de València constituïts, e a cascun de aquells, als quals la present pervendrà. De nós, En Martí Fuster, justícia de la ciutat de València en lo civil. Salut e honor. Per tenor de les presents vos signifficam que Içach Çarrochel.la, juheu de la juheria de la dita ciutat de València, metge de físicha, és estat examinat per los honrats e discrets maestre Jacme Mederes, maestre en arts e en medicina, e En Francesch Cambres, maestre en arts e licenciat en medicina, metges de la ciutat sobredita, examinadors deputats e assignats per nós e per los honrats jurats de la ciutat sobredita de tots los metges de físicha e de cirurgia vinents novellament per pratichar [en] la dita ciutat, viles [e] lochs del dit regne, per los quals lo dit Içach Çar[rochel.la] és estat // trobat abte e sufficient de usar e pratichar de la art de medicina, segons que [a nós] és cert per letra dels dits examinadors, per lo dit Içach Çarrochel.la a nós presentada *que data fuit Valentie .XXXI*ª. *die mensis septembris anni presentis et infrascripta;* per la qual cosa nós, reebut de aquell primerament e abans sagrament sobre los deu manaments de la lig que nostre senyor Déu donà a Moyssé en lo mont de Senaý, per la man dreta de aquell corporalment tocats, segons forma de fur, que bé e lealment se haurà en la dita art de físicha, havem donat e atorgat a aquell licència de usar e pratichar en les dites ciutats, viles e lochs del regne de València de la dita art de físicha sens temor de alcuna pena. E.n testimoni de veritat, manam li n'ésser feta la present carta testimonial ab lo sagell del nostre offici en pendent sagellada. *Data Valentie undecima die octobris anno a nativitate Domini millesimo .CCC°.LXX°. octavo. Subscripsit Iacobus.*

* * *

In the year of our Lord 1378, at terce on Monday the 11th of October, before the honorable Martí Fuster, civil justiciar of the city of Valencia, there appeared Içach Çaroxel.la, a Jew of the said city, who presented a letter from the honorable master Jacme Maderes, master in arts and in medicine, and Francesch Cambres, master in arts and licentiate in medicine (practitioners of the said city, examiners appointed by the honorable *jurats* of the aforementioned city), written on paper, open, and sealed in red wax with the two seals of the said examiners, whose tenor is as follows:

To the honorable civil justiciar of the city of Valencia, or his lieutenant; from us, Jacme Maderes, master in arts and in medicine, and Francesch Cambres, master in arts and licentiate in medicine, practitioners of the said city, examiners appointed by the honorable justiciar and *jurats* of the said city of all the practitioners of physic and surgery newly arrived to practice in the aforesaid city and towns of the kingdom of Valencia; health and honor. By the tenor of these presents we inform you that Yçach Çarrochel.la, a Jew of the said city, appeared before us and, wishing to practice the art of physic in the city, towns, and villages of the said kingdom, has been examined by us in the manner prescribed by the *fur*; and we have found him competent by long and satisfactory experience to practice the said art of physic; wherefore, at the request of the above-named Yçach Çarrochella [for a certification] of his competence, we certify to you by these presents that beyond any doubt you may grant him license to practice the said art of surgery.

Given at Valencia the thirtieth and last day of September, 1378 AD.

When the said letter had been presented, the said Içach Çarrochel.la requested the said honorable justiciar that he grant him a license to practice the art of physic in the said city, towns, and villages of the kingdom of Valencia, and furthermore to draw up a letter for him to each and every official in the said kingdom of Valencia that from henceforth they acknowledge the said Içach Çarrochel.la as a practitioner of physic, and that they allow him to practice the said art without any let or hindrance and without any penalty.

Upon considering the aforesaid letter and the things requested by the said Içach, the said honorable justiciar, on the advice of his assessor, first received an oath from him on the ten commandments of the law that our Lord God gave to Moses on Mount Sinai, to obey everything laid down in the new *fur* of King Alfons under the rubric "De metges," chapters 6 and 7, which were read to him word by word so that he could understand them; and granted the said Içach Çarrochel.la license to practice the said art of medicine in the cities, towns, and villages of the said kingdom of Valencia, without fear of any penalty. And furthermore at the request of the said Içach Çarrochel.la the said honorable justiciar ordered the following certificate to be drawn up:

To all officials in the kingdom of Valencia to whom these presents may come; from us, Martí Fuster, civil justiciar of the city of Valencia; health and honor. We make known to you by the tenor of these presents that Içach Çarrochel.la, a Jew from the Jewry of the said city of Valencia, practitioner of physic, has been examined by the honorable masters Jacme Mederes, master in arts and in medicine, and Francesch Cambres, master in arts and licentiate in medicine, practitioners of the aforesaid city and examiners appointed by us and by the honorable *jurats* of the aforesaid city of all the practitioners of physic and surgery newly arrived to practice in the said city, towns, and villages of the kingdom of Valencia; by whom the said Içach Çarrochel.la has been found to be apt and competent to employ and practice the said art of medicine, as certified to us by a letter from the said examiners presented to us by the said Içach Çarrochel.la, "which is given at Valencia, the 31st day of the month of September of the present year." Whereupon we—having first received from him an oath on the ten commandments of the law that our Lord God gave to Moses on Mount Sinai, while he touched them physically with his right hand, that he would well and loyally engage in the said art of medicine, have granted him license to practice the said art of physic in the said cities, towns, and villages of the kingdom of Valencia, without fear of any penalty. In testimony of the truth we have ordered the present certificate to be drawn up for him, sealed with the seal of our office appended.

Given at Valencia, the 11th day of October, 1378 AD. Subscribed by Jacobus.

5

Valencia, 19 October 1378.

Grant of a license to practice surgery in Valencia and its kingdom to the Valencian Andreu Gras (ARV, Justícia Civil [Lletres], 391, s. fol.).

Anno a nativitate Domini millesimo .CCC^{o}.LXX°. octavo, die martis que fuit .XIX^{a}. mensis octobris. Comparech davant l'onrat micer Jacme Forner, doctor en leys, assessor e lochtinent de l'honrat En Martí Fuster, justícia de la ciutat de València en lo civil, N'Andreu Gras, ciutadà de la dita ciutat, cirurgià, e presentà a aquell una letra dels honrats e discrets En Jacme Maderes, maestre en arts e en medicina, e En Francesch Cambres, maestre en arts e licenciat en medicina, metges de la dita ciutat, examinadors deputats e assignats per los honrats justícia e jurats de la ciutat damunt dita de tots los metges de física e de cirurgia vinents novellament per praticar en la dita ciutat e viles del regne de València, en paper scrita, uberta, e dins aquella ab dos sagells dels dits examinadors en cera vermella sagellada, la tenor de la qual és segons que.s segueix:

A l'honrat e discret lo justícia civil de la ciutat de València, o a son lochtinent. De nós, En Jacme Maderes, mestre en arts e en medicina, e En Francesch Cambres, mestre en arts e licenciat en medicina, metges de la dita ciutat, examinadors deputats e assignats per los honrats justícia [e] jurats de la dita ciutat de tots los metges de física e de cirurgia vi[nen]ts n[ovel]lament per praticar en la dita ciu[tat e] viles del regne de València. Salut e honor. A la discreció de vós per tenor de les presents certifficam ésser comparegut denant nós N'Andreu Gras, ciutadà de la dita ciutat, lo qual, volent usar de art de cirurgia dins les ciutat, viles e lochs del dit regne, és estat per nós examinat segons forma de fur e havem aquell atrobat apte e sufficient per longa e ap[ro]vada experiència de usar e praticar de la dita art de cirurgia, per què, instant e requirent lo dessús dit N'Andreu Gras de la sua suffici[èn]cia, per les presents certifficam per ço q[ue se]ns alcun dubte donets [e] atorguets licència e plen poder a aquell de usar e praticar de la dita art de cirurgia. *Data Valentie .XIIII^a. die mensis octobris anno a nativitate Domini millesimo .CCC^o.LXX°.VIII°.*

Et presentada la di[ta letr]a, lo dit [N'A]ndreu Gras requerí de paraula lo dit // honrat lochtinent de justícia que li donàs licència de usar e praticar de la art de cirurgia en la dita ciutat, viles e lochs del regne de València, com fos apparellat fer tot ço que per fur de València fos tengut e astret de fer, requirén encara que letra li fos manada fer a universes e sengles officials e lochs de senyoria tinents dins lo dit regne de València constituïts, que al dit N'Andreu Gras hajen e tinguen d'açí avant per metge de çirurgia e que de la dita art de cirurgia lo lexen usar e praticar sens temor de alcuna pena e sens alcun contrast o embarch.

Et lo dit honrat lochtinent de justícia, vista e regoneguda la damunt dita letra e les coses en aquella expressades, e hoïdes e enteses les coses per lo dit N'Andreu Gras requestes, de continent reebré (*sic*) sagrament del dit N'Andreu Gras sobre los sants quatre Evangelis de nostre senyor Déu, de la man dreta de aquell corporalment to[cat]s, que bé e lealment se haurà en la dita art de cirurgia e de f[er] tot ço que per fur nou del rey N'Amfós fos e sostengut, donà e atorgà a aquell licència de usar e praticar de la dita art de cirurgia per la dita ciutat, viles e lochs del regne de València [sens] temor de alcuna pena. Et no-res-menys, instant e requirent lo dit N'Andreu Gras, manà ésser feyta la letra següent:

Als honrats e universes e sengles officials e loch de senyoria tinents dins lo regne de València constituïts als quals la present pervendrà, e a cascun de aquells e a lurs lochtinents. De nós, En Jacme Forner, doctor en leys, asses-

[sor] e lochtinent [de] l'honrat En Martí Fuster, justícia de la ciutat de València en lo civil. Salut e honor. A la saviea e discreció d[e cascun de] vós per tenor de les presents signifficam que N'Andreu Gras, ciutadà de València, cirurgià, és estat examinat per los honrats e discrets maestre Jacme Maderes, maestre en arts e en medicina, e En Francesch Cambres, maestre en arts // e licenciat en medicina, metges de la ciutat dessús dita, examinadors deputats e assignats per los honrats justícia e jurats de la dita ciutat de tots los metges de física e de cirurgia vinents novellament per praticar en la dita ciutat, viles e lochs del dit regne de València, per los quals lo dit N'Andreu Gras és estat atrobat abte e sufficient de usar e praticar de la dita art de cirurgia, segons que a nós és cert per letra dels dits examinadors per lo dit N'Andreu Gras a nós en lo present dia de huy, data de la present, presentada, la tenor de la qual és segons que.s segueix: "A l'honrat e discret lo justícia civil de la ciutat de València, etc." *Inseratur ut est supra.* Aprés presentació de la qual, reebut per nós primerament e abans sagrament del dit N'Andreu q[ue], segons forma de fur nou del rey N'Amfós posat sots rúbrica "De metges," que bé e lealment se haurà en la dita art de cirurgia e fer ço que per lo dit fur és ordenat, havem atorgat e [a]torgada licència a aquell de usar e pra[ticar] en la dita ciutat, viles e lochs d[el] dit regne de València, de la [dita art] de cirurgia sens temor de alcuna pena. En testimoni de la qual [cosa manam] li n'ésser feta la present carta testimonial ab lo sagell del nostre offi[ci en] pendent ab çera vermella sagellada. *Data Valentie .XIX^{a}. die mensis octobris anno a nativitate Domini millesimo .CCC^{o}.LXX°. octavo.*

* * *

In the year of our Lord 1378, on Tuesday the 19th of October, before the honorable Jacme Forner, doctor of laws, assessor and lieutenant of the honorable Martí Fuster, civil justiciar of the city of Valencia, there appeared Andreu Gras, a citizen of the said city, surgeon, who presented him with a letter from the honorable Jacme Maderes, master in arts and in medicine, and Francesch Cambres, master in arts and licentiate in medicine, practitioners of the said city, examiners appointed by the honorable justiciar and *jurats* of the aforementioned city of all those practitioners of medicine and surgery newly arrived to practice in the said city and towns of the kingdom of Valencia, written on paper, open, and sealed in red wax on the back with the two seals of the said examiners, whose tenor is as follows:

To the honorable civil justiciar of the city of Valencia, or his lieutenant; from us, Jacme Maderes, master in arts and in medicine, and Francesch de Cambres, master in arts and licentiate in medicine, practitioners of the said city, examiners appointed by the honorable justiciar and *jurats* of the said city of all the practitioners of physic and surgery newly arrived to practice in the aforesaid city and towns of the kingdom of Valencia; health and honor. By the tenor of these presents we inform you that Andreu Gras, a citizen of this city, appeared before us and, wishing to practice the art of surgery in the city, towns, and villages of the said kingdom, has been examined by us in the manner prescribed by the *fur*; and we have well and carefully examined him and have found him competent by long and satisfactory experience to practice the said art of surgery; wherefore, at the request of the above-named Andreu Gras [for a certification] of his competence, we certify to you by these presents that beyond any doubt you may grant him license to practice the said art of surgery. Given at Valencia the fourteenth day of October, 1378 AD.

When the said letter had been presented, the said Andreu Gras requested orally that the said honorable lieutenant justiciar grant him a license to practice the art of surgery in the said city, towns, and villages of the kingdom of Valencia, since he was prepared to do all that he was required to do by the *fur* of Valencia, and also requested that a letter be ordered drawn up for him to each and every official in the said kingdom of Valencia that from henceforth they acknowledge the said Andreu Gras as a practitioner of surgery, and that they allow him to practice the said art of surgery without fear of any penalty and without any let or hindrance.

Upon considering the said letter and the things contained in it, and upon hearing the requests made by the said Andreu Gras, the said honorable lieutenant justiciar thereupon received an oath from the said Andreu Gras on the four holy Gospels of our Lord God, while he physically touched them with his right hand, that he would engage well and loyally in the said art of surgery, and that he would do all that is required by the new *fur* of King Alfons, and granted him license to practice the said art of surgery in the said city, towns, and villages of the said kingdom of Valencia, without fear of any penalty. And furthermore at the request of the said Andreu Gras he ordered the following certificate to be drawn up:

To all officials in the kingdom of Valencia to whom these presents may come, and to each of them or their lieutenants; from us, Jacme Forner, doctor of laws, assessor and lieutenant of the honorable Martí Fuster, civil justiciar of the city of Valencia; health and honor. We make it known to you by the tenor of these presents that Andreu Gras, citizen of Valencia, surgeon, has been examined by the honorable master Jacme Maderes, master in arts and in medicine, and Francesch Cambres, master in arts and licentiate in medicine, practitioners of the aforesaid city and examiners appointed by the honorable justiciar and *jurats* of the said city of all the practitioners of physic and surgery newly arrived to practice in the said city, towns, and villages of the kingdom of Valencia; and that they have found the said Andreu Gras to be competent to practice the said art of surgery, as certified to us by a letter from the said examiners presented to us today by the said Andreu Gras, dated today, whose tenor is as follows: "To the honorable civil justiciar of the city of Valencia, etc. . . . " (here let it be inserted as above). And after this was presented—having first received an oath from the said Andreu that he would well and loyally engage in the said art of surgery according to the terms of the new *fur* of King Alfons under the rubric "De metges," and would do all that is commanded by the said *fur*, have granted him license to practice the said art of surgery in the said city, towns, and villages of the said kingdom of Valencia, without fear of any penalty. In testimony of which thing we have ordered the present certificate to be drawn up for him, sealed in red wax with the seal of our office appended.

Given at Valencia, the 19th day of October, 1378 AD.

6

Valencia, 27 October 1378.

Içach Gabriel, a Jew of Valencia, receives a license to practice medicine in Valencia and its kingdom (ARV, Justícia Civil [Lletres], 391, s. fol.).

Anno a nativitate Domini millesimo .CCC°.LXX°. octavo, die mercurii que fuit .XXVII. mensis octobris. Comparech davant l'onrat En Martí Fuster, justícia de la ciutat de València en lo civil, Içach Grabiel (sic), juheu de la ciutat damunt dita, metge de físicha, e presentà a aquell una letra dels honrats e discrets En Jacme Maderes, maestre en arts e en medicina, e En Francesch de Cambres, maestre en arts e licenciat en medicina, ciutadans de la ciutat dessús dita, examinadors per nós e per los honrats jurats de la sobredita ciutat en l'any present deputats e assignats a examinar los metges que novellament en la ciutat e regne damunt dit volran usar e praticar de art de física e de cirurgia, en paper scrita, uberta, e dins aquella sagellada ab dos sagells de aquells en çera vermella, la tenor de la qual és segons que.s segueix:

A l'honrat e discret lo justícia de la ciutat de València en lo civil, o a son lochtinent. En Jacme Maderes, mestre en arts e en medicina, e.N Francesch de Cambre(s), mestre en arts e licenciat en medicina, ciutadans de la dita ciutat, examinadors per los honrats senyors justí[cia] e jurats de la dita ciutat en l'any present deputats e assignats a examinar los metges que novellament en la ciutat e regne damunt dit volran usar de et praticar de la sciència e art de física e de cirorgia. Salut e honor. A la discreció de vós per tenor de les presents certificam ésser comparegut denant nós Issach Gabriel, juheu de la dita ciutat, lo qual, volent usar e praticar de art de física dins la ciutat, viles e lochs del dit regne, s'és sotsmés al nostre examen, e nós aquell havem examinat bé e diligentment, segons fur, e aquell Issach havem atrobat en los principis de la dita sciència de física introduhit, emperò ab la pràtica de [cu]rar les malalties no ha longament praticat ni usat. E axí certificam que, quant en malaltia fort e gran serà demanat per praticar, si ja altre metge no y haurie primer, que ell sie tengut de demanar altre físich sufficient e antich en pràtica en acompanyat, // si serà en loch que haver-lo pusque, e per ell en demanar mostrat. E sobre açò reebats primerament e abans del dit Issach sa[gra]ment sobre los .X. manaments, que bé e felment e leyal se haurà e praticarà en la manera e forma desús dita de la dita [sciència] de física, per què, instant e requirent lo desús dit Issach de la sua sufficiència, per les presents certificam per ço que sens alcun dupte donets e atorguets licència e plen poder a.quell de usar e praticar en la manera e forma [desús dita] de la dita art de física. *Data Valentie .XVII^a. die [mensis] septembris anno a nativitate Domini millesimo .CCC.LXXVIII°.*

Et presentada la damunt dita letra, lo dit Içach Grabiel requerí de paraula lo dit honrat justícia que li donàs e atorgàs licència de usar e praticar de la dita art de física dins la ciutat, viles e lochs del regne de València, com fos apparellat fer tot ço que per fur de València fos tengut e astret de fer, requirén encara que letra li fos atorgada e manada ésser feyta a universes e sengles officials e lochs de senyoria tinents dins lo dit regne de València constituïts, que d'açí avant hajen e tinguen lo dit Içach Grabiel per metge de físicha e que de la dita art de físicha lo lexen usar e praticar sens temor de alcuna pena, e sens alcun contrast o embarch.

Et lo dit honrat justícia, vista e regoneguda la damunt dita letra e coses en aquella expressades, e hoïdes e enteses les coses per lo dit Içach Grabiel de paraula requestes, de continent reebé sagrament del dit Içach Grabiel sobre los deu manaments de la lig que nostre senyor Déu donà a Moysés en lo munt de Sinaý, per la man dreta de aquell corporalment tocats, per que bé e lealment se haurà en la dita art de físicha e de fer tot ço que per fur nou del rey N'Amfós fos e sia tengut fer e segons continència e manera en la letra dels [dits examina]dors con[ten]guda, donà e atorgà a aquell licència de usar e // praticar de la dita art de físicha en la dita ciutat, viles e lochs del dit regne de València sens temor de alcuna pena. Et no-res-menys manà ésser feyta a aquell la letra testimonial següent:

Als honrats universes e sengles officials e loch de senyoria tinents dins lo regne de València constituïts als quals la present pervendrà, o a lurs lochtinents. De nós, En Martí Fuster, justícia de la ciutat de València en lo civil. Salut e honor. A la discreció de cascun de vós per tenor de les presents significam que Içach Grabiel, metge de físicha, vehín de la dita ciutat, és estat examinat per los honrats e discrets En Jacme Maderes, maestre en arts e en medicina, e En Francesch Cambres, maestre en arts e licenciat en medicina, metges de la dita ciutat, examinadors per nós e per los honrats jurats de la ciutat sobredita en l'any present diputats e assignats a examinar los metges que novellament en la ciutat e regne dessús dit volran usar e praticar de la sciència e art de físicha e de cirurgia, per los quals lo dit Içach Grabiel és estat atrobat abte e sufficient de usar e praticar de la dita art de físicha, segons que a nós és cert per letra dels dits examinadors per lo dit Içach Grabiel en lo present dia de huy, data de la present, a nós presentada, la qual és de la tenor següent: "A l'honrat e discret lo justícia, etc." *Inseratur ut est supra.* Aprés presentació de la qual, reebut per nós de aquell primerament e abans sagrament sobre les deu manaments de la lig que nostre senyor Déu donà a Moysés en lo mont de Sinaý, que, segons forma de fur nou del rey N'Amfós posat sots rúbrica "De metges," bé e lealment se haurà en la dita art de físicha, e fer tot ço àls que per l[o d]it fur és ordenat, e sots virtut del dit sagrament ha promés que sí que entrevedrà en malaltia fort o gran, que ell demanarà altre físich suficient e antich en pràticha en aconpanyat, si serà en loch que aquell haver pogués, e que per ell mostràs en demanar aquell, havem atorgat e donat a aquell licència de usar e praticar de la dita art de medicina en la dita ciutat, viles e lochs del dit regne de València sens temor de alcuna pena. En testimoni de la qual cosa manam li n'ésser feta la presenta (*sic*) carta testimonial ab lo sagell del nostre offici ab çera groga e vermella en pendent sagellada. *Data Valentie .XXVII^{a}. die octobris anno a nativitate Domini millesimo .CCC^{o}.LXX°. octavo. Subscripsit Iacobus.*

* * *

In the year of our Lord 1378, on Wednesday the 27th of October, before the honorable Martí Fuster, civil justiciar of the city of Valencia, there appeared Içach Grabiel (*sic*), a Jew of the aforesaid city, a practitioner of physic, who presented him with a letter from the honorable Jacme Maderes, master in arts and in medicine, and Francesch de Cambres, master in arts and licentiate in medicine, citizens of the aforesaid city, examiners appointed by us and by the honorable *jurats* of the aforementioned city for the current year to examine those practitioners who wish to begin to practice the art of physic and surgery in the city and kingdom aforesaid, written on paper, open, and sealed in red wax with their two seals, whose tenor is as follows:

To the honorable civil justiciar of the city of Valencia, or his lieutenant; Jacme Maderes, master in arts and in medicine, and Francesch de Cambre, master in arts and licentiate in medicine, citizens of the said city, examiners appointed by the honorable justiciar and *jurats* of the said city for the current year to examine all those practitioners who wish to begin to practice the science and art of physic and surgery in the aforesaid city and kingdom; health and honor. By the tenor of these presents we inform you that Issach Gabriel, a Jew of the said city, appeared before us who, wishing to practice the art of physic in the city, submitted himself to our examination; and we have examined him carefully in the manner prescribed by the *fur*; and we have found the said Issach acquainted with the principles of the said science of physic, but he has not long been involved in the practice of treating illnesses. Thus we require that when he is summoned to treat a severe illness, if there is not already another practitioner there, he be required to summon another competent and long-practiced physician to join him, if he can find one, and show that he has done so. And having first received an oath on the Ten Commandments from the said Issach that he would well, faithfully, and loyally engage in the said science of physic and practice in the manner specified above, at the request of the above-named Issach [for a certification] of his competence, we certify to you by these presents that beyond any doubt you may grant him license to practice the said art of surgery in the manner specified above.
Given at Valencia the seventeenth day of September, 1378 AD.

When the said letter had been presented, the said Içach Grabiel orally requested that the said honorable justiciar grant him a license to practice the said art of physic in the city, towns, and villages of the kingdom of Valencia, since he was prepared to do all that he was required to do by the *fur* of Valencia, and asked also that a letter be drawn up for him to each and every official in the said kingdom of Valencia that from henceforth they acknowledge the said Içach Grabiel as a practitioner of physic, and that they allow him to practice the said art without any penalty and without any let or hindrance.

Having read the aforesaid letter and the things stated in it, and having heard the requests made orally by the said Içach Grabiel, the said honorable justiciar then took an oath from the said Içach Grabiel on the ten commandments of the law that our Lord God gave to Moses on Mount Sinai, which he touched physically with his right hand, to engage well and loyally in the said art of physic and to do everything commanded by the new *fur* of King Alfons and in the manner set out in the letter of the said examiners; and granted him license to practice the said art of medicine in the said city, towns, and villages of the said kingdom of Valencia, without fear of any penalty. And furthermore he ordered the following certificate to be drawn up:

To all officials in the kingdom of Valencia to whom these presents may come, or to their lieutenants; from us, Martí Fuster, civil justiciar of the city of Valencia; health and honor. We make it known by the tenor of these presents that Içach Grabiel, a practitioner of physic, an inhabitant of the said city, has been examined by the honorable Jacme Maderes, master in arts and in medicine, and Francesch Cambres, master in arts and licentiate in medicine, practitioners of the said city and examiners appointed by us and by the honorable *jurats* of the aforesaid city to examine the practitioners who wish to begin to practice the science and art of physic and surgery in the city and kingdom aforementioned; by whom the said Içach Grabiel has been found to be competent to practice the said art of physic, as certified to us by a letter from the said examiners presented to us by the said Içach Grabiel today, as dated below, whose tenor is as follows: "To the honorable justiciar, etc." (let it be inserted as above). When this had been presented, we—having first received from him an oath on the ten commandments of the law that our Lord God gave to Moses on Mount Sinai that, in the manner prescribed by the new *fur* of King Alfons under the rubric "De metges," he would well and loyally engage in the said art of medicine and do everything commanded by the said *fur,* and by the same oath promised that if he should encounter a severe illness he would summon another competent and long-practiced physician to accompany him, if he can find one, and show that he has done so—have granted him license to practice the said art of physic in the said city, towns, and villages of the said kingdom of Valencia, without fear of any penalty. In testimony of which we have ordered the present certificate to be drawn up for him, sealed with the seal of our office appended in yellow and red wax.

Given at Valencia, the 27th day of October, 1378 AD. Subscribed by Jacobus.

7

Valencia, 27 November 1378.

Sisto Fort, surgeon of Valencia, receives a license to practice surgery in Valencia and its kingdom (ARV, Justícia Civil [Lletres] 391, s. fol.).

Anno a nativitate Domini millesimo .CCC°.LXX°. octavo, die sabbati hora tertiarum que fuit .XXVII[a]. *mensis novembris.* Comparech davant l'onrat En Martí Fuster, justícia de la ciutat de València en lo civil, En Sisto Fort, cirúrgich, habitant en la dita ciutat, e presentà a aquell una letra dels honrats e discrets En Jacme Maderes, maestre en arts e en medicina, e En Francesch de Cambres, maestre en arts e licenciat en medicina, ciutadans de la dita ciutat, examinadors en l'any present diputats a examinar los metges que novellament en la ciutat e regne damunt dits voldran usar e praticar de sciència e art de físicha e de cirurgia, en paper scrita, uberta, e dins aquella ab dos sagells dels dits examinadors en çera vermella sagellada, la tenor de la qual és segons que.s segueix:

A l'honrat e discret lo justícia de la ciutat de València en lo civil, o a son lochtinent. En Jacme Maderes, mestre en arts e en medecina, e En Francesch de Cambres, mestre en arts e licenciat en medecina, ciutadans de la dita ciutat, examinadors per los honrats senyors justícia e jurats de la dita ciutat en l'any present diputats a [ex]aminar los metges que novellament en la ciutat e regne damunt dits volrran usar e praticar de sciència de art de física e de cirurgia. Salut e honor. A la discreció de vós per tenor de les presents certificam ésser comparegut denant nós En Sisto Fort, habitador de la ciutat, lo qual, volens usar de art de cirurgia dins la ciutat, viles e lochs del dit regne, s'és sotsmés al nostre examen, e nós aquell avem examinat bé e diligentment e aquell havíem trobat apte e suficient, per longa e aprovada [experi]ència de usar e praticar de la dita art de cirurgia; certificam, emperò, que en feyt de pronasticació o desospitació davant lo justícia criminal faedora dels nafrats que curarà, si de les nafres deuen morir o no, o si romandran debilitats en los menbres, lo dit En Sisto Fort deja demanar algun fís[i]ch apte e suficient en acompanyat; e vós rebets primerament e abans del dit En Sisto sagrament que bé, feelment [e] leal se haurà e usarà de la dita art de cirurgia. Per què, instant [e] requirent [lo desús dit En] Sisto Fort de la sua suficiència, per les presents certificam per [ço] que sens algun dupte donets e atorguets licència et plen poder a aquell de usar [e] praticar de la dita art de cirurgia. *Data Valentie tertia die octobris anno a nativitate Domini .M°.CCC°.LXX°.VIII°.*

Et presentada la damunt dita letra, lo dit maestre Sisto Fort requerí de paraula lo dit honrat justícia que li donàs e atorgàs licència de usar e praticar dins la ciutat de València, viles e lochs del regne de aquella, com se proferís apparellat de fer tot ço que per fur de València fos tengut e stret de fer, requirén encara que letra li fos manada ésser feta e liurada a universes e sengles officials e loch de senyoria tinents dins lo dit regne de València constituïts, que d'ací avant aguessen e tinguen per metge de cirurgia lo dit maestre Sisto Fort, e que de la dita art de cirurgia lo lexasen usar e praticar sens temor de alcuna pena, e sens alcun contrast o embarch.

Et encontinent lo dit honrat justícia, vista e regoneguda la dita letra dels dits honrats examinadors dessús presentada, e les coses en aquella expressades, e hoïdes les coses per lo dit maestre Sisto Fort de paraula requestes, de consell de son assessor reebé sagrament del dit maestre Sisto Fort sobre los sants quatre Evangelis de nostre senyor Déu, de la man dreta d'aquell corporalment tocats, que bé e lealment se haurà en la dita art de cirurgia, e fer tot ço que per fur nou del rey N'Amfós fos e sia tengut fer, e segons continència e manera de la dita letra dels dits examinadors, donà e atorgà a aquell licència de usar e praticar de la dita art de cirurgia en la dita ciutat, vil.les e lochs del dit regne sens temor de alcuna pena. Et no-res-menys manà ésser feta a aquell la letra infrasegüent:

Als honrats universes e sengles officials e loch de senyoria tinents dins lo regne de València constituïts als quals la present pervendrà, e a cascun d'aquells o a lurs lochtinents. De nós, En Martí Fuster, justícia justícia (*sic*) de la ciutat de València en lo civil. Salut e honor. A la discreció de cascun de vós per tenor de les presents signifficam [que maestre] Sisto Fort, cirúrgich de la dita ciutat, és estat examinat per [los hon]rats e discrets En Jacme Maderes, maestre en arts e en medicina, e En // Francesch Cambres, maestre en arts e licenciat en medicina, metges de la dita ciutat e examinadors per nós e per los honrats jurats de la ciutat sobredita en l'any present diputats e assignats a examinar los metges que novellament en la ciutat e regne dessús dit volran usar e praticar de la sciència e art de físicha e de cirurgia, per los quals lo dit maestre Sisto Fort és estat atrobat [abte e] sufficient de usar e pratichar de la dita art de cirurgia, segons que a nós és cert per letra dels dits examinadors per lo dit maestre Sisto Fort en lo present dia de huy, data de la present, a nós presentada, la qual és de la tenor següent: "A l'honrat e discret lo justícia, etc." *Inseratur ut est supra.* Aprés presentació de la qual, reebut per nós primerament e abans sagrament del dit maestre Sisto Fort sobre los sants quatre Evangelis de nostre senyor Déu, de la man dreta de aquell corporalment tocats, que, segons forma de fur nou del rey N'Amfós posat sots rúbrica "De metges," bé e lealment se haurà en la dita art de cirurgia, e fer tot ço àls que per lo dit fur és ordenat; e segons forma de la dita e preinserta letra, havem atorgat e donada al dit maestre Sisto Fort licència de usar e praticar de la dita art de cirurgia en la dita ciutat, viles e lochs del dit regne de València sens temor de alcuna pena. [En] testimoni de la qual cosa manam li n'ésser feta la present carta testimonial [ab lo sagell] del nostre offici en pendent ab cera groga e vermella sagellada. *Data Valentie [.XXVII^{a}.] die novembris anno a nativitate Domini millesimo .CCC^{o}.LXX°. octavo.*

* * *

In the year of our Lord 1378, at the hour of terce on Saturday the 27th of November, before the honorable Martí Fuster, civil justiciar of the city of Valencia, there appeared Sisto Fort, surgeon, an inhabitant of the said city, who presented him with a letter from the honorable Jacme Maderes, master in arts and in medicine, and Francesch de Cambres, master in arts and licentiate in medicine, citizens of the said city, examiners for the current year named to examine those practitioners who wish to begin to practice the science and art of physic and surgery in the aforesaid city and kingdom, written on paper, open, and sealed in red wax on the back with the two seals of the said examiners, whose tenor is as follows:

To the honorable civil justiciar of the city of Valencia, or his lieutenant; Jacme Maderes, master in arts and in medicine, and Francesch de Cambres, master in arts and licentiate in medicine, citizens of the said city, examiners appointed by the honorable justiciar and *jurats* of the said city to examine practitioners who wish to begin to practice the science and art of physic and surgery in the aforesaid city and kingdom; health and honor. By the tenor of these presents we inform you that Sisto Fort, an inhabitant of this city, appeared before us and, wishing to practice the art of surgery in the city, towns, and villages of the said kingdom, submitted himself to our examination; and we have carefully examined him and have found him competent by long and satisfactory experience to practice the said art of surgery; however, we specify that in prognostic judgments before the criminal justiciar concerning wounds that he is treating, whether his patients will die from their wounds or not, or whether they will remain weakened in their members, the said Sisto Fort must be accompanied by another competent physician; and you should first of all receive an oath from the said Sisto that he will well, faithfully, and loyally engage in the said art of surgery. Wherefore, at the request of the abovenamed Sisto Fort [for a certification] of his competence, we certify to you by these presents that beyond doubt you may grant him license to practice the said art of surgery.

Given at Valencia the third day of October, 1378 AD.

When the said letter had been presented, the said master Sisto Fort requested orally that the said honorable justiciar grant him a license to practice in the city of Valencia, and the towns and villages of its kingdom, since he was prepared to do all that he was required to do by the *fur* of Valencia, and also requested that a letter be ordered drawn up for him to each and every official in the said kingdom of Valencia that from henceforth they acknowledge the said Sisto Fort as a practitioner of surgery, and that they allow him to practice the said art of surgery without fear of any penalty and without any let or hindrance.

Immediately upon receiving the said letter presented above from the said honorable examiners, and the things contained in it, and upon hearing the requests made orally by the said master Sisto Fort, upon the advice of his assessor the said honorable justiciar received an oath from the said master Sisto Fort on the four holy Gospels of our Lord God, while he physically touched them with his right hand, that he would engage well and loyally in the said art of surgery, and that he would do all that is required by the new *fur* of King Alfons, and according to the terms of the said letter from the said examiners; and granted him license to practice the said art of surgery in the said city, towns, and villages of the said kingdom, without fear of any penalty. And furthermore he ordered the following certificate to be drawn up for him:

To all officials in the kingdom of Valencia to whom these presents may come, and to each of them or their lieutenants; from us, Martí Fuster, civil justiciar of the city of Valencia; health and honor. We make it known to each of you by the tenor of these presents that master Sisto Fort, surgeon of the said city, has been examined by the honorable Jacme Maderes, master in arts and in medicine, and Francesch Cambres, master of arts and licentiate in medicine, practitioners of the said city and examiners appointed for the current year by us and by the honorable *jurats* of the above-mentioned city to examine those practitioners who wish to begin to practice the science and art of physic and surgery in the said city and kingdom; and that they have found the said master Sisto Fort to be competent to practice the said art of surgery, as certified to us by a letter from the said examiners presented to us today by the said master Sisto Fort, dated as below, whose tenor is as follows: "To the honorable justiciar, etc." (here let it be inserted as above). And after this was presented—having first received an oath from the said master Sisto Fort on the four holy Gospels of our Lord God, while he touched them physically with his right hand, that he would well and loyally engage in the said art of surgery according to the terms of the new *fur* of King Alfons under the rubric "De metges," and would do all that is commanded by the said *fur* and according to the terms of the said letter inserted above, have granted the said master Sisto Fort license to practice the said art of surgery in the said city, towns, and villages of the said kingdom of Valencia, without fear of any penalty. In testimony of which thing we have ordered the present certificate to be drawn up for him, sealed in yellow and red wax with the seal of our office appended.

Given at Valencia, the 27th day of November, 1378 AD.

8

Valencia, 23 December 1378.

Hizmel Morcat, a Jew of Valencia, is authorized to practice medicine and surgery in Valencia and its kingdom (ARV, Justícia Civil [Lletres], 391, s. fol.).

Anno a nativitate Domini millesimo .CCC°.LXX°. octavo, die iovis hora vesperorum que fuit .XXIII[a]. *mensis decembris.* Comparech davant l'onrat micer Jacme Forner, doctor en leys, tinent loch de l'honrat En Martí Fuster, justícia de la ciutat de València en lo civil, Hizmel Morcat, juheu de la juheria de la dita ciutat, e presentà a aquell una letra dels honrats e discrets En Jacme Maderes, maestre en arts e en medicina, e En Francesch de Cambres, maestre en arts e licenciat en medicina, ciutadans de la dita ciutat, examinadors per los honrats justícia [e] jurats de la dita ciutat en l'any present, en paper scrita, uberta, e dins aquella sagellada ab dors (*sic*) sagells dels dits examinadors, la tenor de la qual letra és segons que.s segueix:

A l'honrat e discret lo justícia de la ciutat de València en lo civil, o a son lochtinent. En Jacme Mederes, maestre en arts e en medicina, e En Francesch de Cambres, maestre en arts e lecenciat en medicina, ciutadans de la dita ciutat, examinadors per los honrats senyors justícia e jurats de la dita ciutat en l'any present diputats a examinar los m[etges] que novellament en la ciutat e regne de València volran usar e praticar de sciència e art de física e de cirurgia. Salut e honor. A la discreció de vós per tenor de les presents certifficam ésser comparegut denant nós Hizmel Morcat, juheu, habitador de la dita ciutat, lo qual, volent usar e praticar de art de física e de cirurgia [dins la] ciu[tat], viles e lochs del dit regne, sosmés al nostre examen, e nós aquell havem examinat bé e diligentment segons que és acostumat, e aquell dit Huzmel havem atrobat sufficient de usar e praticar de la dita art de cirurgia; attenén emperò que en la sciència de físicha ell longament no ha studiat, ja[tsia] haja praticat en malalties requirents sciència de físicha, per ço certifficam a vós com ell serà demanat en les malalties forts e grans les quals sciència de física serà necessària, que ell sia tengut de menar un físich suficient e abte e antich en speculativa en acompany[nat], si serà en loch que haver-la (*sic*) puscha, e ja per ell en deman[ar mo]strarà. Et sobre açò reebats primerament ab[ans del dit] Hizmel sagrament sobre los deu ma//naments e axí mateix que bé, fellment e leal se haurà, usarà e praticarà de la dita art de física e de cirorgia; per què, instant e requirent [lo] desús dit Huzmel de la sua suficiència, per les presents vos certificam per ço que sens alcun dupte donets e atorguets licència e plen poder a aquell de usar e praticar de la dita art de física e de cirorgia en la manera e forma desús dita. *Data Valentie quartadecima die mensis novembris anno a nativitate Domini millesimo .CCC°.LXX°. octavo.*

Et presentada la damunt dita letra, lo dit I[zmel Mor]cat requerí de paraula lo dit honrat lochtinent de justícia que li donàs e atorgàs licència de usar e praticar de la dita art de físicha e de cirurgia dins la dita ciutat, viles e lochs del regne de València, com ell fos apparellat de fer tot ço que per fur de València fos tengut e astret de fer, requirén encara que letra li fos atorgada e manada ésser feyta a universes e sengles officials e loch de senyoria tinents dins lo dit regne de València constituïts, que d'açí avant hajen e tinguen lo dit Izmel Morcat per metge de físicha e de cirurgia, e que de la dita art de físicha e de cirurgia lo lexen usar e praticar sens temor de alcuna pena e sens alcun contrast o embarch.

Et encontinent lo dit honrat lochtinent de justícia, vista e regoneguda la damunt dita letra e coses en aquella expressades, e hoïdes e enteses les coses per lo dit Hizmell Morcat de paraula requestes, reebé de aquell sagrament sobre los deu manaments de la lig que nostre senyor Déu donà a Moyssé en lo munt de Sinaý, per la man dreta de aquell corporalment tocats, que bé e lealment se haurà en [la dita art] de físicha // e de cirurgia, e que farà tot ço que en los furs del rey N'Amfós és ordenat sots rúbrica "De metges," e segons forma e continència de la dita letra dels examinadors damunt dits, donà e atorgà a aquell licència de usar e praticar en la dita ciutat, viles e lochs del dit regne de València sens temor de alcuna pena. Et no-res-menys atorgà e manà ésser feyta a.quell la carta testimonial següent:

Als honrats universes e sengles officials e loch de senyoria tinents dins les ciutats, viles e lochs del regne de València als quals la present pervendrà, e a cascun de aquells o a lurs lochtinents. De nós, En Jacme Forner, doctor en leys, tinent loch de l'honrat En Martí Fuster, justícia de la ciutat de València en lo civil. Salut e honor. A la discreció e saviea de cascun de vós per tenor de les presents signifficam que Hismel Morcat, juheu de la juheria de València, és estat examinat per los honrats e discrets maestre Jacme Mederes, maestre en arts e en medicina, e En Francesch Cambres, maestre en arts e licenciat [en] medicina, metges de la dita ciutat, examinadors per lo dit hon[rat] justícia e jurats de la ciutat sobredita en l'any present dipu[tats e] elets a examinar los metges que novellament en la ciu[tat e] regne dessús dit volran usar e praticar de la sciència e art [de físi]cha e de cirurgia, per los quals lo dit Hismel Morcat és estat atrobat abte e sufficient de usar e praticar de la dita art de físicha e cirurgia, segons que a nós és çert per letra dels dits examinadors per lo dit Hismel Morcat a nós presentada en lo present dia, data de la present, la qual és de la tenor següent: "A l'honrat e discret lo justícia de la ciutat de València, etc." *Inseratur totam* (*sic*) *ut est supra.* Aprés presentació de la qual, reebut per nós primerament e // abans sagrament del dit Hismel Morcat sobre los deu manaments de la lig que nostre senyor Déu donà a Moysé en lo munt de Sinaý, que bé e lealment se haurà en la dita art de física e de cirurgia, e farà tot ço que en los furs nous del rey N'Amfós, sots rúbrica "De metges," és contengut e ordenat, e encara segons forma de la dita e preinserta letra dels dits examinadors, havem atorgat e donada a aquell licència de usar e praticar de la dita art de física e de cirurgia en la dita ciutat, viles e lochs del dit regne, sens temor de alcuna pena. En testimoni de la qual cosa manam li n'ésser feyta la present carta testimonial ab lo sagell del nostre offici ab çera groga e vermella en pendent sagellada. *Data Valentie .XXIII^{a}. die decembris anno a nativitate Domini millesimo .CCC^{o}. septuagesimo octavo. [Su]bscripsit Iacobus.*

* * *

In the year of our Lord 1378, at the hour of vespers on Thursday the 23rd of December, before the honorable Jacme Forner, doctor of laws, in the place of the honorable Martí Fuster, civil justiciar of the city of Valencia, there appeared Hizmel Morcat, a Jew from the Jewry of the said city, who presented him with a letter from the honorable Jacme Maderes, master in arts and in medicine, and Francesch de Cambres, master in arts and licentiate in medicine, citizens of the said city, examiners for the current year [named] by the honorable justiciar and *jurats* of the said city, written on paper, open, and sealed on the back with the seals of the said masters, whose tenor is as follows:

To the honorable civil justiciar of the city of Valencia, or his lieutenant; Jacme Maderes, master in arts and in medicine, and Francesch de Cambres, master in arts and licentiate in medicine, citizens of the said city, examiners appointed by the honorable justicia and *jurats* of the said city to examine practitioners who wish to begin practice the science and art of physic and surgery in the city and kingdom of Valencia; health and honor. By the tenor of these presents we inform you that Hizmel Morcat, a Jew, an inhabitant of this city, appeared before us wishing to practice the art of physic and surgery in the city, towns, and villages of the said kingdom, and submitted to our examination; and we have well and carefully examined him in the customary manner and have found the said Huzmel competent to practice the said art of surgery; but since he has not studied the science of physic long, although he has treated illnesses requiring the science of physic, we certify to you that should he be called on in severe illnesses where a knowledge of physic is necessary, he should be required to bring a physician competent and long acquainted with theory to accompany him, if it should be in a village where this is possible, and [show that he has done so]. And thereupon, having first received the oath of the said Hizmel on the Ten Commandments that he would well, faithfully, and loyally practice the said art of physic and surgery, at the request of the above-named Hizmel [for a certification] of his competence, we certify to you by these presents that beyond doubt you may grant him license to practice the said art of physic and surgery in the manner and form explained above.

Given at Valencia the fourteenth day of the month of November, 1378 AD.

When the said letter had been presented, the said Hizmel Morcat requested orally that the said honorable lieutenant justiciar grant him a license to practice the said art of physic and surgery in the said city, towns, and villages of the kingdom, declaring himself ready to do all that he was required to do by the *fur* of Valencia, and also requested that a letter be ordered drawn up for him to each and every official in the said kingdom of Valencia that from henceforth they acknowledge the said Izmel Morcat as a practitioner of physic and surgery, and that they allow him to practice the said art of physic and surgery without fear of any penalty and without any let or hindrance.

Immediately upon receiving the said letter and the things contained in it, and upon hearing the requests made orally by the said Hizmell Morcat, the said honorable lieutenant justiciar received an oath from him on the ten commandments of the law that our Lord God gave to Moses on Mont Sinai, while he physically touched them with his right hand, that he would engage well and loyally in the said art of physic and surgery, and that he would do all that is required by the *furs* of King Alfons under the rubric "De metges," and according to the terms of the said letter from the aforesaid examiners; and granted him license to practice in the said city, towns, and villages of the said kingdom of Valencia, without fear of any penalty. And furthermore he ordered the following certificate to be drawn up for him:

To all officials and lords in the cities, towns, and villages of the kingdom of Valencia to whom these presents may come, and to each of them or their lieutenants; from us, Jacme Forner, doctor of laws, lieutenant to the honorable Martí Fuster, civil justiciar of the city of Valencia; health and honor. We make it known to each of you by these presents that Hismel Morcat, Jew of the Jewry of Valencia, has been examined by the honorable master Jacme Mederes, master in arts and in medicine, and Francesch Cambres, master in arts and licentiate in medicine, practitioners of the said city and examiners appointed for the current year by the said honorable justiciar and the honorable *jurats* of the said city to examine those practitioners who wish to begin to practice the science and art of physic and surgery in the said city and kingdom; and that they have found the said Hismel Morcat to be competent to practice the said art of physic and surgery, as certified to us by a letter from the said examiners presented to us today (as dated below) by the said Hismel Morcat, whose tenor is as follows: "To the honorable civil justiciar of the city of Valencia . . ." (here let it be inserted as above). And after this [letter] was presented—having first received an oath from the said Hismel Morcat on the ten commandments of the law that our Lord God gave to Moses on Mount Sinai that he would well and loyally engage in the said art of physic and surgery and would do all that is commanded by the new *furs* of king Alfons under the heading "De metges," and by the terms of the said letter from the said examiners, inserted above, have granted him license to practice the said art of physic and surgery in the said city, towns, and villages of the said kingdom, without fear of any penalty. In testimony of which thing we have ordered the present certificate to be drawn up for him, sealed in yellow and red wax with the seal of our office appended.

Given at Valencia, the 23rd day of December, 1378 AD. Subscribed by Jacobus.

9

Valencia, 27 March 1380.

Pere de Ligalbe, surgeon of Lérida, receives a license to practice surgery in Valencia and its kingdom (ARV, Justícia Civil [Lletres], 414, second quire, fols. 27–28).

Anno a nativitate Domini .M^{o}.CCC^{o}.LXXX°., die mercurii intitulata .XXVII^{a}. marcii. Comparech davant la presència de l'honrat En Berenguer de Rabinats, justícia de la ciutat de València en lo civil, l'onrat En Pere de Ligalbe, cilórgisich (*sic*), e presentà a aquell una letra dels honrats maestre Jacme Maderes, maestre en arts e en medicina, e maestre Vicent Serra, físich, ciutadans de la dita ciutat, patent, en paper scrita, e e.ll dos de aquella sagellada ab los sagells de cascun dels dits maestres, empremtats en cera vermella, la tenor de la qual és *ut sequitur*:

Al molt honrat sènyer lo justícia de la ciutat de València en lo civil, o a son lochtinent. De nós, maestre Jacme Maderes, maestre en arts e en medecina, et mestre Vicent Sera, phísich, ciutadans de la dita ciutat, examinadors diputats e asignats per los honrats justícia e jurats de la dita ciutat per examinar tots e sengles metges de phísica e de cerurgia vinents novelament ha praticar e usar de la dita art en la ciutat de València et regne de aquella. Salut, ab creximent de prosperitat e honor. Sàpia la vostra honrada discreció ésser comparegut davant nós En Pere de Ligalbe, cirúrgich de la ciutat de Leyda, dient e afermant sí voler usar e praticar de la dita art de cirurgia en la dita ciutat de València, e viles e lochs del regne de aquella, requirent que per nós fos examinat; lo qual nós avem examinat bé e diligentment e aquell havem atrobat ésser suficient en la dita art de cirurgia, per què, honrat sènyer justícia, instant e requirent lo dit En Pere de Ligalbe, per la tenor de la present vos certificam de les dites coses, e he.us requerim e pregam en deute de justícia que us plàcia donar licència e fer a aquell carta testimonial sí e segons en semblants fets per vós e vostra cort és acostumat fer, prestat per ell ans e primerament sagrament que bé e lealment usarà e praticarà en la dita art de cirurgia, com nós, sènyer, siam apparellats los vostres justs manaments obeir e enseguir. En testimoni de les quals coses fem-vos fer la present letra testimonial, per nós a ell liurada, ab nostres segells sagellada. Scrita en València a .XXI. de març de l'any de la nativitat de nostre senyor .M.CCC. huytanta.

Et presentada la dita letra, lo dit En Pere de Ligalbe requerí de paraula lo dit honrat justícia que li donàs e atorgàs licència de usar e praticar dins la ciutat de València, viles e lochs del regne de aquella, com se proferís apparellat de fer tot ço que per fur de València fos tengut e astret de fer, requerín encara que letra li fos manada ésser feta e liurada a universes e sengles oficials e lochs de senyoria tinents dins lo dit regne de València constituïts, que d'açí avant haguesen e tinguen per metje en cirurgia lo dit En Pere Ligalbe, que de la dita art de cirurgia lo lexasen usar e praticar sens temor de alcuna pena, e sens alcun contrast e enbarch.

Et encontinent lo dit honrat justícia, vista e regoneguda la dita letra dels dits honrats examinadors desús presentada e les coses en aquella expresades, e hoÿdes les coses per lo dit En Pere de Ligalbe de paraula requestes, de consell de son asesor reebé sagrament del dit En Pere de Ligalbe sobre los sants quatre Evvangel.lis de nostre senyor Déu, de la man dreta d'aquell corporalment tocats, que bé e lealment se haurà en la dita art de cirurgia, e fer tot ço que per fur nou del rey N'Amfós sia tengut fer, e segons continència e manera de la dita letra a les dits examinadors, donà e atorgà a aquell licència de usar e praticar de la dita art de cirurgia en la dita ciutat, viles e lochs del dit regne, sens temor de alcuna pena. Et no-res-menys manà ésser feta a aquell la letra infraseqüent:

Als honrats universes e sengles oficials e loch de senyoria tinents dins lo regne de València constituïts als quals la present pervendrà, e a cascun de aquells o a lurs lochtinents. De nós, En Berenguer de Rabinats, justícia de la ciutat de València en lo civil. Salut e honor. A la discreció de cascun de vós per tenor de les presents significam que En Pere de Ligalbe, cirúrgich, comorant en la dita ciutat, és estat examinat per los honrats e discrets En Jachme Maderes, maestre en arts e en medicina, e En Vicent Serra, físich, metges de la dita ciutat e examinadors per nós e per los honrats jurats de la dita ciutat en l'any present d[ip]utats e asignats a examinar los metjes que novellament en la ciutat e regne desús dit volran usar e praticar de la sciència e art de físicha e de cirurgia, per los quals lo dit En Pere de Ligalbe és estat atrobat abte e suficient de usar e praticar de la dita art de cirurgia, segons que a nós és cert per letra dels dits examinadós // per lo dit En Pere de Ligalbe en lo present dia de huy, data de la present, a nós presentada, la qual és de la tenor següent: "Al molt honrat sènyer lo justícia, etc." *Inseratur ut est supra.* Aprés presentació de la qual, reebut per nós primerament e abans sagrament del dit En Pere de Ligalbe sobre los sants quatre Evvangelis de nostre senyor Déu, de la man dreta de aquell corporalment tocats, que, segons forma de fur nou del rey N'Amfós posat sots rúbrica "De metges," bé e lealment se haurà en la dita art de cirurgia, e fer tot ço àls que per lo dit fur és ordenat e segons forma de la dita e preinserta letra, havem atorgat e donada al dit En Pere de Ligalbe licència de usar e praticar de la dita art de cirurgia en la dita ciutat, viles e lochs del dit regne de València, sens temor de alcuna pena. En testimoni de la qual cosa manam li n'ésser feta la present carta testimonial ab lo segell del nostre ofici en pendent ab cera vermela segellada. *Data Valentie .XVII^a. die marcii anno a nativitate Domini .M^o.CCC^o.LXXX°.*

* * *

In the year of our Lord 1380, Wednesday the 27th of March, before the honorable Berenguer de Rabinats, civil justiciar of the city of Valencia, there appeared the honorable Pere de Ligalbe, surgeon, who presented him with a letter from the honorable master Jacme Maderes, master in arts and in medicine, and master Vicent Serra, physician, citizens of the said city, open, written on paper, and sealed on the back with the seals of each of the said masters imprinted in red wax, whose tenor is as follows:

To the most honorable lord civil justiciar of the city of Valencia, or his lieutenant; from us, master Jacme Maderes, master in arts and in medicine, and master Vicent Sera, physician, citizens of the said city, examiners appointed by the honorable justiciar and *jurats* of the said city to examine each and every practitioner of physic and surgery newly arrived to practice the said art in the city of Valencia; health, with increase of prosperity and honor. May your worship know that Pere de Ligalbe, a surgeon from the city of Lérida, has appeared before us, declaring that he wishes to practice the said art of surgery in the said city of Valencia and the towns and villages of its kingdom, and asking that he be examined by us; and we have carefully examined him and have found him competent in the said art of surgery. Wherefore, honored sir, at the request of the said Pere de Ligalbe, we certify the said things to you by these presents and request in accordance with the law that it please you to grant him license and prepare for him a certificate, as you and your court are accustomed to do in such cases—he first taking an oath that he will practice the said art of surgery well and loyally, as we, lord, are prepared to obey your just orders. In testimony of which things we have drawn up for you the present letter, given by us to him, and sealed with our seals.

Written in Valencia, 21 March 1380 AD.

When the said letter had been presented, the said Pere Ligalbe requested orally that the said honorable justiciar grant him a license to practice in the city of Valencia and the towns and villages of its kingdom, declaring himself ready to fulfill all that he was required to do by the *fur* of Valencia, and also requested that a letter be ordered drawn up for him and addressed to each and every official in the said kingdom of Valencia that from henceforth they acknowledge the said Pere Ligalbe as a practitioner of surgery, and that they allow him to practice the said art of surgery without fear of any penalty and without any let or hindrance.

Immediately upon receiving the said letter presented from the said honorable examiners and reading the things contained in it, and upon hearing the requests made orally by the said Pere de Ligalbe, the said honorable justiciar, at the advice of his assessor, received from the said Pere de Ligalbe an oath on the four holy Gospels of our Lord God, while he physically touched them with his right hand, that he would engage well and loyally in the said art of surgery, and that he would do all that he was required to do according to the new *fur* of King Alfons and under the terms of the letter from the said examiners; and granted him license to practice the said art of surgery in the said city and the towns and villages of its kingdom, without fear of any penalty. And furthermore he ordered the following certificate to be drawn up for him:

To all officials in the kingdom of Valencia to whom these presents may come, and to each of them or their lieutenants; from us, Berenguer de Rabinats, civil justiciar of the city of Valencia; health and honor. We make it known to each of you by these presents that Pere de Ligalbe, surgeon, dwelling in the said city, has been examined by the honorable Jachme Maderes, master in arts and in medicine, and Vicent Serra, physician, practitioners of the said city and examiners appointed for the current year by us and by the honorable *jurats* of the said city to examine those practitioners who wish to begin to practice the science and art of physic and surgery in the said city and kingdom; and that the said Pere de Ligalbe has been found to be competent to practice the said art of surgery, as certified to us by a letter from the said examiners presented to us today by the said Pere de Ligalbe, whose tenor is as follows: (here let it be inserted as above). And after this [letter] was presented, we—having first received an oath from the said Pere de Ligalbe on the four holy Gospels of our Lord God, while he physically touched them, that, in accordance with the terms of the new *fur* of King Alfons under the heading "De metges," he would well and loyally engage in the said art of surgery and would do all that is commanded by the said *fur* and according to the terms of the letter inserted above—have granted the said Pere de Ligalbe license to practice the said art of surgery in the said city, towns, and villages of the said kingdom of Valencia, without fear of any penalty. In testimony of which thing we have ordered the present certificate to be drawn up for him, sealed in red wax with the seal of our office appended.

Given at Valencia, the 17th of March, 1380 AD.

10

Valencia, 20 December 1380.

Grant of a license to operate for hernia anywhere in the kingdom of Valencia, to Tomàs de Maestre Tone, a surgeon from the Mark of Ancona (ARV, Justícia Civil [Lletres], 414, eighth quire, fol. 17).

Anno a nativitate Domini .M°.CCC°.LXXX°., die iovis .XX°. decembris. Denant l'onrat En Berenguer de Rabinats, justícia de la ciutat de València en lo civil, comparegueren los honrats maestre Jacme Mederes, maestre en arts e en medicina, e En Vicent Serra, físich, ciutadans de la dita ciutat, examinadors diputats e assignats per los honrats justícia e jurats de la dita ciutat a examinar tots e sengles metges de phísicha e de cirurgia vinents novellament a praticar e usar de les dites arts en la dita ciutat e regne de aquella, de una part, et maestre Tomàs de Maestre Tone, de la Marcha d'Ancona, de la part altra. Et, instant e requirent lo dit maestre Tomàs, los dits honrats maestres Jacme e En Vicent Serra, examinadors qui dessús, per vigor de un manament a aquells feyt per lo dit honrat a instància del dit maestre Tomàs, feren relació e dixeren de paraula denant lo dit honrat justícia que ells havien vist obrar de les malalties de tal appellades hèrnies, *alias* potresos, al dit maestre Tomàs, et encara reebuda informació sumària de alcunes cures que lo dit maestre Tomàs havia fetes de les dites malalties, et que havien trobat aquell ésser bo e sufficient en la dita art de les dites hèrnies de tal, et que podia e devia usar de aquella, emperò que lo dit maestre Tomàs, ans que començàs o volgués metre mà a fer les dites obres de tal, dega e sia tengut de dir e declarar als pacients dues coses: la primera, lo perill de la mort que s'i pot esdevenir; la segona, que notifique e declar al pacient que deu perdre e li deu ésser tallat lo genitiu, la un o abduy, en què haurà mal. Et que açò fahent, e lo pacient volent-se metre en son poder ab les dites condicions, devia ésser donada licència de usar et praticar de les dites malalties de hèrnies.

Et encontinent lo dit honrat justícia, hoÿda la dita relació dels dits honrats examinadors feta, et a instància e requisició del dit maestre Tomàs de Maestre Tone, et de conseyll de son assessor, reebé sagrament del dit maestre Tomàs sobre los sants Evvangelis de Déu, per la man dreta de aquell corporalment tocats, que bé e lealment se haurà en la dita art de tal de les dites malalties appellades hèrnies, ab les condicions dessús dites, et que farà tot ço que per fur nou del rey N'Anfós és tengut fer, donà e atorgà al dit maestre Tomàs que pogués usar e praticar de la dita art de tal de les dites malalties appellades hèrnia, en la dita ciutat, viles e lochs del regne de aquella. Et resno-menys manà ésser feyta // al dit maestre Tomàs la letra testimonial infrasegüent:

Als honrats universes e sengles officials e lochs de senyoria tinents als quals la present pervendrà o presentada serà, dins lo regne de València, e a cascun de aquells o a llurs lochtinents. De nós, En Berenguer de Rabinats, justícia de la ciutat de València en lo civil. Salut e honor. A la discreció de cascun de vós per tenor de les presents significam que maestre Tomàs de Maestre Tone, de la Marcha de Anchona, cirurgià e maestre de malalties de hèrnies, en altra manera appellades potresos, comorant a present en la dita ciutat, és estat examinat bé e diligentment per los honrats e discrets En Jacme Mederes, maestre en art e en medicina, et En Vicent Serra, phísich, metges de la dita ciutat et examinadors per nós e per los honrats jurats de la damunt dita ciutat en l'any present diputats e assignats a examinar los metges que novellament en la dita ciutat e regne dessús dit volran usar e praticar de la sciència e art de phísicha e de cirurgia, per los quals lo dit maestre Tomàs és estat atrobat abte e suficient de usar e praticar de la dita art de cirurgia de tayl de les dites malalties de hèrnies, *alias* appellades potres, segons que a nós és estat cert per relació dels examinadors feta; aprés de la qual relació, reebut per nós primerament e abans sagrament del dit maestre Tomàs sobre los sants Evvangelis de Déu, per aquell corporalment tocats, que bé e lealment, segons forma de fur nou del rey N'Amfós, se haurà en la dita art de cirurgia de tayl de les dites malalties de hèrnies, et que notificarà als pacients havents aquell mal dues coses: la primera, lo perill de la mort que s'i pot esdevenir en fer la dita obra; la segona, que declararà als pacients que deuen perdre e.ls deu ésser tallat lo genitiu on haurà lo mal, o abduy, si en abduy hauran la dita malaltia, havem atorgada e donada al dit maestre Tomàs licència de usar e praticar de la dita art de cirurgia de tayll de les dites malalties de hèrnies en la dita ciutat, viles e lochs del dit regne de València, sens temor de alcuna pena. En testimoni de la qual cosa, manam li ésser feta la present carta testimonial ab lo segell del nostre offici en pendent ab cera vermella sagellada. *Data Valentie .XXII^a^. die decembris anno a nativitate Domini .M^o^.CCC^o^.LXXX°.*

* * *

In the year of our Lord 1380, Thursday the 20th of December, before the honorable Berenguer de Rabinats, civil justiciar of the city of Valencia, there appeared on the one hand the honorable master Jacme Mederes, master in arts and in medicine, and Vicent Serra, physician, citizens of the said city, examiners appointed by the honorable justiciar and *jurats* of the said city to examine each and every practitioner of physic and surgery newly arrived to practice the said arts in the said city and its kingdom; and on the other hand master Tomás de Maestre Tone, from the Mark of Ancona. And at the request of the said master Tomás, the said honorable masters Jacme and Vicent Serra, the examiners named above, responding to an order given them by the said honorable [justiciar] at the request of the said master Tomás, explained orally to the said honorable justiciar that they had seen the said master Tomás operate on those illnesses called hernias or *potresos*, and had also received accounts of cures that the said master Tomás had brought about of the said illnesses, and that they had found him competent in the said art of operating on the said hernias, and that he could and should employ it; but that the said master Tomás, before beginning or setting his hand to such operations, should be required to make two things plain to his patients: the first, the danger of death that could supervene; the second, that he notify the patient who must have his testicle removed, one or both, whichever is affected. Having done this, if the patient is willing to put himself in his care under these conditions, he should be given license to practice on the said ailments or hernias.

Immediately the said honorable justiciar, having heard the said account given by the said honorable examiners, at the request of the said master Tomás de Maestre Tone, and upon the advice of his assessor, received from the said master Tomás an oath on the holy Gospels of God, while he physically touched them with his right hand, that he would engage well and loyally in practicing the said art of operating on the said ailments called hernias, under the conditions stated above, and that he would do all that he was required to do under the new *fur* of King Alfons; and granted the said master Tomás that he might practice the said art of operating on the said ailment called hernia in the said city and the towns and villages of its kingdom. And furthermore he ordered the following testimonial to be drawn up for the said master Tomás:

To all officials and lords in the kingdom of Valencia to whom these presents may come, and to each of them or their lieutenants; from us, Berenguer de Rabinats, civil justiciar of the city of Valencia; health and honor. We make it known to each of you by these presents that master Tomás de Maestre Tone, of the Mark of Ancona, surgeon and master of hernial complaints (also called *potresos*), dwelling at present in the said city, has been examined carefully by the honorable Jacme Mederes, master in art and in medicine, and Vicent Serra, physician, practitioners of the said city and examiners appointed for the current year by us and by the honorable *jurats* of the above-mentioned city to examine those practitioners who wish to begin to practice the science and art of physic and surgery in the said city and kingdom; and that the said master Tomás has been found by them to be competent to employ and practice the said art of operating surgically on the said hernial complaints or *potres*, as certified to us by the account made by the examiners; and after receiving this account, we—having first received an oath from the said master Tomás on the holy Gospels of God, while he physically touched them, in accordance with the new *fur* of King Alfons, that he would well and loyally engage in the said art of operating for hernial complaints, and that he would first inform patients with such complaints of two things: first, the danger of death that they could run in undergoing the said operation; second, that he would notify those patients who must have an affected testicle removed, or both if the said complaint involved both—have granted the said master Tomás license to practice the said art of surgical operation for the said hernial complaints in the said city, towns, and villages of the said kingdom of Valencia, without fear of any penalty. In testimony of which thing we have ordered the present certificate to be drawn up for him, sealed in red wax with the seal of our office appended. Given at Valencia, the 22nd of December, 1380 AD.

11

Valencia, 9 February 1383.

Bernat Giner, alias Fuster, receives a license to practice medicine and surgery throughout the kingdom of Valencia (ARV, Justícia Civil [Lletres], 459, second quire, fols. 1–2).

Anno a nativitate Domini millesimo .CCC°.LXXX°. tertio, die lune .IXª. februarii. Davant lo honrat En Johan de Cervató, justícia de la ciutat de València en lo civil, comparech En Bernat Giner, en altra manera appellat Fuster, físich cirurgià, et presentà a aquell una letra dels honrats En Jacme Maderes et En Pere Gironés, examinadors en l'any present dels metges cirurgians de la dita ciutat, la tenor de la qual és aytal:

A l'honrat e discret sènyer lo justícia de la ciutat de València en lo civil, o a son lochtinent. De nós, En Jacme Maderes, maestre en arts et en medicina, et En Pere Gironés, bacheller en medicina, ciutadans de la dita ciutat, examinadors en l'any present deputats a examinar los metges qui novellament vénen e volen exercir et praticar en la dita ciutat et regne de València en física et en cirurgia. Salut e honor. Certificam, sènyer, a la vostra discreció, que lo discret En Bernat Giner, *alias* Fuster, és comparegut denant nós e ha request nós que.l deguéssem examinar en física et en cirurgia, lo qual havem examinat en la dita facultat segons forma acostumada, e havem trobat que.l dit En Bernat Gener no és tehòrich, mas ha covinent pràtica et antigua en física et en cirurgia, et per açò longua continuació que ha feyta ab metges en pràtica et en la dita facultat, segons que li'n fan testimonis diverses metges antichs en una carta pública, la qual nós havem vista, havem reputat et reputam aquell, dit En Bernat Gener, ésser abte e sufficient a usar e praticar en la dita ciutat e regne de València de física et de cirurgia, ab les moderació, retenció et forma següents, ço és, que no s'entrametrà ne use en cirurgia de nafres perilloses, axí com nafres de cap, de pits, de budells et d'altres nafres perilloses, et en física de malalties perilloses, axí com fe//bres contínues et frenesis et altres malalties agudes, sens altre coatinent o companyat metge o metges autèntichs o de auctoritat et pus sperts, sots la pena contenguda en lo fur. Per què, instant e requirent lo dit En Bernat Gener, intiman les dites coses ab la present a vós, dit honrat justícia et lochtinent vostre, remetem aquell dit En Bernat et pregam e requirim que donets licència et facultat a ell, dit En Bernat Gener, que puga exercir, usar et praticar en la dita ciutat et regne, et en les dites facultats de físicha et cirurgia, segons forma dessús expressada, rehebent sagrament de aquell que allò servarà et contra no vingua. *Data Valentie .XXII. die ianuarii anno a nativitate Domini millesimo .CCC°.LXXX°. tertio.*

Et presentada la dita letra, encontinent lo dit honrat rehebré (*sic*) sagrament del dit En Bernat Giner sobre los sants Evangelis, que ell que (*sic*) usaria bé e lealment del dit offici de cirurgia et de física, ab les moderació et retenció dessús per los dits examinadors retenguda. Et res-no-menys manà li ésser feyta la letra certificatòria infraseguënt:

Als honrats et discrets universes et sengles officials o loch de senyoria tinents dins lo regne de València constituhits als quals la present pervendrà o presentada serà, o a lurs lochtinents. De nós, En Johan de Cervató, justícia civil de la ciutat de València. Salut e complida honor. Per tenor de les presents certificam-vos que En Bernat Gener, *alias* appellat Fuster, físich e cirurgià, és stat examinat per los honrats En Jacme Maderes, maestre en arts e en medicina, et En Pere Gironés, baxeller en medicina, conciutadans nostres e metges de la dita ciutat, examinadors per nós e per los honrats jurats de la damunt dita ciutat asignats e deputats a examinar los metges volents usar o praticar de medicina en la dita ciutat de València et regne de aquella, per los quals lo dit En Bernat Gener, *alias* Fuster, és stat atrobat abte et sufficient de usar e pra//ticar en art de física o medecina et cirurgia, excepta que ell no use ne s'entrameta en les cures de física et cirurgia següents, ço és, de cirurgia, axí com són nafres de cap et de pits, de budells et de altres nafres perilloses; et de física, de malalties perilloses, axí com són febres contínues e frenesis et altres malalties hagudes, sens altre cohaduït o acompanyat metge o metges autèntichs o de auctoritat pus sp[erts], sots la pena en furs et privilegis contenguda, segons que a nós és cert de totes les dites coses ab letra certificatòria dels dits honrats examinadors, *que data fuit Valentie, .XXIIª. die ianuarii anno a nativitate Domini millesimo .CCC°. LXXX°. tertio,* et presentada a nós per lo dit En Bernat Gener, *alias* Fuster, en lo dia data de la present. Per la qual cosa, avén rehebut de aquell primerament e abans sagrament sobre los sants Evangelis de Déu, per la sua man dreta corporalment tocats, segons forma de furs et privilegis, que bé et lealment se hauria en usar de la dita art de físicha e de cirurgia, havem donat a aquell licència de usar et praticar en la dita ciutat et regne de aquella de la dita art de medicina, ço es, en física et en cirurgia, en e per la manera dessús centada (*sic*) et recomptada, sens temor et incursió o ind[uc]ció de alguna pena que a aquell e béns seus no sia exhigida o levada. En testimoni de les quals coses, manam a aquell ésser feyta la present carta testimonial, sots [. . .]ment del sagell de la nostra cord (*sic*) empendent [sagellada]. *Data Valentie .IXª. die februarii anno a nativitate Domini millesimo .CCC°.LXXX°. tertio.*

* * *

In the year of our Lord 1383, Monday the 9th of February, appeared Bernat Giner, alias Fuster, physician-surgeon, before the honorable Johan de Cervató, civil justiciar of the city of Valencia; and he presented him with a letter from the honorable Jacme Maderes and Pere Gironés, examiners for the current year of surgeon-practitioners in the said city, whose tenor is as follows:

To the honorable lord civil justiciar of the city of Valencia, or his lieutenant; from us, Jacme Maderes, master in arts and in medicine, and Pere Gironés, bachelor in medicine, citizens of the said city, examiners appointed for the current year to practitioners newly arrived and wishing to practice medicine and surgery in the said city and kingdom of Valencia; health and honor. We inform your lordship that Bernat Giner, alias Fuster, has appeared before us and has asked us that we examine him in medicine and in surgery; we have examined him in the said skill in the customary manner, and have found that the said Bernat Gener is not learned, but has long practiced in medicine and in surgery; and given the long involvement that he has had with practicing physicians and in this skill, as a number of practitioners of long standing have certified in a public document that we have seen, we judge the said Bernat Giner to be competent to practice medicine and surgery in the said city and kingdom of Valencia—with the restriction that he not engage in surgery on dangerous wounds (as wounds of the head, the chest, the intestines, and other dangerous wounds) or in medicinal treatment of dangerous illnesses (like continued fevers and frenzy and other acute diseases) unless he is assisted by another expert physician or physicians of authority, under the penalty prescribed by the *fur.* Wherefore, at the request of the said Bernat Giner, notifying you, honored justiciar, or your lieutenant, of the said things, we send on the said Bernat and request that you grant permission to him, the said En Bernat Giner, to exercise, employ, and practice the said skills of medicine and surgery within the said city and kingdom in the manner set out above, taking oath from him that he will fulfill and not contravene it.

Given at Valencia, the 22nd day of January, 1383 AD.

When this letter had been presented, the said honorable [justiciar] took the oath of the said Bernat Giner on the holy Gospels that he would engage well and loyally in the said practice of surgery and physic, with the restriction imposed above by the said examiners. And furthermore he commanded that the following certificate be drawn up for him:

To each and every official in the kingdom of Valencia to whom these presents may come, or to their lieutenants; from us, Johan de Cervató, civil justiciar of the city of Valencia; health and deserved honor. By these presents we inform you that Bernat Giner, also called Fuster, physician and surgeon, has been examined by the honorable Jacme Maderes, master in arts and in medicine, and Pere Gironés, bachelor in medicine, physicians of the said city and our fellow citizens, examiners appointed by us and by the honorable *jurats* of the aforementioned city to examine practitioners wishing to practice medicine in the said city of Valencia and its kingdom; by whom the said Bernat Giner, alias Fuster, has been found competent to practice the art of physic or medicine and surgery, except that he may not use or engage in the following medical and surgical treatments: for surgery, wounds of the head, the chest, the intestines, and other dangerous wounds; for physic, dangerous illnesses like continued fevers and frenzy and other acute diseases—unless he is assisted or accompanied by another physician or physicians, authorized or of greater expertise, under the penalty prescribed by the *furs* and privileges; all of which has been certified to us by a certificate from the said honorable examiners, "which was given at Valencia, the 22nd day of January, 1383 AD," presented to us by the said Bernat Giner, alias Fuster, on the present day. Wherefore we, having first received from him an oath on the holy Gospels of God, while he physically touched them with his right hand as prescribed by the *furs* and privileges, that he will engage well and loyally in practicing the said art of physic and surgery, have given him license to practice the said art of medicine, that is, physic and surgery, in the said city and its kingdom, in the manner described above, without fear or imposition of any penalty that might be imposed on him or his possessions. In testimony of which things we have ordered the present certificate to be drawn up for him, under . . . the pendent seal of our court.

Given at Valencia, the 9th day of February, 1383 AD.

12

Valencia, 23 October 1383.

Francesc Maestre Assensi de Toscana, of Perugia, expert in the treatment of hernias, is authorized to practice his art in the city and environs of Valencia (ARV, Justícia Civil [Lletres], 459, seventh quire, fol. 12).

Anno a nativitate Domini millesimo .CCC^{o}.LXXX°. tertio, die veneris .XXIII^{a}. octobris. Denant l'onrat En Johan de Cervató, justícia de la ciutat de València en lo civil, comparech En Francesch Maestre Assensi de Tosquana, de la ciutat de Perusa, et presentà a aquell una letra dels honrats En Jacme Maderes, maestre en arts e en medecina, e En Pere Gironés, bacheller en medecina, examinadors en l'any present deputats a examinar los metges, de la tenor e continència següent:

A l'honrat e discret sènyer lo justícia de la ciutat de València en lo civil, o a son lochtinent. De nós, En Jacme Marades (*sic*), maestre en arts e en medecina, e En Pere Gironés, baxeller en medecina, ciutadans de la dita ciutat, examinadors en l'any present deputats a exhaminar los metges qui novellament vénen e volen exercir e praticar en la dita ciutat e regne de València en física e en cirurgia. Salut e honor. Certificam, sènyer, a la vostra discreció, que lo discret En Francesch Maestre Assensi de Toscana, de la ciutat de Perusa, en lo dia present és comparegut denant nós, e request nós que.l deguessem examinar en feyt de ruptures o trencadures, *alias* potres, lo qual havem exhaminat en la dita facultat segons forma acostumada e havem trobat e reputat e reputam aquell apte e suficient en praticar, usar e exarcir medecina de les dites ruptures, *alias* trencadures, ab tallar o sens tallar; per què, instant e requirent lo dit En Francesch Maestre Sensi, intiman les dites coses ab la present a vós, dit honrat justícia o lochtinent vostre, remetem aquell dit En Francesch Maestre Assensi, e preguam e requirim que donets licència e facultat a ell que pugua exercir, usar et // praticar en la dita ciutat e regne e (*sic*) de la dita medecina de reptures, *alias* potres, reebut sagrament d'ell que d'altra cosa no s'entrametrà. *Data Valentie vicesima die octobris anno a nativitate Domini .M^{o}.CCC^{o}. LXXX°. tertio.*

Et presentada la dita letra, encontinent lo dit justícia dix que reebia a aquella aytant com per fur e rahó era reebedora, et no empús. Et nores-menys lo dit justícia reebé sagrament del dit En Francesch Maestre Assensi de Toschana sobre los sants quatre Evvangelis de Déu, per virtut del qual, interrogat, respòs e dix que se hauria bé e lealment en lo dit ar(t) de reptures *alias* trenchadures. Et, reebut lo dit sagrament, encontinent lo dit justícia donà licència e facultat al dit En Francesch Maestre Assensi de Toschana, que pogués usar del dit art de ruptures per tota la dita ciutat e terme de aquella.

* * *

In the year of our Lord 1383, Friday the 23rd of October, appeared Francesch Maestre Assensi de Toscana, of the city of Perugia, before the honorable Johan de Cervató, civil justiciar of the city of Valencia; and he presented him with a letter from the honorable Jacme Maderes, master in arts and in medicine, and Pere Gironés, bachelor in medicine, examiners for the current year deputed to examine practitioners, whose tenor and contents are as follows:

To the honorable lord civil justiciar of the city of Valencia, or his lieutenant; from us, Jacme Maderes, master in arts and medicine, and Pere Gironés, bachelor in medicine, citizens of the said city, examiners appointed for the current year to examine practitioners newly arrived and wishing to practice medicine and surgery in the said city and kingdom of Valencia; health and honor. We inform your lordship that Francesch Mastre Assensi de Toscana, of the city of Perugia, has appeared before us today, and has asked us that we examine him on ruptures or hernias, alias *potres;* whom we have examined on this skill in the customary manner, and have found him to be competent to practice treatment for the said ruptures or hernias, with or without cutting; wherefore, at the request of the said Francesch Maestre Sensi, we notify you, honored justiciar, or your lieutenant, of the said things, [and] we send the said Francesch Maestre Assensi to you and request that you grant him license to exercise, employ, and practice the said treatment of ruptures, alias *potres,* within the said city and kingdom, taking oath from him that he will engage in nothing more.

Given at Valencia, the 20th day of October, 1383 AD.

When this letter had been presented, the said justiciar said that he received it as prescribed by the *fur* and by reason, and nothing more; and furthermore the said justiciar took the oath of the said Francesch Maestre de Toschana on the four holy Gospels of God, according to which, questioned, he replied that he would engage well and loyally in the said art of [treating] ruptures or hernias.

When he had received the said oath, the said justiciar immediately gave license to the said Francesch Maestre Assensi de Toschana to use the said art of [treating] ruptures thoughout all the said city and its dependencies.

13

Valencia, 24 January 1388.

Maymó Abdochaxis, Muslim, a barber of Manises, receives a license to treat simple wounds and abcesses, after having been examined and having taken an oath by the Qu'ran to practice the art of surgery well and honestly (ARV, Justícia Civil, 550, fols. 30r–31r).

Anno a nativitate Domini .M°.CCC°.LXXX°.VIII°., die veneris .XXIIII. ianuarii. Denant l'onrat En Jacme Valleriola, justícia de la ciutat de València en lo civil, comparech lo Maymó Abdochaxis, barber del loch de Manizes, e presentà a.quell una letra dels examinadós dels metges, uberta, en paper scrita, sagellada ab dos sagells dels dits examinadós en cera, la un ver(t) e l'altre vermell, la tenor de la qual és *ut sequitur*:

Al molt honrat sènyer lo justícia de la ciutat de València, o a son lochtinent. De nós, En Jacme Maderes, mestre en arts e en medecina, e En Jacme d'Avinyó, batxeller en medecina, ciutadans de la dita ciutat, examinadós en l'any present deputats e assignats per los honrats justícia (e) jurats de la ciutat per examinar tots e sengles metges de phísica e cirorgia vinents nov(e)llament a praticar e usar de la dita art en la ciutat de València e lochs e viles del regne de aquella. Salut, ab creximent de prosperitat e honor. Sàpia la vostra honrada discreció ésser comparegut denant nós Maymó Abdochaxis, barber del loch de Manizes, dient e affermant sí volent usar e praticar de nafres simples, apostemes, lo qual havem bé e deligentment examinat e aquell havem atrobat suficient en les dites nafres simples fetes en la *carni tantum* e en obrir apostemes, e no en pus. Per què, honrat sènyer justícia, instant e requerint lo dit Maymó Abdochaxis, per la tenor de la present vos certificam de les dites coses e us requerim e pregam en deute de justícia que us plàcia donar licència e fer a aquell carta testimonial sí e segons que en semblants feyts per vós e vostra cort és acostumat fer, prestat per ell ans e primerament sagrament que bé e llealment usarà e praticarà en la ciutat de València e en los lochs e regne de aquella de nafres simples feytes en la *carni tantum* e obrir apostemes, e no s'entrametrà de plus, sots les penes contengudes en fur de València, com nós, sènyer, siam apparellats los vostres justs manaments obeir e enseguir. En testimoni de les quals coses fem-vos fer la present letra, per nós a ell liurada, e ab nostres sagells sagellada. *Data* en València a .XXI. dia de jener de l'any de la nativitat de nostre Senyor .M.CCC.LXXX. huit.

Et presentada la dita letra, encontinent lo dit honrat justícia ena(n)tà de rebre sagrament del dit Maymó Abdochxis, barber dessús dit, en la forma següent: //

En Maymó Abd[och]xis, barber, moro, jurà girant la cara ves migjorn per Déu e per l'alchibla, segons zuna e xara dels moros, que bé e lealment s'aurà en la dita art de cirorgia, en per la forma en la dessús dita letra per los dits examinadors contenguda, e servarà totes aquelles coses en aquella contengudes.

Et rebut lo dit sagrament del dit Maymó Abdolo[ch]xis, barber, moro dessús dit, encontinent lo dit honrat justícia donà licència e plen poder al dit Maymó Abdolochxis, moro, de usar e praticar de art de barber o cirorgià dins la ciutat e regne de València sens alguna pena.

Et encontinent lo dit Maymó Abdochis, moro, requerí de paraula lo dit honrat justícia que letra testimonial li fos feta general a tots universes e sengles officials o loch de senyoria tinents, que hajen per metge al dit Maymó Abdochis, moro, e que en praticar e usar en la dita art de cirorgia no li sia feyt algun contrast o enbarch.

Per què de continent lo dit honrat justícia manà ésser feta la letra testimonial en la forma següent:

Als honrats universes e sengles offic[i]als e loch de senyoria tinents dins lo regne de València constituhits als quals la present pervendrà o presentada serà, o a lurs lochtinents. De nós, En Jacme Valleriola, justícia de la ciutat de València en lo civil. Salut e honor. Per tenor de les presents vos significam que Maymó Abdochis, moro, barber del loch de Manizes, és stat examinat per los honrats e discrets En Jacme Maderes, mestre en arts e en medecina, e En Jacme Avinyó, bacheler en medeçina, ciutadans de la dita ciutat, examinadors en l'any present deputats e assignats per nós e per los honrats jurats de la ciutat damunt dita, per los quals lo dit Maymó Abdochis és stat atrobat abte e suficient de usar e praticar de art de cirorgia, ço és, en nafres simples fetes en la carn solament e obrir apostemes, e no empús, segons que a nós és cert // per letr[a] dels dits examinadors per lo dit Maymó Adochixs a nós presentada, *que data fuit Valentie .XXIª. die mensis ianuarie anno a nativitate Domini .Mº.CCCº. LXXXº.VIIIº et infrascripto*, per la qual cosa nós, reebut per aquell primerament e abans sagrament segons zuna e xara de moros, en o per la forma en la dessús dita letra per los dits examinadors contenguda, que bé e lealment se haurà en la dita art de cirurgia, havem donat e atorgat a aquell licència de usar e praticar en la dita ciutat de València e regne de aquella de la dita art de cirurgia en la forma dessús dita sens temor de alguna pena. En testimoni de les quals coses manam li ésser feyta la present carta testimonial ab lo sagell del nostre offici en pendent sagellada. *Data Valentie .XXª. prima (sic) die mensis ianuarii anno a nativitate Domini .Mº.CCCº.LXXX.VIIIº.*

* * *

In the year of our Lord 1388, Friday the 24th of January, appeared Maymó Abdochaxis, a barber from the village of Manises, before the honorable Jacme Valleriola, civil justiciar of the city of Valencia; and he presented him with a letter from the examiners of physicians, open, written on paper, sealed in wax with the two seals of the said examiners (one green and the other red), whose tenor is as follows:

To the honorable lord justiciar of the city of Valencia, or his lieutenant; from us, Jacme Maderes, master in arts and in medicine, and Jacme d'Avinyó, bachelor in medicine, citizens of the said city, examiners appointed for the current year by the honorable justiciar and *jurats* of the said city to examine each and every practitioner of physic and of surgery newly come to practice the said art in the city of Valencia and in the villages and towns of its kingdom; health, with increase of wealth and honor. May your worship know that Maymó Abdochaxis, a barber of the village of Manises, has appeared before us, declaring that he wishes to practice on simple wounds and apostemes, and we have carefully examined him and have found him competent in [treating] simple flesh wounds and in opening apostemes, but nothing more. Wherefore, honored sir, at the request of the said Maymó Abdochaxis, we certify the said things to you by these presents and request in accordance with the law that it please you to grant him license and prepare for him a certificate, as you and your court are accustomed to do in such cases—he first taking an oath that he will practice well and loyally in the city of Valencia and in its villages and kingdom, [treating] simple flesh wounds and opening apostemes but engaging in nothing more, under the penalties set out in the Valencian *fur*, as we, lord, are prepared to obey and follow your just orders. In testimony of which things we have drawn up for you the present letter, given by us to him, and sealed with our seals.

Given at Valencia, 21 January 1388 AD.

When this letter had been presented, the said honorable justiciar immediately proceeded to receive an oath from the said Maymó Abdochxis, the abovementioned barber, according to the following form:

Maymó Abdocxis, barber, Muslim, turning his face towards the south, swears by God and the *qibla*, by the *zuna* and *xara* of the Muslims, that he will engage well and loyally in the said art of surgery, in the manner set out in the above-mentioned letter from the said examiners, and will obey all the conditions contained in it.

When the oath of the said Maymó Abdolochxis, barber, Muslim, had been taken, the said honorable justiciar immediately gave license to the said Maymó Abdolochxis, Muslim, to practice as a barber or surgeon in the city and kingdom of Valencia without any penalty.

And immediately the said Maymó Abdochis, Muslim, requested orally that the said honorable justiciar prepare him a general certificate to each and every official , that they accept the said Maymó Abdochis, Muslim, as a practitioner, and that no let or hindrance be raised against him in practicing the said art of surgery.

Whereupon the said honorable justiciar immediately ordered a certificate to be drawn up in the following form:

To all officials in the kingdom of Valencia to whom these presents may come, or to their lieutenants; from us, Jacme Valleriola, civil justiciar of the city of Valencia; health and honor. By these presents we certify to you that Maymó Abdochis, Muslim, barber of the village of Manises, has been examined by the honorable Jacme Maderes, master in arts and medicine, and Jacme Avinyó, bachelor in medicine, citizens of the said city, examiners appointed for the current year by us and by the honorable *jurats* of the aforementioned city, by whom the said Maymó Abdochis has been found competent to practice the art of surgery—that is, [to treat] simple flesh wounds and to open apostemes, and nothing more—as has been certified to us by a letter from the said examiners presented to us by the said Maymó Adochixs, which "was given at Valencia the 21st day of January 1388 AD *et infrascripto*"; wherefore we, having first received from him an oath by the *zuna* and *xara* of the Muslims, according to the form set out in the above letter from the said examiners, that he will engage well and loyally in the said art of surgery, have granted him license to practice the said art of surgery according to the manner defined above within the city of Valencia and its kingdom, without fear of any penalty. In testimony of which things we have commanded the present certificate to be drawn up for him, sealed with the seal of our office affixed.

Given at Valencia, the 21st day of January, 1388 AD.

14

Valencia, 25 January 1388.

Guillem Vives is authorized to practice certain aspects of the art of surgery, after having been declared qualified by the examiners and having sworn before the justiciar to act honestly in his craft (ARV, Justícia Civil, 550, fol. 33r–v).

Als honrats universes e sengles officials e loch de senyoria tinents dins lo regne de València constituhits als quals la present pervendrà o presentada serà, o a lurs lochtinents. De nós, En Jacme Valleriola, justícia de la ciutat de València en lo civil. Salut e honor. Per tenor de les presents vos significam que En Guillem Vives, de la dita ciutat de Xàtiva, és estat examinat per los honrats e discrets En Jacme Maderes Maderes (*sic*), mestr[e] en arts e en medecina, e En Jacme d'Avinyó, baxeler [e]n medecina, ciutadans de la dita ciutat, examinadors en l'any present deputats e assignats per nós e per los honrats jurats de la ciutat damunt dita, per los quals lo dit En Guillem Vives és stat atrobat abte e suficient de usar e praticar de art de cirurgia, ço és a saber, en nafres simples feites en la superfíciens (*sic*) de la carn *tantum* e en obrir floroncos e curar aquells, e no de més av[an]t, segons que a nós és cert per letra de les dits examinadors per lo dit En Guillem Vives a nós presentada, *que data fuit Valentie vicessima tertia ianuarii anno a nativitate Domini .M^o.CCC^o.LXXX°. octavo et infrascripto*, per la qual cosa nós, reebut per aquell primerament e abans sagrament // sobre los sants Evangelis de nostre se[n]yor Déu, de la man dreta de aquell corporalment toca[ts], segons forma de fur, que bé e lealment se haurà en la dita art de cirurgia en la forma dessús dita, havem donat e atorgat a aquell licència de usar e praticar en la dita ciutat de València e regne de aquella de la dita art de cirurgia sens temor de alcuna pena. En testimoni de les quals coses manam li ésser feyta la present carta testimonial ab lo sagell del nostre offici en pendent sagellada. *Data Valentie .XXV^a. ianuarii anno a nativitate Domini .M^o.CCC^o.LXXX°. octavo.*

* * *

To all officials in the kingdom of Valencia to whom these presents may come, or to their lieutenants; from us, Jacme Valleriola, civil justiciar of the city of Valencia; health and honor.

By these presents we notify you that Guillem Vives, of the said city of Xàtiva, has been examined by the honorable Jacme Maderes, master in arts and in medicine, and Jacme d'Avinyó, bachelor in medicine, citizens of the said city, examiners appointed for the current year by us and by the honorable *jurats* of the aforesaid city; by whom the said Guillem Vives has been found competent to practice the art of surgery—that is, in simple superficial flesh wounds only, and in opening furuncles and treating them, and nothing more—as is certified to us by a letter from the said examiners given to us by the said Guillem Vives, which was "given at Valencia 23 January 1388 *et infrascripto.*" Wherefore we, having first received from him an oath on the holy Gospels of our Lord God, while he physically touched them with his right hand, as prescribed by the *fur*, that he will act well and loyally in the said art of surgery in the manner specified above, have given him license to practice the said art of surgery in the said city of Valencia and its kingdom without fear of any penalty. In testimony of which things we have ordered the present certificate to be drawn up for him, sealed with the pendent seal of our office.

Given at Valencia, 25 January 1388 AD.

15

Valencia, 29 January 1388.

Grant of a license to Andreu Martí of Guinarch (Sinarcas?) to practice hernial surgery (ARV, Justícia Civil, 550, fol. 35r–v).

Als honrats [un]iverses e sengles officials o loch de senyoria tinents dins lo regne de València constituïts als quals la present pervendrà o presentada serà, o a lur(s) lochtinents. De nós, En Jacme Valleriola, justícia de la ciutat de València en lo civil. Salut e honor. Per tenor de les presents vos significam que mestre Andreu Martí, del loch de Guinarch, és estat examinat per los honrats e discrets En Jacme Maderes, mestre en arts e en medicina, e En Jacme d'Avinyó, batxeler en medicina, ciutadans de la dita ciutat, examinadors en l'any present deputats e assignats per nós e per los honrats jurats de la ciutat damunt dita per examinar totes e sengles metges de phísica e de cirurgia volents novellament prati[car e] usar de la dita art en la ciutat de València e regne de aquella, per los quals lo dit mestre Andreu Martí és estat atrobat abte e suficient de usar e praticar de art de cirurgia, ço és, de ruptura dindimal, lo qual és inflació hernial, en la qual lo budell o lo cre[. . .] és dislogat e exit de les parts de dintre a la carn del mirach pròpriament *in dindimo* e *osseo seu testiculorum bursa,* e no de més avant, segons que a nós és cert per letra dels dits examinadors per lo dit mestre Andreu Martí a nós presentada, *que data fuit Valentie .XXVI^a^. ianuarii anno a nativitate Domini .M^o^.CCC^o^.LXXX°.VIII° et infrascripto,* per la qual cosa nós, reebut per aquell primerament e abans sagrament sobre los [s]ants Evangelis de nostre senyor Déu de la man dreta de aquell corporalment tocats, segons forma de fur, que bé e lealment se haurà en la dita art de cirurgia e en la forma dessús dita, e no en àls, havem donat e atorgat a aquell licència de usar e prati[c]ar en la dita ciutat de València e regne de aquella de la dita a[r]t de cirurgia sens temor de alcuna p[e]na. En testimoni de les quals coses manam li // li (*sic*) ésser feyta la present carta testimonial ab [lo] segell del nostre offici en pendent sagellada. *Data Valentie .XXIX°. die ianuarii anno a nativitate [Domini] .M^o^.CCC^o^.LXXXVIII°.*

* * *

To all officials in the kingdom of Valencia to whom these presents may come, or to their lieutenants; from us, Jacme Valleriola, civil justiciar of the city of Valencia; health and honor.

By these presents we notify you that master Andreu Martí, of the village of Guinarch, has been examined by the honorable Jacme Maderes, master in arts and in medicine, and Jacme d'Avinyó, bachelor in medicine, citizens of the said city, examiners appointed for the current year by us and by the honorable *jurats* of the aforesaid city to examine each and every practitioner of physic and of surgery wishing to begin to practice the said art in the said city of Valencia and its kingdom; by whom the said master Andreu Martí has been found competent to practice and employ the art of surgery—that is, in dindimal rupture or hernial swelling, in which the intestine or the *cre*[. . .] is displaced and comes out from the inner parts to the *mirach,* namely *in dindimo* and *osseo seu testiculorum bursa,* and no more —as is certified to us by a letter from the said examiners given to us by the said master Andreu Martí, which was "given at Valencia 26 January 1388 *et infrascripto.*" Wherefore we, having first received from him an oath on the holy Gospels of our Lord God, while he physically touched them with his right hand, as prescribed by the *fur,* that he will engage well and loyally in the said art of surgery in the manner specified above, have given him license to practice the said art of surgery in the said city of Valencia and its kingdom without fear of any penalty. In testimony of which things we have ordered the present certificate to be drawn up for him, sealed with the pendent seal of our office.

Given at Valencia on the 29th day of January 1388 AD.

16

Valencia, 29 January 1388.

Guillem Gaubert of Montauban (France) receives a license to practice surgery in the kingdom of Valencia (ARV, Justícia Civil, 550, fol. 37r–v).

Als honrats universes e sengles officials o loch de senyoria tinents dins lo regne de València constituïts als quals la present pervendrà o presentada serà, o a lus lochtinents. De nós, En Jacme Valleriola, justícia de la ciutat de València en lo civil. Salut e honor. Per tenor de les presents vos significam que mestre Guillem Gaubert, de la ciutat de Muntalbà, prop Tolosa, és stat examinat per los honrats e discrets En Jacme Maderes, mestre en arts e en medicina, e En Jacme d'Avinyó, batxeler en medicina, ciutadans de la dita ciutat, examinadors en l'any present deputats e assignats per nós e per los honrats jurats de la ciutat damunt dita a examinar tots e sengles metges de física e de cirurgia volents novellament praticar e usar de la dita art en la dita ciutat de València e regne de aquella, per los quals lo dit mestre Guillem Gaubert és stat atrobat apte e suficient de usar e praticar de art de cirurgia, segons que a nós és cert per letra dels dits examinadors per lo dit mestre Guillem Gaubert a nós presentada, *que data fuit Valentie .XXVII^{a}. ianuarii anno a nativitate Domini millesimo .CCC^{o}.LXXX°. octavo et infrascripto,* per la qual cosa nós, reebut per aquell primerament e abans sagrament sobre los sants Evangelis de nostre senyor Déu, de la mà dreta de aquell corporalment tocats, segons forma de fur, que bé e lealment se haurà en la dita art de cirurgia, havem donat a aquell licència de usar e praticar en la dita ciutat de València e regne de // aquella de la dita art de cirurgia sens temor de alcuna pena. En testimoni de les quals coses manam li ésser feyta la present carta testimonial ab lo segell del nostre offici en pendent sagellada. *Data Valentie .XXIX^{a}. die ianuarii anno a nativitate Domini .M^{o}.CCC^{o}.LXXX°. octavo.*

* * *

To all officials in the kingdom of Valencia to whom these presents may come, or to their lieutenants; from us, Jacme Valleriola, civil justiciar of the city of Valencia; health and honor. By these presents we notify you that master Guillem Gaubert of the city of Montauban, near Toulouse, has been examined by the honorable masters Jacme Maderes, master in arts and in medicine, and Jacme d'Avinyó, bachelor in medicine, citizens of the said city, examiners appointed for the current year by us and by the honorable *jurats* of the aforesaid city to examine each and every practitioner of physic and of surgery wishing to begin to practice the said art in the said city of Valencia and its kingdom; by whom the said master Guillem Gaubert has been found competent to practice the art of surgery, as certified to us by a letter from the said examiners given to us by the said master Guillem Gaubert, which was "given at Valencia 27 January 1388 *et infrascripto.*" Wherefore we, having first received from him an oath on the holy Gospels of our Lord God, while he physically touched them with his right hand, as prescribed by the *fur,* that he will act well and loyally in the said art of surgery, have given him license to practice the said art of surgery in the said city of Valencia and its kingdom without fear of any penalty. In testimony of which things we have ordered the present certificate to be drawn up for him, sealed with the pendent seal of our office.

Given at Valencia 19 January 1388 AD.

17

Valencia, 20 February 1388.

Joan Cabrera, of Valencia, is granted a licence to practice medicine and surgery in the kingdom of Valencia (ARV, Justícia Civil, 550, fol. 38r–v).

Anno a nativitate Domini .M°.CCC°.LXXX°.VII[I]°., die iovis .XX^a. februarii. Denant l'onrat En Jacme [V]ayllleriola, justícia de la ciutat de València en lo civil, comparech En Johan Cabrera, cirurgià, et a instància e requisició de aquell, lo dit justícia manà ésser feta a aquell la letra següent:

Als honrats universes e sengles officials e loch de senyoria tinents dins lo regne de València constituïts als quals la present pervendrà o presentada serà. De nós, En Jacme Valleriola, justícia de la ciutat de València en lo civil. Salut e honor. Per tenor de la present vos significam que l'honrat En Francesch Despulgues, cavaller, justícia de la dita ciutat en lo civil, precessor nostre en lo dit offici, ab letra sua de la tenor següent— "Als honrats universes e sengles officials e loch de senyoria tinens dins lo regne de València constituhits als quals la present pervendrà o presentada serà, o a lurs lochtinents. De nós, En Francesch Despulgues, justícia de la ciutat de València en lo civil. Salut e honor. Per tenor de les presents vos significam que En Johan Cabrera, habitant en la dita ciutat, és stat examinat per los honrats e discrets maestre Pere Figuerola e maestre Bernat d'Artesa, phísichs de la dita ciutat, examinadós deputats e assignats per nós e per los honrats jurats de la ciutat damunt dita, per los quals lo dit En Johan Cabrera és stat atrobat apte e sufficient de usar e praticar de art de cirurgia, segons que a nós és cert per letra dels dits examinadors per lo dit En Johan Cabrera a nós presentada, *que data fuit Valentie .XI^a. die mensis februarii anno a nativitate Domini .M°.CCC°.LXXX°. septimo et infrascripto,* per la qual cosa nós, reebut de aquell primerament e abans sagrament sobre los sants Evangelis de nostre senyor Déu, de la man dreta de aquell corporalment tocats, segons forma de fur, que bé e lealment se haurà en la dita art de cirurgia, havem donat e atorgat a aquell licència de usar e praticar en la dita ciutat de València e regne de aquella de la dita art de cirurgia sens temor de alguna pena. En testimoni de les quals coses manam li ésser feyta la present carta testimonial ab lo sagell del nostre offici en pendent sagellada. *Data Valentie .XII^a. die februarii anno a nativitate Domini millesimo .CCC^o. LXXX°. septimo.*"—haver donada licència e facult[at] al dit En Johan Cabrera, habitant en la dita ciutat, examinat e sufficient trobat per los honrats e discrets maestre Pere Figuerola e maestre Bernat d'Artesa de usar e praticar de art de cirurgia en la dita ciutat e regne de València, segons que en la desús dita letra havem vist ésser contengut. E en lo dia de huy, data de la present, lo dit En Johan Cabrera sia comparegut denant nós, dient que com ell duptàs per vigor de la desús dita licència en l'any present e d'ací avant usar e praticar de la dita art de cirurgia e de físicha, e per ço ha supplicat e request nós, axí com a president en lo dit offici, e als honrats jurats de la dita ciutat, que ab altra letra nostra donàssem a aquell semblant licència que.l dit nostre predecessor havia donada e atorgada a aquell, e més encara, ampliant la dita licència donàssem a aquell licència de usar e praticar de art de físicha, e nós, vehents les dites coses requestes e supplicades ésser justes e a rahó consonants, per tal, ab tenor de la present, per auctoritat de l'offici del qual usam, de voler dels dits honrats jurats de la dita ciutat, donam e atorgam a vós, dit En Johan Cabrera, licència e plenària facultat de usar e praticar en la dita ciutat e regne de València de les dites arts de cirurgia e físicha sens encorriment de les penes en fur de València sobre açò stablides. En testimoni de les quals coses manam ésser feta e liurada la present letra testimonial ab lo sagell de l'offici a nós comanat en pendent sagellada. *Data Valentie .XX^a. die februarii anno a nativitate Domini .M^o.CCC^o.LXXX°.VIII°.*

* * *

In the year of our Lord 1388, Thursday 20 February, Johan Cabrera, surgeon, appeared before the honorable Jacme Vayllleriola, civil justiciar of the city of Valencia, and at his request the said justiciar commanded the following letter to be drawn up for him:

To all officials in the kingdom of Valencia to whom these presents may come; from us, Jacme Valleriola, civil justiciar of the city of Valencia; health and honor. By these presents we notify you that the honorable Francesch Despulgues, knight, civil justiciar of the said city and our predecessor in the said office, with a letter reading as follows— "To all officials in the kingdom of Valencia to whom these presents may come, or to their lieutenants; from us, Francesch Despulgues, civil justiciar of the city of Valencia; health and honor. By these presents we notify you that Johan Cabrera, an inhabitant of the said city, has been examined by the honorable masters Pere Figuerola and Bernat d'Artesa, physicians of the said city, examiners appointed by us and by the honorable *jurats* of the aforesaid city, by whom the said Johan Cabrera has been found competent to practice the art of surgery, as certified to us by a letter from the said examiners given to us by the said Johan Cabrera, which was 'given at Valencia 11 February 1387 *et infrascripto.*' Wherefore we, having first received from him an oath on the holy Gospels of our Lord God, while he physically touched them with his right hand, as prescribed by the *fur*, that he will act well and loyally in the said art of surgery, have given him license to practice the said art of surgery in the said city of Valencia and its kingdom without fear of any penalty. In testimony of which things we have ordered the present certificate to be drawn up for him, sealed with the pendent seal of our office. Given at Valencia 12 February 1387 AD." —gave license to the said Johan Cabrera, living in the said city and examined and found competent by the honorable masters Pere Figuerola and Bernat d'Artesa, to practice the art of surgery in the said city and kingdom of Valencia, as we have verified in the letter given above. And today, on the date of this letter, the said Johan Cabrera has appeared before us, saying that because he questioned the validity of the above license for the current year for practicing the said art of surgery *and physic* from today henceforth, he wished us as presiding in the said office together with the honorable *jurats* of the said city to grant him another letter of our own, granting him a license similar to that which our said predecessor granted to him; and more, to extend the said license by granting him license to practice the art of physic. And we, seeing these things requested to be just and reasonable, therefore by these presents, by the authority of the office which we perform, by the will of the said honorable *jurats* of the said city, grant to you the said Johan Cabrera license and full permission to practice the said arts of surgery and physic in the said city and kingdom of Valencia without incurring the penalties laid down by the *furs* of Valencia in this regard. In testimony of which things we have ordered the present certificate to be drawn up and given to him, sealed with the pendent seal of the office committed to us.

Given at Valencia, 20 February 1388 AD.

18

Valencia, 13 April 1388.

Jucef Çameja, Jew of Alzira, is authorized to practice medicine throughout the kingdom of Valencia (ARV, Justícia Civil, 550, fols. 39v–40r).

Als honrats universes e sengles officials e loch de senyoria tinents dins lo regne de València consti[tu]ïts als quals la present pervendrà o presentada serà, o a lurs lochtinents. De nós, En Jacme Valleriola, justícia de la ciutat de València en lo civil. Sal(u)t e honor. Per tenor de les presents vos significam que Jucef Çameja, juheu del loch de Alzezira, és stat examinat per los honrats e discrets En Jacme Maderes, maestre en arts e en medicina, e En Jacme d'Avinyó, bacheler en medicina, ciuta//dans de la dita ciutat de València, examinadors, en l'any present d[i]putats e asignats per nós e per l'onrats jurats de la dita ciutat, de phísica, e per los quals lo dit Jucef Çameja és stat atrobat apte e suficient a usar e praticar de la dita art de phísica, segons que a nós és cert per letra dels dits examinadors per lo dit Jucef Çameja a nós presentada, *que data fuit Valentie .X*^{a}. *die aprilis anno a nativitate Do-*

mini millesimo .CCC^{o}.LXXX°. octavo et infrascripto, per la qual cosa nós, reebut per aquell primerament e abans sagrament sobre los deu manaments de la lig que Déus donà a Moysé en lo mont de Sinaý de la man dreta de aquell corporalment toquats, segons forma de fur, que bé e lealment se haurà en la dita art de phísica, havem donat a aquell licència de usar e praticar en la dita ciutat de València e regne de aquella de la dita art de phísica sens temor de alguna pena. En testimoni de les quals coses manam li éser feyta la present carta testimonial ab lo segell del nostre ofici en pendent segellada. *Data Valentie .XIII^{a}. mensis aprilis anno a nativitate Domini .M^{o}.CCC^{o}.LXXX°.VIII°.*

* * *

To all honorable officials in the kingdom of Valencia to whom these presents may come, or to their lieutenants; from us, Jacme Valleriola, civil justiciar of the city of Valencia; health and honor.

By these presents I declare to you that Jucef Çameja, a Jew from the village of Alzira, has been examined by the honorable Jacme Maderes, master in arts and in medicine, and Jacme d'Avinyó, bachelor in medicine, citizens of the said city of Valencia, examiners in physic appointed for the current year by us and by the honorable *jurats* of the said city, and that the said Jucef Çameja has been found competent by them to practice the said art of physic, as is certified to us by a letter from the said examiners given to us by the said Jucef Çameja, "given at Valencia 10 April 1389 *et infrascripto*." Wherefore we, having first received from him an oath on the ten commandments of the law that God gave to Moses on Mount Sinai while he physically touched them with his right hand, as prescribed by the *fur*, that he will act well and loyally in the said art of physic, have given him license to practice the said art of physic in the said city of Valencia and its kingdom without fear of any penalty. In testimony of which things we have ordered the present certificate to be drawn up for him, sealed with the pendent seal of our office.

Given at Valencia, 13 April 1388 AD.

19

Valencia, 16 April 1388.

En Martí Saranyana, bachelor in arts and in medicine, from Xàtiva, presents himself before Jacme Valleriola, civil justiciar of Valencia, with a letter from Jacme de Maderes and Jacme de Avinyó (municipal examiners of physicians and surgeons) in which they certify that they have examined him and determined that he is qualified to practice the art of medicine (ARV, Justícia Civil, 550, fol. 40v [incomplete]).

20

Valencia, 19 February 1389.

The municipal examiners of physicians and surgeons notify the civil justiciar of Valencia that Francesc Descade of Morvedre (=Sagunt) has been examined and found qualified to practice surgery (ARV, Justícia Civil, 593-ter, fol. 27r–v).

Al molt honrat mossén Pelegrí de Montagut, cavaller, justícia de la ciutat de València en lo civil en lo present any. [De] nós, mestre Guillem Çes-Fàbregues e mestre Pere Figuerola, mestres en arts e en medecina, ciutadans de la dita ciutat, e examinadós deputats e assignats per los honrats justícies e jurats de la dita ciutat per examinar tots e sengles metges de físicha e de cirurgia vinents novellament praticar e usar de les dites arts en la ciutat de València e regne de aquella. Salut, ab creximent de prosperitat e honor. Sàpia la vostra hon[rad]a discreció ésser compa(re)gut denant nós En Francesch Descade, habitant en la vila de Murvedre, dient e afermant sí voler usar e pratica[r] de art de cirurgia, requirent que per nós fos examinat. Lo qual nós havem examinat bé e diligentment, lo qual nós havem atrobat suficient en la dita art de cirurgia. Per què, honrat justícia, instant e requirent lo dit En Francesch Descade, per la tenor de la present vos certificham e us requerim e pregam en deute de justícia que us plàcia donar licència e fer aquella carta testimonial, segons que en semblants fets per vós [e] vostra cort és acustu[m]at fer, prestant ans e primerament per ell sagrament de usar e praticar bé e lealment en la dita art. *Data Valentie .XVIIII. februarii anno a nati[vitate] Domini .M.CCC°.LXXX. nono.*

* * *

To the honorable Pelegrí de Montagut, knight, civil justiciar of the city of Valencia for the current year; from us, master Guillem Ça-Fàbrega and master Pere Figuerola, masters in arts and in medicine, citizens of the said city, examiners appointed by the honorable justiciars and *jurats* of the said city for the present year to examine each and every practitioner of the art of physic and surgery newly arrived to practice the said arts in the city of Valencia and its kingdom: greetings, with increase of wealth and honor.

May your worship know that Francesc Descade, an inhabitant of the town of Morvedre, has appeared before us affirming that he wishes to practice the art of surgery, and asking to be examined by us; we have examined him carefully and have found him competent in the said art of surgery. Wherefore, honored justiciar, at the request of the said Francesch Descade, we certify to you by these presents and ask you in accordance with the law that it please you to give him a license and prepare a certificate for him, as you and your court are accustomed to do in such cases, he first of all taking oath to act and practice well and loyally in the said art.

Given at Valencia, 18 February 1389 AD.

21

Valencia, 7 July 1389.

The municipal examiners of physicians and surgeons request the civil justiciar of Valencia to grant a license to extract vesical calculi to Joan Gaschó, who has submitted to an examination and been found qualified (ARV, Justícia Civil, 593-ter, fol. 34r).

Al molt honorable mossén En Pelegrí de Muntagut, cavaller, justícia en lo civil en la ciutat de València.

Molt honorable sènyer: Com algunes malalties sien a les quals comunament sia ignorant remey de medecina, natural rahó requir, per profit de la cosa pública, que si alcú és atrobat qui singularment sàpia la medicina de la dita malaltia, sia admés en praticar d'aquella. Com, donchs, nós, mestre Guillem Ça-Fàbrega e maestre Pere Figuerola, maestres en arts et en medecina, examinadors en lo present any dels metges e cirurgians novellament volents praticar en regne de València, ajam atrobat En Johan [Gaschó] apte e suficient en la cura de la pedra de la vexiga, aq[uel]la trahents sens lesió del pacient, segons que per diligent examinació et experiència per aquell denant nós feta havem atrobat, requirim la vostra saviea que aquest donets licència de praticar e[n] la dita art de medecina tant solament, com d'aquella e no altra l'ajam examinat. En testimoni de la qual veritat posam aquí nostres sagells. Scrita en València dimecres a .VII. de juliol, l'any mill .CCC°.LXXX. e nou.

* * *

To the honorable Pelegrí de Muntagut, knight, civil justiciar in the city of Valencia.

Honorable lord: since there are some maladies for which no medical remedy is generally known, natural reason requires for the public good that if some person is found who knows the treatment for that malady, he should be allowed to treat it. Since therefore we, masters Guillem Ça-Fàbrega and Pere Figuerola, masters in arts and in medicine, examiners for the current year of physicians and surgeons wishing to begin to practice in the kingdom of Valencia, have found Joan Gaschó competent in the treatment of bladder stone, removing it without harm to the patient, as we have determined by careful examination and a demonstration carried out before us, we ask your worship that you give him a licence to practice in that medical art and that one alone, since we have examined him in that and nothing more. In testimony of which truth we affix our seals here.

Given at Valencia, Wednesday 7 July 1389.

22

Valencia, 15 July 1389.

The municipal examiners of physicians and surgeons notify the civil justiciar of Valencia that the barber Pere Fraga, of Valencia, has been examined and found qualified to practice surgery (ARV, Justícia Civil, 593-ter, fol. 36r).

Al molt honorable mossén En Pelegrí de Muntag[u]t, cavaller, justícia de la ciutat de València en lo civil. De nós, En Pere Figuerola e En Guillem Ça-Fàbrega, maestres en arts e en medecina, examinadors de medecina en l'any present. Salut e honor. Com En Pere Fraga, barber, vehí de la dita ciutat, sia per nós novellament examinat en cirurgia, certificam per les presents aquell per nós ésser atrobat apte e suficient a usar de cirurgia tant solament. Et en testimoni de la verita(t) apposam ací nostres sagells. Scrita en València digous a .XV. dies del mes de juliol, l'any mil .CCC°.LXXX°. nono.

* * *

To the honorable Pelegrí de Muntagut, knight, civil justiciar of the city of Valencia; from us, Pere Figuerola and Guillem Ça-Fàbrega, masters in arts and in medicine, examiners of medicine for the current year; health and honor.

Since Pere Fraga, barber, inhabitant of the said city, has recently been examined by us in surgery, we certify by these presents that he has been found by us competent to practice surgery and nothing more. And in testimony of the truth we affix our seals here.

Given at Valencia, Thursday the 15th day of July, 1389.

23

Valencia, 25 August 1389.

The municipal examiners of physicians and surgeons notify the civil justiciar of Valencia that they have examined Joan de Venecia and found him qualified to practice certain aspects of surgery (ARV, Justícia Civil, 593-ter, fol. 29r).

Al molt honorable mossén En Pelegrí de Montagut, cavaller, justícia de la ciutat de València en lo civil. De nós, En Guillem Ça-Fàbrega e

En Pere Figuerola, maestres en arts e.n medicina, examinadors en l'any present d'aquells qui praticar volen novellament en medicina o cirurgia en la ciutat de València e regne de aquella. Salut. Com alcuns casos sien en cirurgia forts difícils e perillosos de praticar, e pochs sien qui aquells gosen temptar, digna cosa és que si alcú, per longa pràtica, és trobàt abte e suficient en aquells, per profit de la cosa pública sia admés en praticar en los dits casos. On, com maestre Johan de Venècia, segons que per examinació plenària havem trobat, sia suficient en aquests tres punts, ço és, en ruptura, la qual cura ab tall, e en pedra de vexiga a traure-la ab tall, e en abatre catarates dels hulls, intimam a vós, senyor, les dites coses, per tal que en aquells solament e no en altres li sia dada licència de praticar, com en totes altres comfesse-s'i no ésser sabent ne volent praticar. Scrita en València a .XXV. dies del mes d'agost, l'any .M.CCC.LXXX. nou, e ací nostres sagells sotsposam.

* * *

To the honorable Pelegrí de Montagut, knight, civil justiciar in the city of Valencia; from us, Guillem Ça-Fàbrega and Pere Figuerola, masters in arts and in medicine, examiners for the current year of those who wish to begin to practice medicine or surgery in the city of Valencia and its kingdom; greetings.

Since there are some cases in surgery very difficult and dangerous to treat, and there are few who dare to attempt them, it is proper that if someone is found to have become competent in them through long practice he should be allowed to treat such cases for the public good. Hence, since master Joan de Venecia is competent in three areas (as we have fully determined by examination), that is, in hernia, which he treats with the knife, and in bladder stone, which he removes by incision, and in removing cataracts from the eyes, we inform you, lord, of these things, so that he may be given a license to treat these things alone and no others, since he acknowledges that he is not knowledgeable in any others and does not wish to treat them.

Written in Valencia on the 25th day of the month of August, 1389, and here we suffix our seals.

24

Valencia, 2 September 1389.

Vidal Benzunana, Jew of Valencia, is declared qualified to practice medicine by the municipal examiners of physicians and surgeons, who notify the civil justiciar that he should be granted a license (ARV, Justícia Civil, 593-ter, fols. 37v-38r).

Al molt honorable mosén En Pelegrí de Montagut, cavaler, justícia de la ciutat de València, o a son lochtinent. De nós, En Guillem Ça-Fàbrega e En Pere Figuerola, mestres en arts e en medecina, ciutadans de la dita ciutat, examinadors en l'any present per los honrats justícia e jurats de la dita ciutat per examinar tots e sengles metges de art de phísica et de cirurgia vinents novellament praticar e usar de la dita art e(n) lochs e vil.les de regne de aquella. Salut, ab creximent de prosperitat e de honor. Sàpia la vostra honrada discreció ésser comparegut denant nós Vidal Benzunana, juheu de València, dient e afermant sí volent usar e praticar de art de físicha, lo qual havem bé e diligentment exhaminat e aquell havem atrobat suficient per praticar de la dita art de phísica. Per ço, de la suficiència e indústria del dit Vidal Benzunana certificant-vos per la present, per què us pregam e requirim en deute de justícia manar fer a.quell letra testamonial, en la qual aquesta sia insertada, prestat per ell // ans e primerament sagrament que bé e lealment usarà e praticarà de la art de físicha en la dita ciutat de València e vil.les e lochs de regne de aquella. En testimoni de la qual cosa fem vos fer la present letra, per nós a ell liurada, ab nostres sagells sagellada a dos dies del mes de setembre, *anno a nativitate Domini .M°.CCC°.LXXX°.IX°.*

* * *

To the honorable Pelegrí de Montagut, knight, justiciar of the city of Valencia, or his lieutenant; from Guillem Ça-Fàbrega and Pere Figuerola, masters in arts and in medicine, citizens of the said city, examiners [appointed] by the honorable justiciars and *jurats* of the said city for the present year to examine each and every practitioner of the art of physic and surgery newly arrived to practice and employ this art in the villages and towns of this kingdom: greetings, with increase in wealth and honor.

May your worship know that Vidal Benzunana, a Jew of Valencia, has appeared before us affirming that he wishes to practice the art of physic; we have examined him carefully and have found him competent to practice the said art of physic. Wherefore we certify to you by these presents the competence and industry of the said Vidal Benzunana, and ask you in accordance with the law that it please you to prepare a certificate for him incorporating this [letter of ours], he first having sworn an oath to practice well and loyally the art of physic in the said city of Valencia and in the towns and villages of that kingdom. In testimony of which thing we have caused the present letter to be drawn up for you and given by us to him, sealed with our seals on the second day of September, 1389 AD.

25

Valencia, 29 November 1389.

The municipal examiners of physicians and surgeons notify the civil justiciar of Valencia that they have examined Johan de Sena and found him qualified to practice three special surgical techniques, and ask that he be given a license to practice his art in Valencia and its kingdom (ARV, Justícia Civil, 593-ter, fols. 43r, 44r).

Al molt honorable mossén Pelegrí de Montagut, cavaller, justícia de la ciutat de València en lo civil. Pere Figuerola (e) Guillem Ça-Fàbrega, maestres en arts // et en medicina, ciutadans de la dita ciutat et examinadors en la sciència de medicina per lo present any constituïts. Salut, ab deguda ho[nor]. Com maestre Johan de Sena se sia a nosaltres presentat que per sguart de nostre ofici deguéssem en tres parts de cirurgia él examinar, so és saber, en deposició de [ca]taratta, e en trencadura, e pedra de vexiga, e [a]quell hajam suficient en nostre examen atro[bat], com les dites coses stiguen més en speriència e hobra manual que no en theòrica de sciència, per què ab deguda reverència e instància a la vostra honorable discreció suplicam que, pres primerament de ell jurament, axí com en vostra honrada cort és acostumat, que lo dit maestre Johan vullats acceptar e a aquell de les dites coses donar licència e praticar e usar en la dita ciutat e regne, e a ell fer carta segons la solemnita[t] en la dita cort acostumada. *Scriptum Valentie die dominica .XXVIII. mensis novembris anno a nativitate Domini .M^{o}. CCC^{o}.LXXXIX°.*

* * *

To the honorable Pelegrí de Montagut, knight, civil justiciar of the city of Valencia; Pere Figuerola and Guillem Ça-Fàbrega, masters in arts and in medicine, citizens of the said city appointed as examiners in the science of medicine for the present year; health, with proper honor.

Since master Johan de Sena has presented himself to us that we might examine him by virtue of our office in three parts of surgery— namely removal of cataract, hernia, and bladder stone— and since we have found him competent in our examination, since the said things pertain more to experience and manual activity than to scientific understanding, we ask your worship with due deference that, first taking an oath from him as your honorable court is accustomed to do, you accept the said master Johan and give him a certificate of these things and license to practice in the said city and kingdom, and to prepare a document for him according to the procedures of the said court.

Written at Valencia, Sunday, 28 November 1389 AD.

26

Valencia, 20 December 1389.

The municipal examiners of physicians and surgeons ask the civil justiciar of Valencia to grant a license to practice surgery to Francesc Moliner, who has been examined and found qualified (ARV, Justícia Civil, 593-ter, fol. 39v).

Al molt honorable mossén Pelegrí de Montagut, (justícia) de València en lo civil, de nós, maestre Pere Figuerola e maestre Guillem Ça-Fàbrega, examinadors en medicina en lo present any. Salut e honor. Com En Francesch Moliner, menor de dies, sia stat per nós examinat en art de cirurgia e aquell hajam trobat su[ficient] en tot ço que.s pertany a la sua art, per tal requerim la vostra saviea a aquell donar licència de praticar segons que per fur e rahó conexerets ésser fahedor. En testimoni de la qual cosa posam aquí nostres seguells. Scrit en València dilluns a .XX. dies del mes de deembre, l'any .M.CCC.LXXXIX.

* * *

To the honorable Pelegrí de Montagut, civil justiciar of Valencia; from us, masters Pere Figuerola and Guillem Ça-Fàbrega, examiners in medicine for the current year: health and honor.

Since Francesc Moliner the younger has been examined by us in the art of surgery, and since we have found him competent in all that pertains to his art, we therefore ask your worship to grant him a licence to practice in the manner that you know is warranted by law and reason. In testimony of which thing we here affix our seals.

Written in Valencia, Monday, the 20th day of December, 1389.

27

Valencia, 21 March 1390.

The civil justiciar of Valencia grants a license to Toríbio Gonçàlvez to treat hernias, at the recommendation of the municipal examiners of physicians and surgeons (ARV, Justícia Civil, 616-bis, fols. 21v-22r).

Als honrats universes e sengles oficials e loch de senyoria tinents dins lo regne de València constituhits als quals la present pervendrà o presentada serà, o a lurs lochtinents. De nós, En Guillem Estrany, justícia de la ciutat de València en lo civil. Salut e honor. Per tenor de les presents vos certificam que En Toríbio Gonçàlvez és estat examinat per los honrats e discrets En Bernat d'Artessa e En Gabriel Dezcortell, maestres en arts e en medecina, ciutadans de la dita ciutat, examinadors en l'any present deputats e asignats per nós e per los honrats jurats de la damunt dita ciutat a examinar tots e sengles metges de física e de serorgia volents novellament praticar e usar de la dita art en la dita ciutat e regne de aquella, per los quals lo dit En Toríbio Gonçàlvez és estat atrobat apte e suficient de usar e praticar de art de trencadura, segons que a nós és cert per letra dels dits examinadors per lo dit En Toríbio Gonçàlveç a nós presentada, la qual és de la tenor següent:

Molt honorable justícia: Notificam a la saviea vostra nosaltres haver bé e deligentment deligentment (*sic*) examinat En Toríbio Gonçàlveç, lo qual volrà praticar en la ciutat de València e regne de aquella de malaltia apellada trencadura, per què, com lo dit En Toríbio Gonçàlveç ajam trobat abte e suficient de praticar de la dita malaltia e com aquell encara, per descàrech // nostre, ajam volgut venir obrar en presència de nosaltres, lo qual ha obrat e curat de la sobredita malaltia a Minguiquo Aznar, fadrí de .XIIII. ans, fill d'En Domingo Aznar, del loch de Novalixes, terme de Exèrica, per què, com les dites coses sien e són veres, suplicam a vós per deute de justícia que aquell vullats prestar vostra acturitat e donar licència que la desús dita malaltia puxa usar e praticar tant solament e no de altra en la ciutat de València e en lo regne de aquella, e de altra malaltia de cerurgia no gos praticar ni presumesca, rebent d'él sagrament que contra les dites coses no farà. Aparelats tota veguada nosaltres per vos complir les vostres justs manaments en semblants coses e.n altres obehir, en testimoni de veritat aposam en la present letra los sagells nostres. Scrita en València, disabte, a .XVIII. de març de l'any .M.CCC. noranta. Maestre Bernat d'Artesa, maestre Gabriel Dezcortell, examinadors en l'any present.

Per la qual cosa nós, reebut de aquell primerament e abans sagrament sobre los sants Evvangelis de Déu per les sues mans corporalment tocats, segons forma de fur, que bé e lealment se haurà en la dita art de trencadura, havem donat aquell licència de usar e praticar en la ciutat de València e regne de aquella de la dita art de trencadura sens temor de alguna pena. En testimoni de les quals coses manam li ésser feta la present carta testimonial ab lo sagell del dit ofici en pendent sagellada. *Data Valentie .XXI^{a}. marcii anno a nativitate Domini .M^{o}. CCC^{o}.LXXXX°.*

* * *

To all officials in the kingdom of Valencia, or to their lieutenants, to whom these presents may come; from us, Guillem Estrany, civil justiciar of the city of Valencia; health and honor. By these presents I certify to you that Toríbio Gonçàlvez has been examined by the honorable Bernat d'Artesa and Gabriel Dezcortell, masters in arts and in medicine, citizens of the said city, appointed by us and by the honorable *jurats* of the aforesaid city as examiners for the current year to examine each and every practitioner of physic and of surgery wishing to begin to practice the said art in the said city and its kingdom; and that the said Toríbio Gonçàlvez has been found competent to practice the treatment of hernia, as certified to us by a letter from the said examiners given to us by the said Toríbio Gonçàlveç, whose tenor is as follows:

Most honored justiciar: we inform your worship that we have well and diligently examined Toríbio Gonçàlveç, who wishes to treat the malady called hernia in the city of Valencia and its kingdom, and that since we found the said Toríbio Gonçàlveç competent to treat the said malady, and since we wished him to operate in our presence, to discharge us of responsibility, and he did treat the aforesaid malady in Minguiquo Aznar, a boy of 14 years, the son of Domingo Aznar of Novalixes in Jérica, therefore, since the said things are true, we request that in accordance with the law you give your consent and grant him license to treat the aforesaid malady alone, and nothing else, within the city of Valencia and its kingdom—nor may he practice or presume to any other surgical complaint—receiving from him an oath that he will not contravene these conditions, we being always ready to fulfill your just commands in these and other matters. In testimony of the truth we affix our seals to the present letter.

Written in Valencia, Saturday, the 18th of March 1390. Master Bernat d'Artesa, master Gabriel Dezcortell, examiners for the current year.

Wherefore we, having first received from him an oath on the holy Gospels of God touched physically by his hands, in the manner prescribed by the *fur*, that he will well and loyally carry out the said treatment of hernia, have given him licence to practice the said treatment of hernia in the city of Valencia and its kingdom without fear of any penalty. In testimony of which things we have commanded that the present certificate be made for him, sealed with the seal of the said office affixed.

Given at Valencia, 21 March 1390 AD.

28

Valencia, 26 October 1390.

The municipal examiners of physicians and surgeons recommend to the civil justiciar of Valencia that he grant the Jew Vidal Albar a license to practice medicine (ARV, Justícia Civil, 616-bis, fols. 22v-23v).

A l'honrat En Guillem Strany, justícia de la ciutat de València en lo civil en lo present any. De nós, maestre Bernat de Artesa e maestre Guabriel Dezcortell, físichs, examinadors diputats e assignats per los honrats justícia e jurats de la dita ciutat per examinar tots e sengles metges de físiqua e silorgia vinents novellament praticar e usar de les dites arts en la ciutat de València e regne de aquella. Salut, ab acreximent de prosperitat e honor. Sàpia la vostra honrada discreció ésser comparegut denant nós Vidal Albar, juheu, requerint que per nós fos examinat en la dita física, lo qual havem examinat bé e diligentment, e encara més havem legida una letra en la qual se conté que en *Barchinona* és estat e diligentment examinat per maestre Bernat Oriol e per aquell ja en la dita ciutat havie obtenguda licència. Per què, honrat sènyer justícia, instant e requirent lo dit Vidal Albar, per la tenor de la present vos certificam les dites coses e us requerim e pregam en deute de justícia, que us plàcia donar licència e fer a aquell carta testimonial, segons que en semblants fets per vós e vostra cort és acostumat fer, prestat ans e primerament per ell sagrament sobre.lls .X. manaments usar e praticar bé e lealment de la dita art de física, com nós, sènyer, siam apparellats los vostres justs manaments obeir. En testimoni de les quals coses fem-vos la present // letra testimonial ab nostres sagells sagellada. *Data Valentie die mercurii .XXVI^a. octobris anno a nativitate Domini .M^o.CCC^o.LXXXX°.*

* * *

To the honorable Guillem Strany, civil justiciar of the city of Valencia for the present year; from us, master Bernat de Artesa and master Guabriel Dezcortell, physicians, appointed by the honorable justiciars and *jurats* of the said city as examiners to examine each and every practitioner of physic and surgery newly arrived to practice these arts in the city and kingdom of Valencia: health and increase in wealth and honor.

May your worship know that Vidal Albar, Jew, has appeared before us asking that he be examined by us in the said physic; we have examined him carefully, and moreover have read a letter stating that he has been living in Barcelona, was thoroughly examined [there] by master Bernat Oriol, and therefore has already obtained a license in that city. Wherefore, honored sir, at the request of the said Vidal Albar, we certify to you by these presents the aforesaid facts and ask you in accordance with the law that you grant him a license and prepare a certificate for him, as you and your court are accustomed to do in similar cases, he having first of all taken oath on the Ten Commandments to practice well and loyally the said art of physic, as we, lord, are prepared to obey your just commands. In testimony of which things we have prepared for you the present certificate sealed with our seals.

Given at Valencia, Wednesday, 26 October 1390 AD.

29

Valencia, 15 November 1390.

The municipal examiners of physicians and surgeons recommend to the civil justiciar of Valencia that he grant Guillem Metge a license to practice surgery (ARV, Justícia Civil, 616-bis, fol. 33r).

A l'honrat lo senyor En Guillem Strany, justícia de la ciutat de València en lo civil en lo present any. De nós, maestre Bernat Artesa e maestre Gabriel Dezcortell, físichs e exhaminadors diputats e assignats per los honrats justícia e jurats de la dita ciutat per eximenar (*sic*) tots e sengles metges de física e celorgia vinents novellament praticar e usar de les dites arts en la ciutat de València e.n regne de aquella. Salut e creximent de prosperitat e honor. Sàpia la vostra discrecció ésser comparegut denant nós En Guillem Metge, celorgià, ciutadà de València, dient e affermant sí voler usar e praticar de art de cirurgia, requirent que per nós fos exhaminat, lo qual nós havem bé e deligenment exhaminat e aquell havem atrobat suficient en art de cirorgia. Per què, honrat justícia, instant e requirent lo dit En Guillem Metge, per tenor de la present vos certificam e us requerim e pregam en deute de justícia que us plàcia donar licència e fer a.quell carta testimonial, segons que en senblants fets per vós e vostra cort és acostumat fer, prestat ans e primerament per él sagrament de praticar bé (e) lealment de la dita art, e que no s'entrametrà en res de phísica, com nós, sènyer, siam apparellats los vostres justs manaments obeir. En testimoni de les quals coses fem-vos la present letra testimonial ab nostres sagells sagellada. *Data Valentie* dimarts a .XV. de novembre de l'any de la nativitat de nostre Senyor .M.CCC.LXXXX.

* * *

To the honorable Guillem Strany, civil justiciar of the city of Valencia for the present year; from us, master Bernat de Artesa and master Guabriel Dezcortell, physicians and examiners appointed by the honorable justiciars and *jurats* of the said city to examine each and every practitioner of physic and surgery newly arrived to practice these arts in the city and kingdom of Valencia: health and increase in wealth and honor.

May your worship know that the surgeon Guillem Metge, a citizen of Valencia, has appeared before us stating that he wishes to practice the art of surgery, and asking that he be examined by us; we have examined him carefully and have found him competent in the art of surgery. Wherefore, honored sir, at the request of the said Guillem Metge, we certify to you by these presents the aforesaid facts and ask you in accordance with the law that you grant him a license and prepare a certificate for him, as you and your court are accustomed to do in similar cases, he having first of all taken oath to practice the said art well and loyally, and not to involve himself at all in physic, as we, lord, are prepared to obey your just commands. In testimony of which things we have prepared for you the present certificate sealed with our seals.

Given at Valencia, Tuesday, 15 November 1390 AD.

30

Valencia, 21 November 1390.

The municipal examiners of physicians and surgeons recommend to the civil justiciar of Valencia that he grant a license to practice medicine to Haabram Cofen Crespín, a Jew of Elx (ARV, Justícia Civil, 616-bis, fol. 34r-v).

A l'honrat En Guillem Strany, justícia de la ciutat de València en lo civil en lo present any. De nós, maestre Bernat d'Artesa e maestre Guabriel Dezcortell, físichs, examinadors deputats e assignats per los honrats justícia e jurats de la dita ciutat per examinar tots e sengles metges de phísica e de cilorgia volents novellament pratichar e usar de les dites arts en la ciutat de València e regne de aquella. Salut ab acreximent de prosperitat e de honor. Sàpia la vostra honrada discreció ésser comparegut denant nós Haabram Cofen Crespín, habitador del loch e vila de Elch, dient e affermant sí voler usar e pratichar de art de phísicha, requerint aquí per nós fos examinat, lo qual havem examinat bé e diligentment e aquell havem atrobat ésser suficient en físiqua. Per què, honrat sènyer justícia, instant e requirent lo dit Haabram Cofen Crespín, per la tenor de la present vos certificam les dites coses e us requerim e preguam en deute de justícia que us plàcia donar a.quel licència de físicha o fer carta testimonial, segons que per vós e vostra cort és acostumat fer, prestat ans e primerament per ell sagrament de pratichar bé e lealment de la dita art de phísicha, com nós, sènyer, siam apparellats los vostres justs manaments hobeir. En testimoni de les quals coses fem-vos fer la present letra testimonial ab nostres sagells sagellada. *Data* en València a .XXI^{a}. de noembre, *anno a nativitate Domini .M^{o}.CCC^{o}.LXXXX°.*

* * *

To the honorable Guillem Strany, civil justiciar of the city of Valencia for the present year; from us, master Bernat de Artesa and master Guabriel Dezcortell, physicians appointed by the honorable justiciars and *jurats* of the said city as examiners to examine each and every practitioner of physic and surgery wishing to begin to practice these arts in the city and kingdom of Valencia: health and increase in wealth and honor.

May your worship know that Haabram Cofen Crespín, an inhabitant of the town of Elx, has appeared before us stating that he wishes to practice the art of physic, and asking that he be examined by us; we have examined him and have found him competent in the art of physic. Wherefore, honored lord, at the request of the said Haabram Cofen Crespín, we certify to you by these presents the aforesaid facts and ask in accordance with the law that you grant him a license for physic and prepare a certificate for him as you and your court are accustomed to do, he first of all taking oath to practice the said art of physic well and loyally, as we, lord, are prepared to obey your just commands. In testimony of which things we have prepared for you the present certificate sealed with our seals.

Given at Valencia, 21 November 1390 AD.

31

Valencia, 9 December 1396.

Grant of a license to practice medicine in the city and kingdom of Valencia to Pere Ferràndiz, a native of Alzira living in Castillo de Garcimuñoz (ARV, Justícia Civil, 718-bis, fols. 16r-18r).

Anno a nativitate Domini millesimo .CCC^{o}.XC^{o}. sexto, die sabbati .IX^{a}. mensis decembris. Denant l'onrat En Johan de Torragrossa, justícia de la ciutat de València en lo cevil, comparech En Pere Ferràndiz, natural de la vila de Algezira e vehí del Castell de García, e presentà a aquell huna letra dels honrats mestre Pere Figuerola e de mestre Vicent Serra, examinadors dels metges l'any present, uberta, en paper scrita, sagellada ab dos sagells dels dits examinadors ab cera vermella, la tenor de la qual és *ut sequitur*:

Al molt honorable sènyer En Johan de Torragrossa, justícia de la ciutat de València en lo cevil en l'any dejús scrit. Nós, mestre Pere Figuerola e maestre Vicent Serra, per vós examinadors dels metges en aquell mateix any, notificam a vós, sènyer honorable justícia, que com En Pere Ferràndiz sia per nós diligentment examinat en art de medecina de phísica, e aquell haver trobat suficient a usar de la dita art. En testimoni de la qual cosa metem-hi nostres sagells. Scrita en València l'any de la nativitat de nostre Senyor mil .CCC.LXXXX. sis, a nou dies del mes de deembre.

E presen[t]ada la dita la dita (*sic*) letra, encontinent lo dit hon[ra]t justícia reebé sagrament del dit En Pere Ferràndiz, metge físich que dessús, per virtut del qual féu promissió e obligació següent: //

En Pere Ferràndiz, metge físich qui dessús, jurà sobre los sants Evvangelis de Déu, de la sua man dreta corporalment tocats, que bé e lealment se aurà en la dita art de phísica e, sots pena encara de cent morabatins, no participarà en los salaris dels apothecaris, e que no rebrà encara algú o alguna qui sia greument malalt si donchs primerament lo malalt no aurà confessat, sinó en tal cas de perill de mort que la triga fos perillosa, e ladonchs no sia feta la segona visitació tro lo pacient haja confessat. Et axí mateix jurà *ut supra* que les receptes que dictarà, ha[j]a a dictar en romanç, declarant los noms de les erbes e de les altres coses medicinals en lur nom comú e vulgar. Et axí mateix, haja a declarar los noms del pes o mesura de les dites coses, en manera que.s puxa clarament entendre per la gent popular, segons forma de fur, e servar totes aquelles coses en aquell contengudes.

Et rebut lo dit sagrament del dit En Pere Ferràndiz, metge dessús dit, encontinent lo dit honrat justícia donà e atorgà licència e plen poder al dit En Pere Ferrà(n)diz de usar e praticar de art de física dins la ciutat e regne de València sens alguna pena, manan li ésser feta letra testimonial de les dites coses *prout sequitur*: //

Als honrats universes e sengles officials e loch de senyoria tinents dins lo regne de València constituïts als quals la present pervendrà o presentada serà, o a lurs lochtinents. De nós, En Johan de Torragrossa, justícia de la ciutat de València en lo cevil. Salut e honor. Per tenor de les presents vos significam que En Pere Ferràndiz, natural de la vila de Algezira, ara dient-se vehí del Castell de García Munyoç, és stat examinat per los honrats e discrets mestre Pere Figuerola e mestre Vicent Serra, maestres en ar[t]s e en medecina de la dita ciutat, examinadors diputats e assignats per nós e per los honrats jurats de la ciutat damunt dita, per los quals lo dit En Pere Ferràndiz és stat atrobat apte et // suficient de usar e praticar en art de phísica, segons que a nós és cert per letra dels dits examinadors per lo dit En Pere Ferràndiz a nós presentada, la qual és de la tenor següent: (*here follows the text of the letter already given above*). Per la qual cosa nós, reebut de aquell primerament e abans sagrament sobre los sants Evvangelis, per aquell de la sua man dreta corporalment tocats, segons forma de fur, que bé e lealment se aurà en la dita art de phísica, havem donat e atorgat a aquell licènciat (*sic*) de usar e praticar en la dita ciutat de València e regne de aquella de la dita art de phísica sens temor de alguna pena. En testimoni de les quals coses manam li ésser feta la // present carta testimonial ab lo sagell del nostre offici en pendent. *Data Valentie .IX^{a}. mensis decembris anno a nativitate Domini .M^{o}.CCC.LXXX(X)^{o}. sexto.*

Presents testimonis foren a les dites coses, En Bernat Taverner e En Ramon del Mas, scrivents en la dita cort.

* * *

In the year 1396 AD, Saturday 9 December, appeared before the honorable Johan de Torragrossa, civil justiciar of Valencia, Pere Ferràndiz, a native of the town of Alzira but living in Castillo de Garcimuñoz; who presented a letter from the honorable masters Pere Figuerola and Vicent Serra, examiners of physicians for the year, open, written on paper, sealed in red wax with the two seals of the said examiners, whose tenor is as follows:

To the honorable lord Johan de Torragrossa, civil justiciar in the city of Valencia for the year written below; we, master Pere Figuerola and master Vicent Serra, examiners of physicians for the same year, certify to you, lord justiciar, that Pere Ferràndiz has been carefully examined by us in the medical art of physic, and has been found competent to practice the said art. In testimony of which fact we affix our seals.

Written in Valencia in the year 1396 AD, on the ninth day of December.

Having been given the said letter, the said honorable justiciar immediately took the oath of the above Pere Ferràndiz, practitioner of physic, by which he made the following promise:

En Pere Ferràndiz, the above practitioner of physic, swears on the holy Gospels of God, touching them physically with the right hand, that he will perform well and loyally in the said art of physic and, under penalty of 100 morabatins, will not share in the fees of apothecaries; and will not treat anyone who is seriously ill, man or woman, if the patient has not first made confession, except in a potentially fatal case where a delay would be dangerous, and then he will not make a second visit until the patient has confessed. Likewise he swears in the same manner that he will give prescriptions for medicines in the vulgar tongue, naming herbs and other medicinal things by their common or popular names. Likewise he shall give weights and measures of the said things in a manner that can be readily understood by the common people, in the manner prescribed by the *furs*, and to obey all the things contained therein.

Having received the said oath from the said Pere Ferràndiz, the practitioner named above, the said honorable justiciar granted licence and full authority to the said Pere Ferràndiz to practice the art of physic in the city and kingdom of Valencia without any penalty, ordering a certificate of these things to be drawn up for him as follows:

To all officials in the kingdom of Valencia, or their lieutenants, to whom these presents may come; from us, Johan de Torragrossa, civil justiciar of the city of Valencia; health and honor. By these presents I make known to you that Pere Ferràndiz, a native of the town of Alzira now calling himself an inhabitant of Castillo de Garcimuñoz, has been examined by the honorable masters Pere Figuerola and Vicent Serra, masters in arts and in medicine of this city, examiners appointed by us and by the honorable *jurats* of the aforesaid city; and that the said Pere Ferràndiz has been found competent to practice the art of physic, as has been certified to us by a letter from the said examiners presented to us by the said Pere Ferràndiz, whose tenor is as follows: [here follows the text of the letter already given above]. Wherefore we—having first received his oath upon the holy Gospels while he physically touched them with his right hand, in the manner prescribed by the *furs*, that he will act well and loyally in the said art of physic—have given him license to practice the said art of physic in the said city and kingdom of Valencia without fear of any penalty. In testimony of which facts we have commanded that the present certificate be drawn up for him, with the seal of our office attached.

Given at Valencia, 9 December 1396 AD.

Bernat Taverner and Ramon del Mas, scribes of the said court, present as witnesses to these things.

IV

Jewish Appreciation of Fourteenth-Century Scholastic Medicine

By Luis García-Ballester, Lola Ferre and Eduard Feliu

FOR MOST OF THE MIDDLE AGES, Jewish physicians maintained a reputation within Latin Christian society that was altogether disproportionate to their numerical presence. The importance of medicine as a calling within the Jewish community, able to draw on the learning of the Greco-Arabic tradition, set Jewish medicine apart from the empirical practice that was nearly universal in the West during the twelfth and thirteenth centuries; it continues to enjoy this high reputation among present-day historians.[1] What has not been fully appreciated is that by the fourteenth century this situation had been to some extent reversed—that the Latin system of medical learning had so developed as to establish itself, in the eyes of at least a few Jewish practitioners, as a model to be imitated and a resource to be exploited.[2]

I. SOURCES OF LEARNING

The intellectual life of the three great Mediterranean cultures of the Middle Ages —Judaic, Christian, and Islamic—was molded by religion; the development of

We would like to thank David Romano, Angel Sáenz-Badillos, Saul Jarcho, Miguel Pérez, Ron Barkai, and Joseph Shatzmiller for criticism and for help with the Hebrew text; and Lola Badia for supplying us with valuable bibliographical references.

[1] Joseph Shatzmiller has studied the social and intellectual world of the Provençal Jewish physicians with particular care: see, e.g., his "Notes sur les médecins Juifs en Provence au Moyen Age," *Revue des Etudes Juives,* 1969, *128*:259–266; "Rationalisme et orthodoxie religieuse chez les Juifs provençaux au commencement du XIVe siècle," *Provence Historique,* 1972, *22*:261–286; "Contacts et échanges entre savants juifs et chrétiens a Montpellier vers 1300," in *Juifs et judaïsme de Languedoc, XIIIe siècle–début XIVe siècle,* ed. Marie-Hembert Vicaire and Bernhard Blumenkranz (Toulouse: Edouard Privat, 1977), pp. 337–344; "Livres médicaux et éducation médicale à propos d'un contrat de Marseille en 1316," *Mediaeval Studies,* 1980, *42*:463–470; "In Search of the 'Book of Figures': Medicine and Astrology in Montpellier at the Turn of the Fourteenth Century," *Association for Jewish Studies Review,* 1982/83, *7/8*:383–407; "On Becoming a Jewish Doctor in the High Middle Ages," *Sefarad,* 1983, *43*:239–250; "Doctors' Fees and Their Medical Responsibility: Evidence from Notarial and Court Records," in *Gli atti privati nel tardo Medioevo: Fonti per la storia sociale,* ed. Paolo Brezzi and Egmont Lee (Rome: Istituto di Studi Romani, 1984), pp. 201–208.

[2] The influence of Latin scholastic medicine on the Jewish medical tradition is only one aspect of a much larger problem that still needs to be studied—the impact of scholastic thought generally on Jewish intellectual history. The first to examine this problem was Shlomo Pines, "Scholasticism after Thomas Aquinas and the Teaching of Hasdai Crescas and His Predecessors," *Proceedings of the Israel Academy of Sciences and Humanities,* 1967, *1*(10):1–101; see also Isadore Twersky, "Joseph ibn Kaspi: Portrait of a Medieval Jewish Intellectual," in *Studies in Medieval Jewish History and Literature,* ed. Twersky (Cambridge, Mass.: Harvard Univ. Press, 1979), pp. 231–257, on pp. 235–236.

natural philosophy (and medicine) in all three was conditioned by issues that were more theological than philosophical.[3] Each claimed authority from a divine revelation, and therefore each encountered difficulty in reconciling revelation with Greek thought, specifically with Aristotelian thought. Aristotelian rationalism encouraged the formulation of a logically consistent theology, which could easily come into sharp conflict with those who considered themselves the only ones capable of interpreting the divine word, or simply with those who defended alternative approaches to understanding the relationship between man and God.

Within Latin Christendom, the university world was able during the thirteenth century (not without difficulty) to harmonize Aristotelian thought and Christian doctrine, somewhat as Maimonides had done for Judaism at the end of the twelfth century and as the *muᶜtazilites* and *mutakallimin* had tried to do for Islam still earlier.[4] Albertus Magnus (ca. 1200–1280) and Thomas Aquinas (1225–1274) symbolize the assimilation of Greek natural philosophy and metaphysics by Christian theology that established Aristotle's teachings as the starting point for all intellectual investigations.[5] In turn, the acceptance of Aristotle facilitated the systematic study of the enormous medical corpus of Galenic writings, which (together with works of the great representatives of Arab Galenism—Haly Abbas, Avicenna, Albucasis, Averroes) began to enter the universities in the last third of the thirteenth century.[6] During the next hundred years, a scholastic Galenism was founded on the texts of the "new Galen," and Latin medicine in late medieval Europe was thereby able to claim for itself a new status as *scientia,* with an associated elevation in social prestige.

The same forces worked upon the Jewish intellectual community to produce three occasionally discernible tendencies: "The Rabbis, whose main interest was in questions of Halakhah and Talmudic exegesis, the Kabbalists, whose main concern was theosophical speculation, and the philosophical group, whose major intellectual interests were secular in nature."[7] The Talmudic and kabbalistic

[3] See David C. Lindberg, "Science and the Early Christian Church," in *God and Nature: Historical Essays on the Encounter between Christianity and Science,* ed. D. C. Lindberg and R. L. Numbers (Berkeley/Los Angeles: Univ. California Press, 1986), pp. 19–48 (revision of an article published in *Isis,* 1983, *74*:509–530); Edward Grant, "Science and Theology in the Middle Ages," in *God and Nature,* pp. 49–75; Joseph Sarachek, *Faith and Reason: The Conflict on the Rationalism of Maïmonides* (1935; rpt. New York: Hermon Press, 1970); and A. I. Sabra, "The Appropriation and Subsequent Naturalization of Greek Science in Medieval Islam: A Preliminary Statement," *History of Science,* 1987, *25*:223–243.

[4] Sarachek, *Faith and Reason;* and Isadore Twersky, "Aspects of the Social and Cultural History of Provençal Jewry," *Journal of World History,* 1968, *2*:185–207. For Islamic culture see S. Munk, *Mélanges de philosophie juive et arabe* (rev. ed., Paris: J. Vrin, 1955), pp. 318–324; and Seyyed Hossein Nasr, *An Introduction to Islamic Cosmological Doctrines: Conceptions of Nature and Methods Used for Its Study by the Ikhwān al-Ṣafāᵓ, al-Bīrūnī, and Ibn Sīnā* (Cambridge, Mass.: Belknap Press of Harvard Univ. Press, 1964).

[5] M.-D. Chenu, *Introduction à l'étude de Saint Thomas d'Aquin* (Montreal: Institut d'Etudes Médiévales, 1954); Albert Zimmermann, ed., *Thomas von Aquin: Werk und Wirkung im Licht neuerer Forschungen* (Berlin/New York: Walter de Gruyter, 1988); James A. Weisheipl, ed., *Albertus Magnus and the Sciences: Commemorative Essays, 1980* (Toronto: Pontifical Institute of Mediaeval Studies, 1980); and G. Meyer and A. Zimmermann, eds., *Albertus Magnus Doctor Universalis, 1280–1980* (Mainz: Matthias-Grünewald Verlag, 1980).

[6] Nancy G. Siraisi, *Taddeo Alderotti and His Pupils: Two Generations of Italian Medical Learning* (Princeton, N.J.: Princeton Univ. Press, 1981); Luis García-Ballester, "Arnau de Vilanova (c. 1240–1311) y la reforma de los estudios médicos en Montpellier (1309): El Hipócrates latino y la introducción del nuevo Galeno," *Dynamis,* 1982, 2:97–158; and Marie-Thérèse d'Alverny, "Pietro d'Abano traducteur de Galien," *Medioevo,* 1985, *11*:19–64.

[7] Lawrence V. Berman, "Greek into Hebrew: Samuel ben Judah of Marseilles, Fourteenth-Century

commentaries constructed a system of thinking and of understanding of man and the world with its own logic and terminology, different from the Aristotelian way of reasoning: "The historical Kabbalah (in Provence and Catalonia) represented an ongoing effort to systematize existing elements of Jewish theurgy, myth, and mysticism into a full-fledged response to the rationalistic challenge."[8] Even so, antirationalist authors were influenced by the Greek-Islamic natural philosophy embraced by rationalists.[9] In Muslim Spain, where Jewish intellectual life was especially vigorous, the Almohad conquest of the mid-twelfth century added a new element of religious intolerance that weighed heavily on the Jewish minority, particularly on the rationalist group therein, and many families chose to leave the peninsula, either for Muslim lands in the eastern Mediterranean (like Maimonides' family, which went first to the Maghreb and then to Egypt) or for Christian territories in the North (like Judah ibn Tibbon, who moved to southern France).[10]

Jewish intellectual life, wherever it was diffused, had still to deal with the tension between a wholehearted acceptance of divine revelation and the attitude of those we have labeled "rationalists." Critics of the latter group objected that familiarity with the Greco-Arab philosophical tradition (Aristotle, Ptolemy, Galen, Avicenna, Averroes) would lead away from Orthodox Judaism.[11] In particular, various passages from Revelation were in sharp conflict with doctrines established in accordance with logic or at least commonly accepted within Greek natural philosophy as elaborated by Islamic scientists; this further complicated the situation of Jewish rationalists, who had to decide whether to follow a literal or an allegorical interpretation of such passages. The recourse (by men like Maimonides, in the last third of the twelfth century) to the Aristotelian corpus and its commentators (e.g., al-Farabi or Averroes) to clarify the philosophical problems posed by such contradictions led to intellectual achievements that in turn only intensified the antirationalist polemic.[12]

Philosopher and Translator," in *Jewish Medieval and Renaissance Studies*, ed. Alexander Altmann (Cambridge, Mass.: Harvard Univ. Press, 1967), pp. 289–320, on pp. 289–290, 293. On this division of Jewish society into three rival social groups see the Hebrew grammar of Profiat Duran (Perpignan, ca. 1340/45–1414), *Maᶜase Efod* (Vienna, 1865), pp. 4–10.

[8] Moshe Idel, *Kabbalah: New Perspectives* (New Haven, Conn.: Yale Univ. Press, 1988), p. 253.

[9] Here we employ the terms *antirationalist* and *rationalist* for the sake of convenience, although they are overly simplistic. See Isadore Twersky, "Rabbi Abraham Ben David of Posquières: His Attitude to and Acquaintance with Secular Learning," *Proceedings of the American Academy for Jewish Research*, 1957, *26*:161–192, on pp. 164, 184–185; and Charles Mopsik, *Lettre sur la sainteté: Le secret de la rélation entre l'homme et la femme dans la cabale* (Paris: Verdier, 1986), pp. 32–34, 48–49.

[10] Judah ibn Tibbon described the conditions of Jewish learning in Provence when he arrived there as an exile from Spain in the middle of the twelfth century: "Also in the lands of the Christians there was a remnant for our people. From the earliest days (of their settlement) there were among them scholars proficient in the knowledge of Torah and Talmud, but they did not occupy themselves with other sciences because their Torah-study was their (sole) profession and because books about other sciences were not available in their region"; cited and trans. by Twersky, "Aspects of the Social and Cultural History" (cit. n. 4), p. 195.

[11] Shatzmiller, "Rationalisme et orthodoxie" (cit. n. 1), p. 281; and Berman, "Greek into Hebrew" (cit. n. 7), p. 303.

[12] The polemic has given rise to a considerable literature: see Sarachek, *Faith and Reason* (cit. n. 3); Georges Vajda, *Introduction à la pensée juive du Moyen Age* (Paris: J. Vrin, 1947), pp. 119ff.; Vajda, *Recherches sur la philosophie et la kabbale dans la pensée juive du Moyen Age* (Paris: Mouton, 1962), pp. 118ff.; Daniel Jeremy Silver, *Maimonidean Criticism and the Maimonidean Controversy, 1180–1240* (Leiden: E. J. Brill, 1965); Charles Touati, "La controverse de 1303–1306 autour des études philosophiques et scientifiques," *Rev. Etud. Juives*, 1968, *127*:21–37; and Joseph Shatz-

The debates over Maimonidean teachings were still very much alive in the heart of the Jewish communities of Provence and the Spanish Mediterranean at the beginning of the fourteenth century, when the events culminating in the expulsion of Jews from France (1306) led to a reinforcement of the rationalists and an intensification of the controversy in cities such as Gerona and Barcelona.[13] The members of this group thought of themselves as faithful to the tradition of Maimonides, as belonging to a "sect of philosophers," "interested in rational speculation, the [true] congregation of believers." Natural philosophy had become for them a way of life—indeed almost a religion, with its own "prophets" (*nebi*ᵓ*im*): Greek, Muslim, and Christian natural philosophers and doctors.[14]

Jewish intellectuals had by now something of a philosophical literature available to them in Hebrew, for during the thirteenth century most of Aristotle's works had been translated into that language, along with the commentaries of Averroes, but traditionally it was their knowledge of Arabic that had given them access to the classical texts.[15] It was of course not only Jewish philosophers who recognized the richness of the sources still available only in Arabic; Christian scholars did as well. At Montpellier, Arnau de Vilanova used his knowledge of Arabic to correct passages in the standard Latin translations of medical works;[16] scholars who could not read Arabic asked students who could to translate works of possible interest to them.[17] But it was the Jews who still had the reputation for interest in and mastery of the Arabic-language material, especially those living in the Crown of Aragon or on the frontiers of Islam in southeastern Spain. Guillem de Béziers, who came from Montpellier to teach medicine at the newly created University of Lerida in 1301, asked its founder, King James II of Aragon, to provide him with "quosdam libros arabicos medicinales quos aliqui judei habent," in order to emend the texts that he had found on arriving at the new *studium*.[18] It was men like Samuel ben Judah (1294–ca. 1340) who kept this reputation alive: in 1324 he traveled from Marseilles to Murcia (on the Spanish coast, south of Valencia), recently conquered from Islam by Christians, simply to find a trustworthy Arabic text of Alexander of Aphrodisias's *De anima*.[19]

---

miller, "Towards a Picture of the First Maimonidean Controversy" (in Hebrew), *Zion,* 1969, *34*:126–144. See too the penetrating paper by Twersky, "Joseph ibn Kaspi" (cit. n. 2), esp. pp. 233–234.

[13] Touati, "La controverse de 1303–1306." Yitzhak Baer, *History of the Jews in Christian Spain,* 2 vols. (Philadelphia: Jewish Publication Society of America, 1978), Vol. I, p. 301, reports the *herem* (ban) drawn up by Solomon ben Adret and other religious leaders in Catalonia against scholars interested in Greek philosophy. Rabbi Moses ben Nahman (Nahmanides) of Gerona was a vigorous defender of traditionalism in the debates: see *ibid.,* pp. 102ff.; David Berger, "Nahmanides' Attitude toward Secular Learning and Its Bearing upon His Stance in the Maimonidean Controversy" (M.A. thesis, Columbia Univ., 1965); and Shatzmiller, "Rationalisme et orthodoxie" (cit. n. 1), and literature cited there.

[14] See the various remarks by Samuel ben Judah in the epilogues to his translation from the Arabic of Averroes' *Epitome of Plato's Republic* and of his correction of Jacob ben Makhir's translation of Jabir ibn Aflah's *Epitome of the Almagest,* quoted in Berman, "Greek into Hebrew" (cit. n. 7), pp. 309, 310, 312–313.

[15] Twersky, "Aspects of the Social and Cultural History" (cit. n. 4), pp. 201–202.

[16] Arnau de Vilanova, *Commentum supra tractatum Galieni de malicia complexionis diverse,* ed. Luis García-Ballester and E. Sánchez Salor, in *Arnaldi de Villanova Opera medica omnia,* ed. L. García-Ballester, J. A. Paniagua, and M. R. McVaugh, Vol. XV (Barcelona: Univ. Barcelona, 1985), p. 192, lines 15–18.

[17] Roger Bacon is a famous case in point; see his *Compendium studii,* Ch. 8, in *Fr. Rogeri Bacon Opera quaedam hactenus inedita,* ed. John Serren Brewer (London, 1859), pp. 467–468, 471–472.

[18] Antoni Rubió y Lluch, *Documents per l'història de la cultura catalana mig-eval,* Vol. II (Barcelona: Institut d'Estudis Catalans, 1921), pp. 13–14.

[19] Berman, "Greek into Hebrew" (cit. n. 7), p. 318.

Yet by this time the fame of Jewish scholars as masters of Arabic was no longer fully deserved, as a closer look at that same Samuel ben Judah makes plain. In his prologue to his Hebrew translation of Averroes' *Middle Commentary on the Nicomachean Ethics* Samuel speaks regretfully of his "limited grasp of the Arabic language" and remarks wistfully, "I trust to study it intensively again."[20] After translating Averroes' summary of Plato's *Republic,* he asks any reader who knows Arabic as well as Hebrew to forgive the defects of his translation and to improve it wherever possible, though he admits that such knowledge would be "unique and exceptional."[21] Embedded now in a Christian world, the Jewish community of the western Mediterranean was losing its familiarity with Arabic,[22] and with it its easy access to a rich philosophical and medical heritage. By the second half of the fourteenth century, so distinguished a scholar as Hasday Crescas (ca. 1340–ca. 1411) could no longer read Arabic and was forced to study Aristotle through Hebrew translations of Averroes' commentaries.[23]

A possible alternative for Jewish scholars was natural-philosophical or medical literature in the Romance vernacular. The vitality of medieval Catalan or Provençal is manifested in a variety of medical treatises on practical subjects, surgery and recipes, and such texts did circulate within the Jewish medical world of the fourteenth century: witness the thick marginal glosses in Hebrew that festoon several chapters in the Catalan translation (produced in Mallorca in 1305) of the *Surgery* of Teodorico Borgognoni;[24] or the intercalation of Romance vernacular words in a Hebrew recipe collection from Catalonia, probably also of the fourteenth century.[25] Learned texts from the Christian university world sometimes

[20] *Ibid.,* p. 305.

[21] He acknowledged, "It is not impossible—rather it is possible, nay, it is unavoidable—that whoever examines my translation of the two parts of this science will be perplexed about some passages on account of the badness of the translation, which is a result of my limited grasp of the Arabic language." *Ibid.,* p. 308.

[22] Lawrence V. Berman, "Ibn Rushd's *Middle Commentary on the Nicomachean Ethics* in Medieval Hebrew Literature," in *Multiple Averroès* (Paris: Belles Lettres, 1978), pp. 287–322, on p. 299. An anonymous Hebrew translation of Averroes' *Fasl al-Magal* (a general approach to the role of philosophic speculation in religion) was probably produced by a Provençal Jew who lived in the first years of the fourteenth century and "whose native tongue was not Arabic nor had achieved great prowess in that language": N. Golb, "The Hebrew Translation of Averroes' *Fasl Al-Magal," Proc. Amer. Acad. Jewish Res.,* 1956, *25*:91–113; 1957, *26*:41–64, on pp. 92–95. See also David Romano, "La transmission des sciences arabes par les juifs en Languedoc," in *Juifs et judaïsme de Languedoc,* ed. Vicaire and Blumenkranz (cit. n. 1), pp. 363–386, on p. 379.

[23] Harry A. Wolfson, *Crescas' Critique of Aristotle* (Cambridge, Mass.: Harvard Univ. Press, 1929), p. viii. In the last years of the thirteenth century, Solomon ben Adret had difficulties finding in Barcelona an experienced translator from Arabic into Hebrew to translate Maimonides' *Commentary on the Mishna,* as Rome's Jewish community had asked him to do. He sent a messenger to Aragon (Huesca, Saragossa), where he found Jews skilled in Arabic. See Fred Rosner, *Maimonides' Commentary on the Mishna: Tractate Sanhedrin* (New York: Sepher-Hermon Press, 1981), pp. xi–xii.

[24] The *Surgery* of Teodorico Borgognoni was translated at least twice into Catalan in the first decade of the fourteenth century. One translation was made by Maestre Bernat (fl. 1305), physician of James II of Mallorca (1275–1311) (MS Graz, Universität-Bibliothek 342, fols. 4–282). All chapter titles were translated into Hebrew, with a summary in Hebrew at fol. 25v. The other was made by Guillem Correger, a Valencian surgeon (fl. 1288–1308) (MS Paris, Bibliothèque Nationale, Fons Espagnol 212, fols. 1–89). There is a manuscript fragment in the Municipal Archive in Barcelona (Capsa B-109 [2]) related to the Graz copy; see Antonio Contreras, *La difusión medieval de la* Cyrurgia *de Teodorico Borgognoni (1205–1298) en los paises de habla catalana: La versión catalana de Guillem Correger, Libro I (cirugía general), según el MS Paris Bibliot. Nat., fons espagnol 212, fols. 1–18v* (Tesis de Licenciatura en Medicina) (Santander: Univ. Cantabria, 1986). Contreras and García-Ballester are preparing a critical edition of the Catalan version, to be published in 1992 (Barcelona: Els Nostres Clàsics).

[25] Gregorio del Olmo Lete and José R. Magdalena Nom de Deu, "Documento hebreo-catalán de farmacopea medieval," *Anuario de Filología,* 1980, *6*:159–187. For a nonexhaustive list of medical

were translated from Latin into Romance and then translated from Romance into Hebrew. Three treatises, at least, by the Montpellier master Bernard de Gordon —his *Tractatus de prognosticis* (*de crisi*) (*Haqdamat ha-yedi*ᶜ*ah*); his chef d'oeuvre, the *Lilium medicine* (*Shoshan ha-refu*ᵓ*ah*); and his *De phlebotomia* (*Ha-ma*ᵓ*amar ba-haqazah*)— and one by Arnau de Vilanova (his *Regimen sanitatis ad regem Aragonum* [*Hanhagat ha-beri*ᵓ*ut*]) passed into Hebrew by this route, very much as Arabic texts had earlier been wont to undergo Latinization via an intermediate language.[26] But such Hebrew versions suffered from the compounding of error and obscurity inevitable in two-stage translation, and this made it preferable to turn, where possible, to the Latin original.[27] The ignorance of Latin by the Jewish translator was another reason for the low quality of a translation. The translator of the *De phlebotomia* admitted that his ignorance of Latin had made it impossible to verify quotations from Galen and had rendered his translation less valuable.[28]

In fact, a knowledge of Latin in the medieval Jewish world was increasing as its familiarity with Arabic withered. The intellectual tide was turning; the Latin West was becoming the creative power. Few Jews could read Avicenna's *Canon* in the original Arabic any longer, and the Hebrew translation was defective enough that "reading it keeps us from the truth," as a contemporary critic put it, even though it circulated more widely than any other medical text in Hebrew.[29] The "rediscovery of learning" by Christian Europe and the success of its universities meant that a wide variety of scientific literature was now fairly easily available in Latin, and prohibitions against its sale to Jews were not systematically enforced.[30] Mosse Aventida, a Jewish physician of Monzón in Aragon, had copies of the *Canon* and the *Practica* of Ibn Sarabi (Serapion) in his library (1381), not in Arabic but "in latino xristianico scripti"; in the first half of the next century, Bendich de Borriano (d. 1441), a Jewish physician of Arles, bequeathed

---

works translated into Provençal see Clovis Brunel, *Bibliographie des manuscrits littéraires en ancien provençal* (Paris, 1935; rpt. Geneva: Slatkine, 1973), pp. 38 (no. 121, *Chirurgie* d'Albucasis), 102 (no. 355, surgical treatises). We suspect some medical works belonging to the Jewish physician Astruc de Sestiers (d. 1439) may have been written in Romance; unfortunately the notarial description does not include the incipit. See Danielle Iancu-Agou, "L'inventaire de la bibliothèque et du mobilier d'un médecin juif d'Aix-en-Provence au milieu du XVe siècle," *Rev. Etud. Juives,* 1975, *134*:47–80, on p. 51 (nos. 120, 130, 134, 145, 154).

[26] On these texts see Moritz Steinschneider, *Die hebraeischen Übersetzungen des Mittelalters und die Juden als Dolmetscher* (Berlin, 1893; rpt. Graz: Akademische Druck- u. Verlagsanstalt, 1956), pp. 778–787. To give an example of the dissemination of such works: the library of the Jewish physician Astruc de Sestiers contained Hebrew translations from the Latin (or conceivably Romance) of works by three Montpellier academics of the fourteenth century—the *Regimen sanitatis* (*Hanhagat ha-beri*ᵓ*ut*) of Arnau de Vilanova, the *Introductorium iuvenum* (*Maishir ha-mathilim*) of Gérard de Solo, and the *Lilium* (*Shoshan ha-refu*ᵓ*ah*) of Bernard. See Iancu-Agou, "L'inventaire de la bibliothèque," nos. 146, 162, and 176, on pp. 59–61. On the *Lilium*'s translator, Bonsenyor Salamon (d. ca. 1415 in Perpignan), see Richard W. Emery, "Documents Concerning Some Jewish Scholars in Perpignan in the Fourteenth and Early Fifteenth Centuries," in *Michael: On the History of the Jews in the Diaspora,* ed. Shlomo Simonshon and Joseph Shatzmiller (Tel-Aviv: Diaspora Research Institute, 1976), pp. 27–48, on pp. 43–45.

[27] See Appendix D, lines 113–114. Here and subsequently the reader is referred to the Hebrew texts included (with their English translations) as appendixes to this article.

[28] The treatise was translated in 1378 by an anonymous translator in the Catalonian town of Castelló d'Empúries: Steinschneider, *Die hebraeischen Übersetzungen* (cit. n. 26), p. 787.

[29] Benjamin Richler, "Manuscripts of Avicenna's *Kanon* in Hebrew Translation, a Revised and Up-to-Date List," *Koroth,* 1982, *8*:145*–168*; see Appendix D, lines 40–43.

[30] Appendix D, lines 119–121.

to his brother-in-law Salamies Manelli (also a physician) copies of the *Canon* in both Hebrew and Latin.[31] But while most Mediterranean Jews could read or at least speak the Romance vernacular, Latin was known only to a minority, and this gave rise to a remarkable feature of the intellectual reversal of the fourteenth century: a new impulse to translate Latin medical and natural-philosophical texts directly into Hebrew.

This countercurrent has so far been noted only in scattered cases, like that of the Castilian Jew Meir Alguadez ben Solomon, who retranslated the *Nicomachean Ethics* in the 1390s from Latin because the Hebrew version Samuel ben Judah had prepared directly from the Arabic, seventy years before, was incomprehensible; for Meir Alguadez, Latin was more precise and articulate as a language of translation.[32] In this article, therefore, we mean to draw attention to a series of Jewish translators from the western Mediterranean whose careers encompassed the fourteenth century and who shared an admiration for the learned medical tradition at the Christian *studium* of Montpellier: Estori bar Moses ha-Parhi (1306), translator of the *Tabula antidotarii* of Armengaud Blaise (fl. 1290–1310) (see Appendix A); Israel ben Joseph Caslari (1327), translator of the *Regimen sanitatis* of Arnau de Vilanova (d. 1311) (Appendix B); Joseph bar Judah ha-Sefardi, translator of the *Regimen sanitatis* of Arnau de Vilanova (Appendix C); Leon Joseph of Carcassonne (fl. 1394–1402), translator of the *Practica super nono Almansoris* of Gérard de Solo (fl. 1335) (Appendix D); and Abraham ben Meshullam ben Solomon Abigdor (1379), translator of the *Introductorium* of Bernard Alberti (fl. 1340) (Appendix E). Each of these translators prefixed a personal statement as an introduction to his work, explaining (in varying detail) why he had undertaken the task. Difficult to transcribe and translate, and of course partaking of the self-justifying rhetoric characteristic of almost all prefaces, these introductions are nevertheless remarkably revealing, individually and as a whole, for they show that the intellectual reversal was not merely a response to the shifting fortunes of Arabic and Latin. A few members of the Jewish intellectual community, we will see, had with time come to feel that the well-structured scholastic training provided by the Latin *studia* had a power their own schools no longer possessed. As the century advanced, the interest of medical translators shifted from obviously practical works by Christians especially famous for their medical practice and distinguished clientele, to theoretical, typically academic productions by university masters. These fourteenth-

[31] "Item tercius et quintus libri Avicenne in latino xristianico scripti. Item alius liber scriptus in latino xristianico vocatus Sarampio. . . . Item [lego] quartam et quintam particulas sive libros Avicenne in uno volumine in papiro descriptos lictera ebrayca; item primum (et) quartum librum Avicenne in pergameno in uno volumine lingua latina scripto; item tercium librum sive particulam Avicenne in pergameno lingua latina descriptum." Rubió y Lluch, *Documents* (cit. n. 18), Vol. II, p. 247. Cited by Danielle Iancu-Agou, "Une vente de livres hébreux à Arles en 1434: Tableau de l'élite arlésienne au milieu du XVe siècle," *Rev. Etud. Juives*, 1987, *146*:5–62, on p. 55.

[32] "Die Übersetzung aus dem Arabischen war ihm umverständlich, darum schien es ihm zweckmässig, das Buch aus dem Lateinischen zu übersetzen, vielleicht würden sie dadurch verständlicher [*yoter mebu ᵓarim*], 'da wir unter christlichen Weisen wohnen,' welche jene Bücher studirt haben, auch Commentare derselben sich (bei ihnen) finden, welche alles Dunkle erläutern. Dennoch säumte Meïr, sein Vorhaben auszuführen, aus verschiedenen Gründen. Ein Übersetzer müsse beide Sprachen gründlich verstehen, die Gabe besitzen, die Worte des Vf. in einer anderen Sprache wiederzugeben, er müsse ruhig an einem Orte arbeiten können; diese 3 Bedingungen haben ihm gefehlt, und das Lateinische ist weitläufig [*we-lashon nosrí arukhah*]." Steinschneider, *Die hebraeischen Übersetzungen* (cit. n. 26), p. 210.

century translations are, in fact, an attempt to recapture for medieval Jewish medicine not only learned texts but an underlying approach and habit of mind.

II. THE NORMS OF THE HEBREW TRANSLATORS

The dependence of the Jewish minority upon translations of scientific works made it particularly sensitive to the requirements that translations had to meet, and translators routinely commented on the set of norms they felt compelled to observe. Such norms often recalled the instructions laid down in 1199 by Maimonides himself, when he advised Samuel ibn Tibbon of Arles on the translation of the *Guide of the Perplexed* from Maimonides' original Arabic into Hebrew.[33] They can be summarized as follows: the translator should possess a total mastery of the two languages; he should have a thorough understanding of the material he is translating; he must not translate rigidly, word for word; and he must make sure that the constructions of the translation are perfectly understandable. This purely technical advice was still essential for Jewish translators from Latin two hundred years later, but the very different social context in which they lived made them add new requirements to those set out by the master. Samuel ben Judah, the first translator of the *Nicomachean Ethics,* noted the urgency of seeking out at whatever pains a manuscript containing an accurate text, error free, as he himself had done in his trip to Murcia in 1324.[34] He insisted, too, that the translator needed a knowledge not only of the subject he was translating but of all the sciences, for all intellectual disciplines are interrelated. Consequently, the translator could not work in isolation; he should consult other books and other scholars, Jews and Christians.[35]

Fifty years later, Meir Alguadez remarked on a further requirement for the intellectual labor of translation: peace and tranquillity.[36] The increasingly harsh conditions, including expulsion, imposed by Christianity upon its internal Jewish communities during the fourteenth century rendered intellectual development therein particularly difficult.[37] But even forced displacement could have its com-

[33] Maimonides, *Qobetz Teshubot ha-RaMBaM we-iggerotaw* (Leipzig, 1859; rpt. Farnborough, 1969), pp. 26–29; M. Sonne, "Maimonides' Letter to Semu'el b. Tibbon according to an Unknown Text in the Archives of the Jewish Community of Verona" (in Hebrew), *Tarbiz,* 1939, *10*:135–154, 309–332. There are English versions by H. Adler, "Translation of an Epistle Addressed by R. Moses Maimonides to R. Semu'el ibn Tibbon," *Miscellania of Hebrew Literature,* 1975, *1*:219–227; L. D. Stitskin, *Letters of Maimonides, Translated and Edited with Introductions and Notes* (New York: Yeshiva Univ. Press, 1977), pp. 130–136, 197–198; and Franz Kobler, *Letters of Jews through the Ages,* 2 vols. (New York: East & West Library, 1978), pp. 208–213. These two last versions are incomplete. A Spanish translation is given by Maria J. Cano and Dolores Ferre, *Cinco epístolas de Maimónides* (Barcelona: Riopiedras Ediciones, 1988), pp. 111–124.

[34] Berman, "Greek into Hebrew" (cit. n. 7), p. 318.

[35] "I thought and conceived the desire to correct this translation again together with the Christian philosophers, especially the first part of it because they have the separate treatises of the philosopher on that part together with their explanation by Abu Nasr al-Farabi. . . . He [the translator] must be well educated, not only in the science or art which he is translating but also in all sciences conventionally recognized as such, or most of them, because of the interconnectedness of all of the sciences and arts one with the other, since one always uses analogies taken from other sciences." *Ibid.,* pp. 308, 309.

[36] See the passage from Steinschneider, *Die hebraeischen Übersetzungen* (cit. n. 26), quoted above, n. 32.

[37] See the remarks in Appendixes A (line 16) and D (line 79). Samuel ben Judah alludes to the expulsion of the Jews from France, Burgundy, and Languedoc in 1322 in the following passage: "I promised to correct the translation of this science with the help of Christian philosophers but was unable [to do so] on account of the magnitude of the annoyances and persecutions which have

pensations by bringing exiles into contact with new and intellectually stimulating circles of scholars. Estori bar Moses ha-Parhi was among those forced out of France in the expulsion of 1306, only to find a welcome in the Jewish community of Barcelona, as well as, apparently, from some Christians. There he must have encountered Armengaud Blaise, formerly a master at Montpellier but from 1301 to 1306 in the service of James II of Aragon in the Catalan capital, and also Armengaud's *Tabula antidotarii,* which he found "more precious than fine gold, mother-of-pearl, and onyx" and translated in the following year.[38]

At the very end of the century, two new requirements for the Jewish translator and scholar were identified by Leon Joseph of Carcassonne, who was expelled from France in 1394 and settled at Perpignan (in the Crown of Aragon), where he is found practicing medicine in 1414. Sometime thereafter he converted to Christianity, adopting the name "Leonardus Benedictus"; he died before February 1418.[39] Leon's introduction to his translation of Gérard de Solo's *Practica super nono Almansoris* is a particularly personal statement, undoubtedly the most reflective and most illuminating of the texts we are here considering; it will be worthwhile concentrating most of our attention henceforth on it. The first of the new conditions identified by Leon is the necessity of appreciating the scholastic method, based on the *questio* and the *disputatio* and using dialectical reasoning to guarantee the necessary truth of conclusions.[40] The other requirement, on which Leon places even more stress, is sociocultural rather than technical: the necessity of freedom of discourse within the Jewish communities themselves, freedom from the very real tyranny of "those learned in the Torah, who . . . from the strength of their hands and from their many ruses make the mass of the common people believe . . . that these sciences [natural philosophy and theoretical medicine] and those who are concerned with them are sundered from the community of those who possess the Torah." Lacking such freedom, the rationalist minority has been forced to carry on its studies "in secret . . . 'in the clefts of the rocks and in the secret places' " (Song of Sol. 2:14).[41] With these observations, Leon Joseph brought into the open an issue that he found of great concern: Why, he asked, do the Jews no longer display intellectual creativity in the sciences (medicine), and what can be done to change this?

III. ADMIRATION OF THE SCHOLASTIC TEACHING METHOD

Part of the answer lay, for Leon, in the system of intellectual training. Within the Jewish community, medical education had always followed what we might call

overtaken us on the part of this nation which exiles us." Berman, "Greek into Hebrew" (cit. n. 7), p. 310. See also Yom Tov Assis, "Juifs de France réfugiés en Aragon (XIIIe–XIVe siècles)," *Rev. Etud. Juives,* 1983, *142*:285–322, on p. 315.

[38] Appendix A, line 13. Michael R. McVaugh and Lola Ferre are preparing an edition of the Latin original together with the Hebrew translation. Samuel ben Judah's journey to Murcia and his contact with new Arabic manuscripts may also be connected with the expulsion of the Jews in 1322; see Assis, "Juifs de France," p. 317.

[39] Emery, "Documents Concerning Jewish Scholars" (cit. n. 26), pp. 40–43. Leon's son, Astruc Leo, was also a physician at Perpignan.

[40] Appendix D, lines 70–71. On the intellectual impact of Latin scholasticism on Jewish philosophy (as distinct from medicine) see A. Altmann, "Judaism and World Philosophy," in *The Jews: Their Role in Civilization,* ed. L. Finkelstein (New York: Schocken Books, 1971), pp. 65–115; and Pines, "Scholasticism after Aquinas" (cit. n. 2).

[41] Appendix D, lines 29–31, 24–25.

an "open" model. Under this model, anyone might pass on medical knowledge who had it to impart, faithful to personal standards and outside any institutional framework. In such an open system, teaching activity reflects the interests of an individual teacher, not the requirements of a set curriculum; and the success of education, a student's qualification for practice, can be tested only by his success at curing his patients—it is ultimately the patient who will judge who is a physician and who is not. Where books for technical instruction are relatively scarce, as in medieval Judaism (and Islam),[42] the open system built around the master-disciple arrangement further encourages the oral transmission of knowledge and consequently a tradition of empirical and familiar medical practice.

The model that stood opposed to the open system, institutionalized education, was represented for Leon Joseph by the new Latin university, the *studium generale;* the system of certification it offered was closed to non-Christians. At the beginning of the fourteenth century, the medieval university held the monopoly on systematic medical education, and within a few decades it was attempting to add to this a monopoly on medical practice: to claim, that is, that only those individuals who had been trained at a university should be permitted to practice medicine. But while Christian society did indeed begin in the early fourteenth century to increase its efforts to supervise anyone claiming a medical occupation, these measures were never more than a dim ideal; the European university system was still inadequate to turn out the number of professionals necessary to meet the demands of late-medieval society.[43]

For the Jewish (and Muslim) communities of the western Mediterranean, the open model prevailed throughout the fourteenth century, though we have very little documentation to help us understand how it actually functioned then.[44] But this did not prevent them—or at least their rationalist minority—from admiring the very different institutional model of the Christians. Partly this was a consequence of power relationships. Both in Provence and in the Crown of Aragon, a would-be Jewish (or Christian) physician had by law to pass an examination; a Jew would confront a mixed tribunal of Christian and Jewish physicians in a scholastic ritual, with *questiones et responsiones, disputationes, rationes et argumentationes* requiring a mastery of medical authorities. Thus the Jewish physician who wanted to practice among Christians had to be acquainted with the methods and contents of scholastic medicine. Indeed, the ritual of the examination played a role of acculturation for those Jewish physicians who aspired to be respected by Christian authorities.[45]

[42] At the end of his *Middle Commentary on the Ethics,* Averroes "states that only the first four books of the *Ethics* were available to him in Andalusia until Abuᵓ Amr ibn Martin brought the integral text of the *Ethics* from Egypt." Berman, "Ibn Rushd's *Middle Commentary*" (cit. n. 22), p. 291. See also Berman, "Revised Hebrew Translation of Averroes' *Middle Commentary on the Nicomachean Ethics,*" in *Seventy-Fifth Anniversary Volume of the Jewish Quarterly Review* (Philadelphia: Dropsie College, 1967), p. 106, n. 4.

[43] Luis García-Ballester, Michael R. McVaugh, and Agustín Rubio Vela, *Medical Licensing and Learning in Fourteenth-Century Valencia* (Transactions of the American Philosophical Society, 79.6) (Philadelphia, 1989).

[44] Examples of the scattered documentation upon which we must depend are L. Barthélemy, *Les médecins à Marseille avant et pendant le Moyen-Age* (Marseilles, 1883), pp. 31 (28 Aug. 1326), 32 (7 Mar. 1431); P. Pansier, "Les médecins juifs à Avignon aux XIIIe, XIVe et XVe siècles," *Janus,* 1910, *15*:421–451, on pp. 442, 443; and Antonio de la Torre and Jordi Rubió i Balaguer, *Documentos para la historia de la Universidad de Barcelona,* Vol. I (Barcelona: Univ. Barcelona, 1971), document 46.

[45] P. Hildenfinger, "Documents relatifs aux juifs d'Arles," *Rev. Etud. Juives,* 1900, *41*:62–97, on p.

Further, power relationships aside, the Latin faculties of medicine seemed to be particularly effective centers of learning, to judge both from the quality and quantity of knowledge they generated and from the achievements of particular individuals trained there. The individual Christian physician as well as the institutional model was becoming an object of admiration: famous practitioners like Armengaud or Arnau (who "surpassed all his predecessors"[46]) early in the century, eminent teachers in the second half. It is again Leon Joseph who provides the telling vignette.

> In his time [Jean de Tournemire] [fl. 1380] was at the head of all the scholars of Montpellier. . . . I saw him with my own eyes and I spoke to him. He was a man who was pleasant to talk to. His behavior was not like that of the other scholars of his generation, who scorned those Jews who practiced the art of medicine. . . . His book speaks of the limbs and of the faculties, and of the illnesses that occur in them. It asks and answers, it explains and clarifies. He teaches like a father to a son, true and proper words, which are pleasing and agreeable to whoever listens.[47]

The existence of such teachers seemed to explain to Leon why, throughout the fourteenth century, progress in the science of medicine had obviously been restricted to men with an academic formation.

The learned medicine of the universities was of course in its content not at all foreign to Jewish scholars and certainly not distinguishably Christian. Its Galenic outline, articulated by the Arabs, was the common intellectual property of all three Mediterranean cultures.[48] It was not so much the content of medicine as the manner in which it was pursued at the universities, its systematic development out of Aristotelian methodology and philosophy, that excited admiration and a desire to study. Leon Joseph confessed, "I directed my attention toward the study of and research into the profane sciences, which are . . . as many as the days of the week [i.e., the seven liberal arts], and each one has its own subject matter. . . . In my eyes, the merits of these sciences were above all praise. This explains my zeal . . . to master them."[49] But to do so it had been necessary to seek the setting of a Christian *studium*. Likewise, when, after years of medical practice, Abraham Abigdor wanted to be able to answer the fundamental questions of medicine, he found no other solution than to direct himself to Montpellier in order "to hear the science of medicine [*hokhmat ha-refu*ᵓ*ah*]"[50]—that is,

67, n. 4; English trans. by Cecil Roth, "The Qualifications of Jewish Physicians in the Middle Ages," *Speculum*, 1958, *28*:834–843, on pp. 839–840. Unfortunately, the translation has not preserved the scholastic terminology; see García-Ballester, McVaugh, and Rubío, *Medical Licensing* (cit. n. 43).

[46] Appendix B, lines 47–48.

[47] Appendix D, lines 132–138.

[48] While the diffusion of Galenism through the Latin West is relatively well understood (see n. 6), its spread within the Jewish world is not. It is one thing to identify Hebrew translations of Galen's writings, quite another to speak confidently about their circulation. It seems that the Alexandrine canon of Galen's work was translated into Hebrew by Simson ben Salomo (fl. 1322) in the early fourteenth century (Steinschneider, *Die hebraeischen Übersetzungen* [cit. n. 26], pp. 653–656), but we find very few copies of the Hebrew Galen in the libraries of Jewish physicians. Everything seems to suggest that Jewish Galenism was based on the Arabic encyclopedists, particularly Avicenna. See Danielle Iancu-Agou, "Préoccupations intellectuelles des médecins juifs au Moyen Age: Inventaires de bibliothèques," *Provence Hist.*, 1976, *26*:21–44, on pp. 36–38; Vajda, *Recherches sur la philosophie* (cit. n. 12), pp. 120–137; and Richler, "Manuscripts of Avicenna's *Kanon*" (cit. n. 29).

[49] Appendix D, lines 2–7.

[50] Appendix E, lines 10–11.

scholastic medicine founded upon natural philosophy. For to penetrate this scientific medical world, the liberal arts were a necessary tool; without them it was impossible to begin to learn, since scholastic learning required a preliminary mastery of definitions and distinctions, of the nature of the syllogism, and so forth.[51] These intellectual materials formed the core of medical instruction in the medieval university, which turned around the reading (*lectio*) of medical writings of Greek and Arabic authorities.

The content of the *lectio* in scholastic medicine during the period we are discussing was quite broad. It could include anything from the simple exposition of words or sentences, explanation of meaning, to the most intricate exegesis, but it always involved a detailed dissection of the passage in question.[52] In the course of this analysis, particular problems (*questiones*) might emerge that needed to be resolved. Subsequently, during the fourteenth century, these *questiones* became a new literary form independent of the *lectio;* and this in turn gave rise to academic medical *disputationes,* in which students and auditors were invited to participate. In medicine, as in scholastic education generally, the *questio* became a flexible, effective tool permitting university masters to identify problems, treat them in depth, and develop and defend new replies. In fact, we can follow the changing intellectual concerns of fourteenth-century scholastic medicine by tracing a chain of *questiones* through contemporary commentaries, where they may be found noted down in the margins of manuscripts or extracted into separate lists. *Questiones* reveal that apparently abstruse speculative issues in pathology —for example, the nature of fever and the mode of its production—were not merely subjects of debate in narrow professional circles but topics of lively interest to which students of all levels as well as masters were exposed and might contribute. Thus this institutionalized system of medical education combined the tools of analysis with a method of scientific communication in such a way as to encourage cohesion within a broad academic community.

This allows us to understand still better the enthusiasm that the system aroused in a few Jewish intellectuals like Abraham Abigdor and Leon Joseph, to understand why they chose to travel to Montpellier "to hear the science of medicine from the mouths of Christian doctors and scholars."[53] One of the reasons why the latter physician chose to translate into Hebrew particular works by Gérard de Solo and Jean de Tournemire was precisely that they made, in his opinion, perfect use of the *questio* technique. Indeed, Leon was so taken by this literary form that he enhanced his translation of Gérard's *Practica super nono Almansoris* by adding

> in some chapters questions and answers following the disputes [*questiones, disputationes*] that I have found recorded, scattered here and there, some attributed to this

[51] Chenu, *Introduction à l'étude de Thomas d'Aquin* (cit. n. 5); P. Glorieux, "L'enseignement au Moyen Age: Techniques et méthodes en usage à la Faculté de Théologie de Paris, au XIIIe siècle," *Archives d'Histoire Doctrinale et Littéraire du Moyen Age,* 1968, *43*:65–186; Brian Lawn, *The Salernitan Questions: An Introduction to the History of Medieval and Renaissance Problem Literature* (Oxford: Clarendon Press, 1963); and John Marenbon, *Later Medieval Philosophy (1150–1350): An Introduction* (London/New York: Routledge & Kegan Paul, 1987).

[52] Roger French, "A Note on the Anatomical Accessus of the Middle Ages," *Medical History,* 1979, *23*:461–468, on p. 465.

[53] Appendix E, line 11.

> same learned author, others to another eminent and authoritative scholar; others I drew up as well as I was able to when I could find nothing suitable that discussed the problem of that chapter. . . . In the case of each question that is not from the book you will find at the beginning ALYH [*Amar Leon Yosef Ha-maᶜtiq* = Here speaks Leon Joseph, the translator], which are the initials of my name, so that you may know it is an addition.[54]

To Leon we owe a particularly eloquent eulogy of the scholastic method:

> Consequently, I found great benefits in this [the study of the liberal arts], because in general their discussions on these sciences [natural philosophy, law, medicine] do not stray from the subject matter; [the Christians] leave out nothing when it is a question of debating the truth or falsehood of a proposition; they are very rigorous concerning the questions and answers of a debate, which are linked together in such a way as eventually to bring out the truth by means of an analysis of opposing points of view, "like a lily among thorns" [Song of Sol. 2:2].[55]

IV. RESISTANCE TO CLASSING MEDICINE AS LEARNING

These translators' enthusiasm for scholastic medicine was not, however, universally shared by their contemporaries. Inevitably, the intellectual divisions within the Jewish community, the debates between rationalists and antirationalists or traditionalists, had found some reflection in its attitudes toward medicine. Its religious leaders contended that the medical knowledge necessary for the practitioner who tries to cure his patients is, first and foremost, a skill (*tahbulah*), not a science; neither the study of natural philosophy nor a grounding in medical theory is needed in order to heal. Social stimuli encouraged a utilitarian approach to medicine, an instrumentalist view of medical knowledge.[56] Indeed, if Abraham Abigdor and Leon Joseph are to be believed, an empirical medicine was the norm within the community. Medicine was simply not generally understood to be a way of obtaining knowledge of nature and of man, while the open system of education further encouraged a pragmatic approach to the art of healing.

The historian looking back at the fourteenth century finds occasional instances of what these men bemoaned, the decreasing cultivation of the sciences, broadly considered, by the Jewish communities of the western Mediterranean in this period, from Provence around the coast to the frontier with the kingdom of Granada. Some Jewish intellectuals were already beginning to fear an inferiority at the beginning of the fourteenth century. Writing from Montpellier to Solomon ben Adret just before his death, the philosopher-translator Jacob ben Makhir ibn Tibbon (Profatius) advised him that

> we need to convince the Gentiles of our knowledge and understanding [of natural philosophy], so that they cannot say that we lack all science and wisdom. We must

[54] Appendix D, lines 155–161.

[55] *Ibid.*, lines 68–72.

[56] This utilitarian approach, which did not reject the use of rational medicine, was shared by, e.g., Solomon ben Adret, who recommended the use of "experimental [empirical] medicine [*refuᵓah nisyonit*]," since the utility of remedies—even charms—was demonstrated by experience. See Ron Barkai, "L'ús dels salms en la màgia jueva de l'édat mitjana i el renaixement: El llibre *Shimush Tehilim*," in *La Càbala* (Barcelona: Fundació Caixa de Pensions, 1989), pp. 17–57, esp. pp. 28–30. For a similar movement in medieval Islam see the appealing article by Sabra, "Appropriation of Greek Science" (cit. n. 3), p. 241.

follow the lead of the Gentiles—at least, of the most learned ones. They have translated scientific works into their various languages, even when the content of these works is at odds with their faith. They respect scholarship and scholars, no matter what creed they may profess.[57]

It was not only the Jews who were conscious of this difference; it was commented upon also by Christian scholars as part of their defense of Christianity. Some put it down to a deficient education. The absence of the liberal arts from the training of those in the Jewish community who wanted to pursue an intellectual activity meant that the Jews (through their most conspicuous intellectual representatives) were prevented from discussing certain topics (be they natural philosophy, medicine, or theology and law), as well as deprived of an analytical tool of proven value. Ramon Llull had this in mind when he asserted in 1313 that "the Jews are a people intellectually coarse, for they have no knowledge of the liberal arts. Therefore, when anyone wishes to speak with them or to discuss scientifically [*subtiliter*] the faith, the seven sacraments, or the ten commandments, they cannot understand what is said to them. . . . Without [the liberal arts] it is impossible to understand anything, even to follow an argument."[58]

But their silence could also be seen by contemporary Christian critics as an indication that Jews were incapable of achievement in natural philosophy or medical theory. Leon Joseph attacked this second interpretation vigorously. "If these and other sciences should remain beyond our reach, it is not because our intelligence is inferior to that of the Christians, for we possess the same capacity for understanding; indeed, it is the circumstances that have kept us apart . . . exile and oppression. . . . For this reason the Christians have continued to advance in the profane sciences while we have continued to lose ground as a consequence of distress and oppression."[59] Thus Leon argued that the failure of Jewish natural philosophy should be explained by a combination of social circumstances that had produced intellectual sterility: in part their exile and their

[57] Given in French translation by Shatzmiller, "Contacts et échanges" (cit. n. 1), p. 337. The letter was published by Abba Mari ben Moïse, *Minhat genaot* (Pressburg, 1838), letter 39, p. 85; we have checked our English translation with the Hebrew text. Shatzmiller, who is stressing the positive exchanges between Jewish and Christian scholars in Montpellier around 1300, expresses surprise at ibn Tibbon's attitude. "Mais une autre idée, qui peut paraître singulière, se dégage encore de ce texte: les connaissances diffusées dans le monde chrétien doivent aussi être acquises par les Juifs. Et l'effort scientifique des Gentils est présenté comme un modèle" (p. 338). As we see, ibn Tibbon follows a model of scientific progress still based on translations from the Arabic. Among his reasons, he does not include Jewish ignorance of the tools of scholasticism—techniques that Jewish rationalists would discover later.

[58] "Iudaei sunt homines grossi intellectus, quia non uescuntur artibus liberalibus, nec eas sciunt. Et propter hoc, quando quis cum eis loquitur, subtiliter disputando de fide, de septem sacramentis et de decem preceptis, id, quod eis dicitur non intelligunt . . . per quam subtilitatem queant intelligere et percipere rationes." Ramon Llull, *Summa sermonum in civitate Maioricensi . . . composita,* in *Raimundi Lulli Opera latina,* ed. Fernando Rodriguez Reboiras and Abraham Soria Flores, Vol. XV (Turnhout: Brepols, 1987), p. 122. Three years before (1310), in Montpellier, Llull had written, "Judaei sunt homines sine scientia et quando catholicus disputat cum ipsis rationabiliter, non intelligunt rationes"; see P. E. Longpré, "Le *Liber de acquisitione terrae sanctae* du Bienheureux Raymond Lulle," *Criterion,* 1927, *3*:264–278, on p. 274. For Llull, of course, words like "subtiliter" and "rationabiliter" in this context entail the Aristotelian way of reasoning *secundum artes liberales;* see Eusebio Colomer, "Las *Artes liberales* en la concepción científica y pedagógica de Ramón Llull," in *Arts libéraux et philosophie au Moyen Age* (Montreal: Institut d'Etudes Médiévales; Paris: J. Vrin, 1969), pp. 683–690.

[59] Appendix D, lines 77–81.

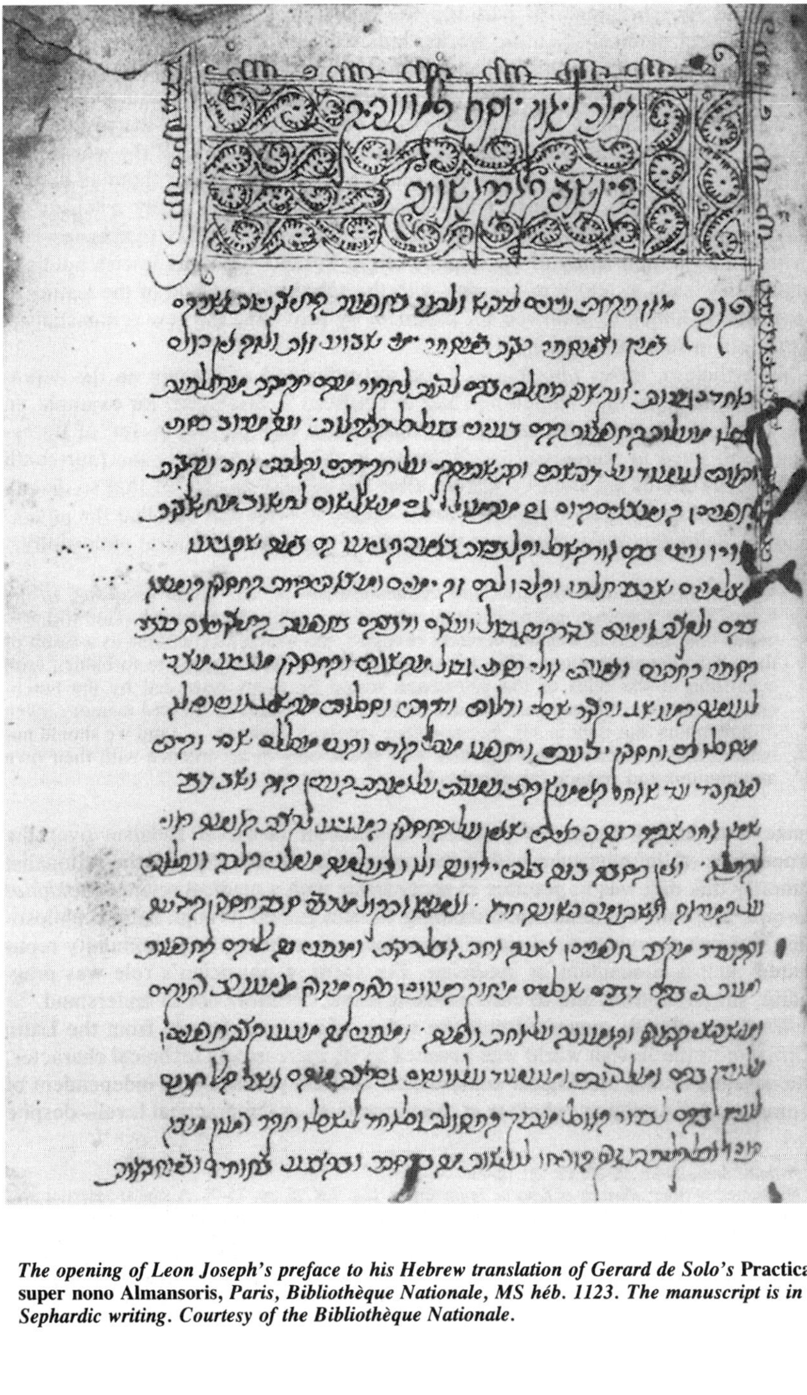

The opening of Leon Joseph's preface to his Hebrew translation of Gerard de Solo's* Practica super nono Almansoris, *Paris, Bibliothèque Nationale, MS héb. 1123. The manuscript is in Sephardic writing. Courtesy of the Bibliothèque Nationale.

oppression by Christians, in part too the inadequacy of the existing Hebrew translations of medical-scientific works, but, most important, the absence of intellectual freedom within the Jewish community. For him, the proven success of the Christians' scholastic medicine was the best reason for condemning the rigidity of the traditionalists within the Jewish community, those "learned in the Torah," whose "words concerning the profane sciences were like 'the words of a sealed book' [Isa. 29:11] . . . and [the sciences] are as far from them as east is from west." Besides, properly understood, scholasticism is really a legacy of earlier Judaism: dialectic was "employed by our own scholars [*hakhamim*] in earlier times in their study of the science of the Torah," and thus Jewish intellectual history leads to and is in keeping with the scholastic method of the Latins.[60] Leon clearly hoped to reinforce his argument by providing the new scholasticism with roots in Jewish tradition.

Nevertheless, those who felt as Leon did remained noticeably on the defensive. The hostility they sometimes had to confront is displayed, for example, in the words of the Talmudic scholar and rabbi Isaac bar Sheshet Perfet, of Barcelona, who lived in Saragossa and Valencia in the second half of the fourteenth century. In one of his letters—written after the upheavals of 1391 that so deeply affected that generation of Spanish Jews—Isaac bar Sheshet extolled the advantages of Talmudic instruction over the study of medicine or natural philosophy.

> We should not judge the laws and commandments of our Torah according to the views of the scientists and physicians, who, if they are to be believed—God forbid—assert that the Torah was not divinely revealed, the which they assume as a result of their false demonstrations. One who interpreted the laws relating to forbidden food according to the rules of the physicians would be richly rewarded by the butchers. . . . But we, for our part, should be loyal to our sages of blessed memory, even if they tell us that right is left, because they received the truth . . . and we should not believe the Greek and Arab scholars who speak only in accordance with their own assumptions and certain experiments.[61]

Isaac thus brings home the potential division in medieval Judaism over the proper role of the physician within the community. Evidently, for the rationalist minority this role was to practice in accordance with a medical science (*hokhmat ha-refu᾿ah*) built up on an understanding of man gained through natural philosophy, but just as evidently some of the religious leaders of the community repudiated such a conception of medicine. For them, a physician's role was pragmatic, simply to treat and to cure, nothing more; certainly not to understand.

We have already suggested that the reflux of medical thought from the Latin Christian to the Jewish world was assisted by its increasingly technical character, the absence of any ideological component. Medical practice was independent of a practitioner's religion, whether at the theoretical or the practical level—despite

[60] *Ibid.*, lines 19–21, 25–32; 12, 21; 72–73.

[61] Quoted by Baer, *History of Jews in Spain* (cit. n. 13), Vol. II, pp. 75–76. A similar assertion was made by Jacob ben Sheshet Gerundi in his polemic against Maimonideanism: "In their madness [the rationalists] follow the science of the Greeks. . . . It is illicit to learn something from the Gentiles." Quoted by Vajda, *Recherches sur la philosophie* (cit. n. 12), pp. 357–358. For illustrations of the complexity of the traditionalists' intellectual world see Twersky, "Rabbi Abraham Ben David" (cit. n. 9); Twersky, "Aspects of the Social and Cultural History" (cit. n. 4); and Shatzmiller, "Rationalisme et orthodoxie" (cit. n. 1), pp. 265–266.

the attempts of the medieval Church to christianize medical activity by, for example, requiring physicians to see to it that dying patients made a last confession, or by simply prohibiting Christians from seeing Jewish physicians.[62] Theoretical medicine as discussed and developed within the universities maintained its autonomy, with a curricular-technical dependence upon the arts faculty but none at all on theology. Doubtless Jews were formally prohibited from enrolling in the *studia,* but they could still find a certain acceptance there, as Leon Joseph did from Jean de Tournemire. This ideological neutrality could have enabled the transfer of a mature Latin Galenism into Judaic society, normally so jealous of its religious identity. Indeed, Leon saw no objection even to translating that portion of Gérard de Solo's commentary in which that author set out his belief in the Holy Trinity; he could not be blamed for translating this, Leon insisted, for those few words at the outset of Gérard de Solo's proemium were merely a personal statement by the Christian author that in no way affected the really interesting part of the *Practica,* its strictly medical content.[63]

It was therefore not the nominally "Christian" character of Latin medical theory that impeded its transmission; its lack of doctrinal character made it all the easier to be accepted by that group of Jews wishing to assimilate the achievements of scholasticism. After 1400, in fact, some Jewish scholars would find those achievements increasingly attractive.[64] How large, how widespread that group was is not something that can be answered here; we are far from wishing to generalize from such a limited number of texts. For the moment, all that the prefaces edited here can prove is that at least a few Jewish physicians in the western Mediterranean found that Latin scholastic medicine opened a new perspective to them during the fourteenth century.

[62] For papal letters and conciliar decrees against the practice of medicine within the Christian community by Jewish physicians see Solomon Grayzel, *The Church and the Jews in the Thirteenth Century* (rev. ed., New York: Hermon Press, 1966), pp. 74–75, 332–337.

[63] Appendix D, lines 168–173. Leon Joseph alludes to the following words from Gérard de Solo's work: "Invoco igitur Deum Patrem qui scit omnia qui sua potentia poterit meam indigentiam relevare cum ab eo dependeat tota celi natura. . . . Invoco Deum Filium qui sua sapientia et excellentia me gubernet quia ipse patris sapientia et a quo omnis sapientia et excellentia me gubernet et a quo omnis sapientia derivatur. Tertio invoco Spiritum Sanctum qui est amicitia et charitas patris." Gérard de Solo, *Nonus liber Almansoris cum expositione Gerardi de Solo* (Venice, 1505), proemium, fols. 13va–b.

[64] B. and C. Lagumina, *Codice diplomatico dei Giudei di Sicilia,* 3 vols. (Salerno, 1884–1895), no. 491, Vol. I, pp. 28–29 (17 Jan. 1466); cited by H. Bresc, *Livre et société en Sicile (1299–1499)* (Palermo: Centro di Studi Filologici e Linguistici Siciliani, 1971), p. 67, n. 1. See also Cecil Roth, *The History of the Jews of Italy* (Philadelphia: Jewish Publication Society of America, 1946), p. 241.

Appendixes follow

APPENDIX A

Prologue to the translation by Estori bar Moses ha-Parhi of Armengaud Blaise's *Antidotarium*[a1]

1 The translator, Estori bar Moses ha-Parhi, says:

13 . . . Then it was I came upon a book written in the language of the Christians, more precious than fine gold, mother-of-pearl, and onyx, which treats of the art of medicine. The usefulness of this book is no trifling matter for one who is wracked in pain, it is as much a treasure to the humble as to the great, / a treasure of which the sage Christian named Armengaud Blaise from Montpellier is the author. It was handed to me here in Barcelona, in the year of my slavery, at the beginning of my new exile, and there I translated it from their language to our own blessed language, thanks to the benevolent care of God for us, His people. After having translated it, I did not wish to publish it for some time, but on the arrival of the Nasi[a2] in the community of wise and judicious men, he asked for a book, and I mentioned this trifle to him, this treatise, which I presented and expounded unto him. /

The theme of this book is self-explanatory. An introduction is unnecessary. That which goes before is the first and the last.

APPENDIX B

Prologue to the translation by Israel ben Joseph Caslari of Arnau de Vilanova's *Regimen sanitatis ad regem Aragonum*[b]

The translator says: It is known to him who is interested in the various branches of the art of medicine, and more so to him who reaches the natural roots, that is to say, the principles and foundations of this art, that there is nothing within the sections relating to the regulation and conservation of health that does not belong to the field of / analogical speculation in the art of medicine; the principles and the roots of his knowledge are taken, in general, from propositions that are to be found in natural science. There is no doubt of their certainty. For most of the nutritive substances that conserve our health have been known by way of analogy, selecting—by means of flavor or smell, for dryness or wetness—those fit from those unfit; all these are attained by one who possesses medical science, he obtains them by analogy, / in accordance with natural principles, as we have said.

On the other hand, most of the things that are found in the sections relating to the restoration of health come from the field of scientific experiment, the object of which is not verified, in any case, by way of analogy. For the character of most medicines and remedies aimed at restoring health is known by way of experimental speculation, especially those products that cure diseases by their tertiary powers or / specific qualities, that is to say, the faculty inherent in the form of the medication or the remedy.

Thus the reason for the large quantity of books and for the repetition of texts that are found concerning the conservation and regulation of health and [concerning] the nutritive substances, is the same reason that explains the multiplicity of books and the repetition of texts that exist concerning the restoration of health and the details of medical treatments. The reason for the first part and for the repetition of texts that can be found in it is that temperaments vary in accordance with / the climates in which the books are written.

[a1] MS Parma, R. 347 (13 pages); see Steinschneider, *Die hebraeischen Übersetzungen* (cit. n. 26), p. 778. We have translated only line 1, which contains the translator's name, and lines 13–21, which are directly connected with the theme of our article.

APPENDIX A

הקדמה לאשתורי בר משה הפרחי

בה אלי ספר מלשון אחרת, יקר מזהב ומפז דר וסוחרת על מלאכת הרפואה, הלא הוא כלל קצר יועיל לכאב לב, אוצר לקטן יעשה ולגדול, אוצר מיחוס לחכם נוצרי שמו מא" ארמנגב בלדי דמונפשליר, מסרו בידי פה ברצלונה שנת שעבודי תחלת גלותי החדשה ושם הוצאתיו מלשונם ללשוננו המאושר כיד השם הטובה עלינו עמו. היה אחר העתקתו ימים אחדים לא רציתי לפרסמו. ובבא הנשיא לכלל אנשים חכמים ונבונים, דרוש דרש ספר וספור וספור הקומץ הזה אליו הקרבתיו ולפניו הצגתיו.

ענין הספר מבואר בעצמו לא יצטרך אל הקדמה. הקודם הראשון והוא אחרון. ישביענו מתורתו ישתבח שמו!

APPENDIX B

הקדמה [לישראל בן יוסף כשלרי]

אמר המעתיק כבר נודע לכל מי שיעיין בסדורי מלאכת הרפואה יותר למי שהשיג השרשים הטבעיים שהם התחלות ויסדות למלאכה ההיא, כי אין אחד מהדברים הנכנסים בחלקי שמי[ר]ת] הבריאות והנהגתו יותר מגדר העיון ההקשי אשר במלאכת הרפואה, וההתחלות והשרשים בידיעתו, בכללות לקוחות מהקדמות מצויות בחכמה הטבעית, אין ספק באמתתה.

וזה כי רוב המזונות שהם שומרים הבריאות נודעו על דרך ההקש, ויובדלו הנאותים מהבלתי נאותים או מטעמם או מריחם או מיבשם או מספוגיותם; וכל אלו הדברים נמשכים ונותנים בהקש לבעל חכמת הרפואה עם התחלות טבעיות כמו שבארנו.

ואמנם הדברים הנמשכים בחלקי השבת הבריאות הם רובם מגדר החכמה הנסיונית, אשר לא יתאמת ענינה בכלל על דרך ההקש. וזה כי רוב הסמים והתרופות המיוחדים להשיב הבריאות נודע ענינם על דרך העיון הנסיוני ובפרט אותם הדברים אשר ירפאו החלאים בכחותם השלישיות או בסגולה רוצה לאמר הכח הנמשך אחר צורת הסם או התרופה, ועל כן סבת רוב הסדורים והשנות המאמרים הנמצאים בחלק שמירת הבריאות והנהגתו ובמסעדים המזוניים, הסבה העצמה ברבוי החבורים והשנות המאמרים אשר חוברו בחלקי השבת הבריאות ופרטי הרפואות, לפי שסבת החלק הראשון והשנות המאמרים המחברים בה היא לפי שסבת המזגים אם לפי טבע האיקלימים אשר חוברו המאמרים בהם.

[a2] President of the rabbinic tribunal.

[b] MS Florence, Mediceo-Laurentiana Library Pl. 88, C. 36. The name of the translator into Hebrew does not appear in the prologue. Steinschneider (*Die hebraeischen Übersetzungen*, p. 779) attributes it to Israel Caslari, to whom the translation of the *Regimen sanitatis ad regem Aragonum* contained in this manuscript belongs.

In fact, remedies are repeatedly talked about, because they need to be tried continually. Each one of the scholars in medicine tries to verify on his own account, not to accept verification by others, the actions of the medicines [and] the limit of their form, called their occult nature; and each one writes a book on what he has proved, as happens in the science of the stars with those aspects that have already been described, / as explained in the *Almagest*.

I say, then, that texts written on the theme of medicines and remedies will be useful to us, and will be preferable to those that discuss the nutritive substances that conserve the health, for these change, sometimes a lot and sometimes a little. In effect, most of the things that conserve health bring about [different] changes in different men; many do not have any purpose. / On the other hand, the efficacy of the medicines and remedies that act as we have described, in accordance with their image, change, in any case, only a little. In this sense, we already know that scammony purges yellow bile and that turpeth purges phlegm; this was determined by the ancients, and it does not appear that it has ever happened that someone should have taken scammony without something similar to the nature of saffron having them come out of his body; and no one has ever taken turpeth without something of the nature of / phlegm having come out of his body.

With this we mean to say that, with respect to remedies, it is not necessary to write as many treatises as we must do with nutritive substances and foods in relation to the conservation of health. It could almost be said that every man needs a text written for himself; for this reason kings and magnates are accustomed to ask their doctors to write a text for them with the diet they should follow. So I myself, the translator of this book, / ask forgiveness for having meddled in an art which is not mine, translating this book, which is the first that has been written to date—although I know well that Rabbi Moises [Maimonides], of blessed memory, wrote a treatise on the theme.

In reality I have two reasons for doing so: the first is that this text is written taking into account the nature of [this] country, for its author is Master Arnau de Vilanova who was in Barcelona, in the service of the King of Aragon; the second is that this book was written according to the customs and habits of the Christians, / in whose lands we live. The great personages always asked him to compose diets, and in order to lighten the task, he composed this work.

I have deemed it fit to translate it, thus adding it to the similar work by the sage I have mentioned [Maimonides], because the author was a great scholar; his wisdom was so great and his science of medicine so high, that he surpassed all his predecessors, to such a point that the common people considered him a prophet. The truth must be accepted for itself; and the truth must be received from him who speaks it.

APPENDIX C

Prologue to the translation by Joseph bar Judah ha-Sefardi of the Catalan version (by Berenguer Ça Riera) of Arnau de Vilanova's *Regimen sanitatis ad regem Aragonum*[c]

I saw that this guide [to good health] was excellent and beneficial for two reasons: on the one hand for the merit of the man who wrote it, and on the other for the excellence of the man for whom it was written.

With / respect to the man who wrote it, you must know that he was a Christian writer called Master Arnau de Vilanova, a great scholar and brilliant physician, who lived among us in this our land. He knew the natural things of these lands and their temperament, and most of the guides that the ancients had written in Arabia, the temperament of their land, their nature, their food, their drink, and their customs, which are not the same as the temperament of our land, our nature, our

[c] New York, Jewish Theological Seminary, Elkan Nathan Adler (ENA) Collection Bill. The manuscript is not described in Steinschneider, *Die hebraeischen Übersetzungen*. We have not been able to

ואמנם השנות הדבור בתרופות הוא לנסות הדברים תמיד, וכל אחד ואחד מחכמי הרפואה ינסה ויתאמת לו הדבר, לא יתאמת לזולתו מהדברים הנמשכים אחר פעולת הסמים, מצד צורתם הנקרא טבע נעלם, ויחבר כל אחד ספר ממה שנסה, כמו בחכמת הכוכבים מהמבטים אשר נכתבו על זה הצד כמו שמבאר באלמגסטי.

והנה אומר כי יספיקו לנו המאמרים המחוברים בעניני התרופות והסמים מאשר המחוברים בעניני המזונות השומרים הבריאות, והם מקבלים התחלפות על הרוב ואחרים על המעט, וזה כי רוב הדברים השומרים הבריאות, יקיפו באישים המתחלפים התחלפויות רבים, אין תכלית להם והתרופות [ו]הסמים הפועלים על דרך שבארנו, כרמות כוללים, לא יתחלף ענינם כי אם על צד הפחות; ויתר דמיון זה כי כבר נוסה שהאשקמוניאה תמשוך המרה הכרכומית והטורביט ימשוך הבלגם; וזה הניחו הראשונים ולא נראה לעולם מי שלקח אשקמוניאה שלא יצא מגופו תחלה מה שידמה לכרכומות וטבעה, ולא מי שלקח הטורביט שלא יצא מגופו מה שהיה מטבע הבלגם.

כונתנו בזה שלא נצטרך לחבר בעניני התרופות מאמרים שונים כהצטרכנו בעניני המזונות ומסעדים בהנהגת הבריאות כמעט שאומר יצטרך בזה לכל איש ואיש מאמר מחובר לעצמו, ולכן מדרך המלכים ואנשי המעלה לצוות רופאיהם לחבר אליהם מאמר מסדר הנהגתם. ע"כ מעתיק זה הספר אומר מתנצל בהיותי אוחז אומנות שאינה שלי להעתיק זה המאמר הראשון המחובר עד היום, גם כן ידעתי חבר בזה הרס" ז"ל.

אמנם לי בזה שני טעמים, האחד כי זה המאמר נעשה לפי טבע הארץ כי מחברו היה משטרא ארנבט רוילה נובא ועמד עם המלך דארגון בברצלונא, השני כי המאמר הזה חבר לפי מנהג הנצרי וחוקותם אשר אנחנו שרויים על ארמתם, ונבקש להם תמיד מגדוליהם לסדר להם הנהגתם ולמען הקל הטורח חדש מאמר, בזה ראיתי להעתיקו מצורף אל זה החכם הנז[כר] אשר חברו, חכם מאר וגדלה חכמתו, ונתעלה בחכמת הרפואה מכל אשר היו לפניו עד שההמון חשבוהו לנביא והנה יקובל האמת מצד עצמו.

קבל האמת ממי שאמרו.

APPENDIX C

הקדמה ליוסף בר יהודה הספרדי

הנהגת הבריאות לחכם הנצרי משטרו ארנב רוילא נובא

בראותי הנהגה הזאת רבת המעלה והתועלת לשני פנים, האחד לפי ערך האיש המחבר אותה והשני לפי גודל מעלת האיש אשר חוברה אליו. אם לפי ערך האיש המחבר אותה, דע כי המחבר הזה היה נצרי, שמו מש" ארנב רוילה נובא, חכם גדול ורופא מובהק היה ביננו ובארצנו זאת. ידע טבעי הארצות האלה ומזגם ורוב הנהגות הבריאות אשר לראשונים חוברו בארץ הערב, ומזג ארצם וטבעם ומאכלם ומשתם ומנהגם בלתי שוה למזג ארצנו

identify this translator. He may have belonged to the Jewish community of Castelló d'Empúries in Catalonia.

food, our drink, and our customs. On the great dignity of the man / for whom it was written, you must know that he was the powerful lord King of Aragon, and may his kingdom be exalted and extolled!

It is well known that this author [Arnau] applied all his effort, all his capacity of understanding, and all his science in order to be able to compose this guide with honesty and great discernment, with fine and subtle reflection, and with the aim of making it useful, as is fitting to the great dignity of the king who asked him for it. Thus when I perceived its excellence and utility I felt stimulated, I, Joseph bar Judah ha-Sefardi (may I be remembered in the next world), / and I translated it from the Christian language to the Hebrew language—in spite of being conscious of my slight intelligence and my defective knowledge of both languages—so that it should be beneficial to us, unfortunate Jews, who live in exile in the land of the Christians.

APPENDIX D

Prologue to the translation by Leon Joseph of Carcassonne of Gérard de Solo's *Practica super nono Almansoris*[d1]

Thus says Leon Joseph, the translator, who lives in Carcassonne. Many years ago I directed my attention toward the study of and research into the profane sciences, which are several in number and nature; in number they are as many as the days of the week, and each one has its own subject matter. / I had placed my confidence in them in order to undertake various pieces of research. In my eyes, the merits of these sciences were above all praise. This explains my zeal and wish to know them and to master them. I therefore followed in the footsteps of the learned men of our own times, as well as those of the recent and distant past who have had such concerns, so that they should illuminate my way with the light of their intelligence and understanding; I said to myself that they must have achieved the level that had been acquired by those perfect men / long since disappeared.

But I realized that the lack of knowledge that they, and some of my people at this time, found themselves submerged in was great and immense, and that their words concerning the profane sciences were like "the words of a sealed book."[d2] Thus I said unto myself: perhaps my wish is greater than my intelligence, and the defect is mine for not being able to fathom the concepts, and it is my own lack of intelligence, the weakness of my spirit and my ignorance, that do not allow me to understand their words, and not their ignorance and their lack of knowledge, for they are the most learned among all men / and I am nothing but the lowest of their class. I was perplexed until, after many attempts, I understood the truth of the situation and "the thing once again was full of sense, after having been without any meaning,"[d3] for I perceived that said lack [of knowledge] on the part of one sector of [our] nation was by no means strange. Its cause was not unknown and I was not unaware of the [Talmudic] law which referred to it,[d4] and I was surprised by what I saw, and felt considerable uneasiness because of this misfortune.

Then I heard a voice telling me that there was not one single cause, but many, for the lack and absence of this knowledge / among some of our scholars. Sciences defeated them because their subject matter is more rational than in the bosom of our people, and they [the sciences] are as far from them as east is from west, and all the more so from the fundamentals of the Torah and of religious faith.

For this reason, some of our scholars refrained from studying them, from learning about them, and from investigating their aims; but others among them, who by

[d1] MS Paris, Bibliothèque Nationale, Héb. 1123. The Hebrew prologue was published in Hebrew by A. Neubauer and E. Renan, "Les écrivains juifs français," *Histoire littéraire de la France*, Vol. XXXI (Paris, 1893), pp. 770–778. The highly defective transcription was accompanied by a French

וטבענו ומאכלנו ומשתנו ומנהגנו. ואם לפי גודל מעלת האיש אשר חוברה אליו, דע כי האיש הזה היה האדון רם ונשא התנשא מלכותו מעלה מעלה מלך ארגון ירום הודו. וידוע כי המחבר הזה שם כל כחו והשגתו והחכמתו לעשות ההנהגה הזאת ביושר ובתשיה גדולה ובעיון דק וטוב ובתכלית התועלת, כפי מה שראוי לפי גודל מעלת המלך אשר בקש אותה ממנו. ולכן בראותי מעלתה ותועלתה נתעוררתי, אני יוסף בר יהודה הספרדי, זלה"ה, והעתקתי אותה מלשון נצרי אל לשון עברי עם היות כי ידעתי קוצר דעתי וחוסר השגתי בשתי הלשונות למען תהיה לתועלת לנו היהודים האמללים הגולים בארצותהם.

הנהגת הזאת נחלקת ליח׳ השערים.

APPENDIX D

הקדמה לליאון יוסף

אמר ליאון יוסף המעתיק, היושבי קארקאשונה: הנה מאז פקחתי עינים לדרוש ולתור בחכמות החיצוניות אשר הם במין ובמספר רבות, במספר ימי שבוע זאת, ולזה אין כולם כאחר בגדרות.

ונקשרה תוחלתי בהם לדעת לחקור מהם חקירות מתחלפות; גדלו מעלות החכמות ההם בעיני בעל כל התהלות. וזה מרוב כספי ותאותי לעמוד על דרישתם והתשוקקי על חקירתם. והלכתי אחרי עקבות חכמינו הנמצאים היום גם מאתמול גם משלשום לחשוב מחשבות ויאורו עיני בהם אור השכל והלבבות באמרי: הגיעו הם במה שהגיעו [ה]שלמים שכבר חלפו והלכו להם זה ימים.

ומצאתי היות החסרון הנמצא בהם ולקצת אומתי בדור הזה גדול ועצום, ודבריהם בחכמות החצוניות כדברי הספר החתום ואמרתי: אולי כספי גדול מהשגתי, והחסרון מגיע מצדי לעומק המושג וקצור שכלי ודלותי ודקותי וסכלותי מהשיג ענינם לא מסכלותם וחסרון ידיעתם, ויחכמו מכל האדם, והנני מכללם שריד. והיתי כמחריד עד שאחר האימוץ הרב עמדתי על אמתת הענין הזה, ושב דבר שמן אחר שהיה רזה, כי ראיתי שאין על החסרון המגיע לקצת האומה ראוי חהפ[לי]א. ואין הסבה בזה בלתי ידוע ולא נתעלמה ממני הלכה, ונפלאתי על המראה ואשתומם רשעה חדא. ואמצא את קול מדבר סבת חסרון הידיעה וההעדר מקצת חכמינו, איננה אחת אבל רבות. ומפני זה אליהם החכמות רמות כי בהם דברים שכליים, מחוק המוננו כרחק מזרח ממערב רחוקים ומשרשי התורה והאמונה על אחת וכמה.

ומפני זה מנעו קצת חכמינו מלעיין בהם ומלדעתם ומעמוד על ענינם;

---

translation of certain fragments. We have considered it opportune to produce a new edition from the original Hebrew, together with an English translation of the entire text.

[d2] Isa. 29:11.

[d3] See Judah Halevi, *The Kuzari (Kitab al-Khazari): An Argument for the Faith of Israel*, trans. from the Arabic by Hartwig Hirschfeld (New York: Schocken Books, 1964), Pt. 1, para. 28.

[d4] See Babylonian Talmud (henceforth **BT**), *Baba Kamma* 82b.

the mercy of God studied them with the intention of selecting what was fit to eat from what was only fit for throwing away, applied their intelligence to this research—"he found a pomegranate; he ate the fruit within, and the peel he threw away"[d5]—and decided to do so in secret / and unknown to others, "in the clefts of the rocks and in the secret places."[d6] They had no right to propound this science in the squares and streets, or to discuss it, to show themselves to be favorable toward it, nor to conduct public debates with the aim of reading the complete truth, for knowledge of the truth can only be attained by means of the contrary. And all this [they did] for fear of the tongues of the foolish among the people, for they are but few and the others form the majority. Also for fear of those learned in the Torah, who proscribed the superfluous from our souls; whose power over wise men comes not from strength nor from the breadth of their knowledge, / but rather from the strength of their hands and from their many ruses that make the mass of the common people believe whatever they think, that is to say, that these sciences and those who are concerned with them are sundered from the community of those who possess the Torah. Such are the virtues of those who insult and tell lies about learned men!

I saw what they wrote about *The Guide of the Perplexed* and what they did [to its author] in those times, even though he was an eminent man and most expert in the Torah, a thousand, nay even ten thousand, times more than they were.[d7] Reason / and truth were on his side and his deeds support this; as a result, divisions increased and the lack [of learning] grew considerably among one part of our community [. . .],[d8] for the following reason: the majority of books concerning these sciences were written by men of other peoples, such as the Greeks, the Ismaelites, or the Christians, and other believers in religions that are different from the religion of the Jews, and those books reached us through translators. It is possible that some of them did not have / a full and perfect command of the language or languages and translated one word by another because of the image and likeness; or they may have omitted one thing or added another because they lacked a deeper knowledge of the language in question; or the books from which they were translating may have contained errors and these then passed into the books that were being translated as a result of a lack of understanding or through exhaustion. And the first error was followed by another even more serious one, as those who studied with those books built "with the line of confusion and the plummet of chaos."[d9] / When they realized their error and noticed their doubt, they redoubled their efforts to clarify the text or texts just as they were written, and on these weak and unstable foundations they built their castles. Anybody who endeavors to write a commentary and elucidate those texts moves further away from the truth and never finds it, and this is never suspected. I know that this is what happened to a wise man of my nation who explained certain / expressions of the books of the learned Avicenna on the basis of an initial translation that was really distant from the truth at many points, with the result that he wrote a book that was acclaimed correct and held up as an example and model. Likewise, another scholar, after the former, explained the words of Avicenna according to his own opinion and the text that he had.[d10] And the people followed him, believing that he was right and that his words were meaningful. Until God sent us the learned rabbi Joseph Lorki, who illuminated / our eyes with his latest translation, that which is closest to the truth. Then the commentators realized that the first translation was of no value, the matters were clear and simple, and they themselves were confused and ashamed.

Behold, then, that we saw with our own eyes that learned Jews had empty hands and lacked arguments. If those wise men were alive in our day, they would also be embarrassed today and ashamed of their opinions before God most awful and most mighty. We should surely not be surprised at this, for the cause is the corruption / of the translations.

On seeing the obstacle that these causes represented and aware that the afore-

[d5] BT *Hagigah* 15b.
[d6] Song of Sol. 2:14.

גם קצת מהם אשר האל חננם לעיין בהם לברור האוכל מתוך הפסולת וכל אחד לשכלו חקר רמון מצא תוכו אכל קליפתו זרק הוכיחו לעשות זה ב[ה]סתר ובהצנע, בחוחים ובמחבואות לא היו רשאים להרביץ החכמה בשוקים וברחובות ולהתוכח בהם להראות פנים להם ולהושיב ישיבה ברבים להמציא האמת על בוריו כי לא יודע האמת כ"א בהפכו, וזה מפחדם מלשון המון הסכלים, כי הם מתי מעט והנה הרבים, מצורף לזה מיראת התורנים אשר מיתר החרימו מנפשנו אשר ידם תקפם על המעיינים לא בכחם ורב ידיעתם רק לחוזק ידיהם, ורוב נכליהם להיות עדת ההמון ההוא נשמע אליהם בחשבם היות החכמת ההם, והמעיינים בהם יוצאים מכלל בעלי התורה. אלה מדות החסרים והמדברים על החכמים תועה.

והנה ראיתי הכתוב על ספר מורה הנבוכים ואת אשר עשו לו בימים הראשונים עם היותו גאון ונסמך התורה יותר מהם לאלפים ורבבה, והצדק והאמת אתו ומעשיו מוכיחין אותו ו[מפני] זה גדל החסרון והפליג, ההעדר בקצת האומה אחר ההשתתפות [בהיותה] על זה סבה: כי רוב ספרי החכמות ההם חברום חכמים מבני העמים כיונים ובני ישמעאל או הנוצרים ויתר המאמינים אשר דתיהם [שונות] מדת היהודים.

והגיעו הספרים אלינו ע"י המעתיקים ואולי הם או קצתם לא היו בקיאים בלשון ההוא או הלשונות על השלמות. והחליפו מלה אחת באחרת, בצלם או בדמות, או חסרו מהם או הוסיפו לחסרון ידיעתם בלשון ההוא, ידיעה בעצמות, או נפל בספרים אשר העתיקו ממנו טעות ומפני זה נפלה השגיאה בספרים ההם וקיצור ההשגה והלאות. ונמשך מהטעות ההוא טעות אחר גדול מזה כי יבנו עליו קו-תוהו ואבני-בוהו המעיינים בספרים ההם בהרגישם בטעות ההוא ובספק ההוא בהעמיקם לבאר הלשון או הלשונות כמו הם כתובים ועל יסוד רעוע וחלוש מגדליהם בונים וכל אשר יתקרבו לפרש ולבאר הלשונות ההם יתרחקו ועל האמת לעולם לא יפגשו ובדבר הזה אין בו חשש.

והנה ראיתי זה בחוש ובמוחש, שקרה לאחר מחכמי אומתי שביאר לשונות מספרי החכם בן סינא בהעתקה הראשונה, האמתית הרחוקה מן האמת במקצת המקומות עד שחבר מהם ספר, קראו ראוי להיות והעמידו למופת ולאות גם חכם אחר קם אחריו וביאר לשונות בן סינא כפי דעתו והלשון הנמצא אתו. וילכו העם אחריו עד שהיו לומדים מספרו בחשבם, נמקו עמו וטעם לדבריו עד ששלחנו האל החכם ר" [יו]סף לורקי, אשר האיר עיננו עם העתקתו האחרונה, האמיתית בקרוב ואז נמצאו המבארים ראשונה ככלום, ויתבררו ויתלבנו הדברים ונשארו בושים ונכלמים.

והנה ראינו בענינינו כי אין כל מאומה בידיהם ונסתמו טענותיהם. ואם היו החכמים ההם חיים כהיום, הנה כמונו היום, יבושו ויחפרו מדעותיהם ודבריהם מאל נורא ואיום; אמנם אין זה מן הפליאה כי מאת שבוש ההעתקה היתה להם נסבה.

ובראותי אלה הסבות המונעות, וידעתי לימוד החכמות הנזכרות אשר

[d7] The allusion is to the so-called Maimonidean controversy. See note 12 above.

[d8] The meaning of the two words in the original here is hopelessly obscure.

[d9] Isa. 34:11.

[d10] Leon's first reference is to the translation of Avicenna's *Canon* by Nathan ha-Meʾati, produced in Rome between approximately 1279 and 1283. His second reference is perhaps to Zerahiah Gratian, who carried out another (unfinished) translation of the *Canon* in Barcelona or Rome between 1270 and 1290.

mentioned sciences were known among the Christians—[God] is awful and marvellous; who could make him sustain us in our poverty!—I said to myself: I shall study their language [that of the Christians] a little, I shall attend their schools and houses of study, I shall follow their footsteps so that I am able to make use of whatever I might learn from their words and a little of the truth of their books, both for myself and for any other person; / I shall study what the most perfect among them studied, if time allows me to and no accident or hindrance should prevent me from doing so, and if my intelligence is able to cope with this and is not bewildered. Consequently, I found great benefits in this, because in general their discussions on these sciences do not stray from the subject matter; they leave out nothing when it is a question of / debating the truth or falsehood of a proposition [*lit.*, certain thing]; they are very rigorous concerning the questions and answers of a debate, which are linked together in such a way as eventually to bring out the truth by means of an analysis of opposing points of view, "like a lily among thorns."[d11] The way of studying that they practice today as regards these sciences is the same as that followed by our own scholars in earlier times in their study of the science of the Torah. I refer to that saying of the Talmud [on the scholars of Pumbedita who were able] to make an elephant pass through the eye of a needle,[d12] or as Rabbi Dosa said: "I have a younger brother who is a devil, who calls himself [Jonathan]; with his talent he is able to make whatever / was prohibited permissible. And he has more than three hundred arguments to prove that the rival of a daughter may marry the brothers."[d13] And those conclusions of Rabbi Meir and his companion that the religious law that has to be followed was not that of the latter but the restrictive measures of the former. And the school of Shammai, as it appears in the appropriate place. If these and other sciences should remain beyond our reach, it is not because our intelligence is inferior to that of the Christians, for we possess the same capacity for understanding; indeed, it is the circumstances that have kept us apart, and the memory of them has been erased as a result of exile and repression, and in the same way their pleasure, splendor, / and wealth [have been erased]. For this reason, the Christians have continued to advance in the profane sciences while we have continued to lose ground as a consequence of distress and oppression.

When I lived among the Christians, I was of an inferior condition in their eyes, for there is none of our nation who is honored in their eyes except him who is a physician and who cures them of their ills; in such a case, he sits at the table of kings and remains standing before them, whether he be of humble birth or / of high rank, owing to his knowledge of medical science, which follows that of physics and law, for physical science has as its end man and his form, and it is here that medicine begins, the object of which is man.

I understood this and I took it as my model, and I said unto myself: I shall go in search of Jewish physicians and I shall beg them to have mercy on me and to teach me their science in exchange for a small payment or free of charge, for the money of my purse has been exhausted. Thus I went forth to seek them and I found / that they were lacking nothing except that one science, for the two reasons that have already been explained and for another two, which make four. Not one less, nor one more. The majority of those who practice the art of medicine among my people do not intend to fathom the depths of their object; even if they were able to go into it in greater depth, they do not wish to tire their intelligence with this, and they mutter: this science is not a true science, but rather a skill; and with a "sound of tumult"[d14] everybody wishes to turn it into a means of existence. / They make an ideal of it, and they say that a learned physician is he who asks large amounts of money and does not heal free of charge; this man, called an expert physician, with his deceits and frivolities makes it appear as if he knows or, sometimes, he introduces himself as if he were so-and-so, son of so-and-so. How many physicians do we see, lacking understanding, who have gathered treasures of gold and silver, without ever having passed a single examination; whereas others who have always been in pursuit of books have obtained knowledge, but have not earned a penny? For this and other reasons, they have not whiled away their time in the study of /

בין הנוצרים ידועות, נורא מאד ונפלא ומי יכילנו שעמד על ענינו ויקיפנו. אמרתי בלבי: אלמד מעט מידיעת לשונם ואשב בישיבותיהם ובית עיונם ואלך אחרי עקבותם למען אוכל להועיל לעצמי ולזולתי בהשיגי דבריהם וקצת מאמתת ספריהם.

ואשקיף במה שהשקיפו השלמים מהם אם הזמן יספיק בזה [ולא] ימנעני מונע ומקרה ואם השכל יכול להשקיף עליו ולא יטרידהו [הפ]חוז ממנו ואליו ומצאתי התועלת בזה גדול ורב, להיות רוב משאם ומתנם בחכמות ההם, לא סרו במה שראוי לעיין בהם, דבר מהם לא יחסר בהיותם מתפלל[פ]לים על אמתתם ואף בהעמדת שקריותיהם ומדקדקים בשאלותיהם ותשובותיהם על צד הויכוח להוציא האמת ממרכז הפכו בבארם כל דבר בשני הפכים כשושנה בין החוחים. והנה חק עיונם היום באלה החכמות כחק חכמינו ברורות הקדומות בלמדם חכמת התורה, רוצה לומר תלמודה דמעילי "קופא דמחטא", כמאמר דוסא, אח קטן יש לי בכור, שטן שמו, יודע להתיר האיסור בחידודו. ויש לו שלש מאות וכמה תירוצים על צרת הבת שמותרת לאחים. ובפלפול ר" מאיר וחבירו שאין הלכה כמותו רק בגזרותיו ושמאי ובית דינו כמו שנרא זה במקומו והנה נמנעה ממנו ידיעת החכמות בכיוצא בזה לא שיהיה שכלנו למטה משכליהם כי גם לנו לבב כמו הם, אמנם מנעונו הסבות אשר קדר זכרונם על גלותינו ולחצנו ורוב תענוגם הודם והמונם. ומפני זה המה עלו בחכמות החיצוניות מעלה מעלה. ואנחנו ירדנו מטה לרוב הטרדות המעיקות.

וכאשר ארך זמן עמידתי עמהם והייתי שפ[ל] בעיניהם כי אין באומתינו מי שיהיה מכובד בעיניהם אם לא יהיה הרופא אשר ירפאם מחוליהם והוא יעלה על שולחן מלכים ולפניהם יתיצב יהיה שפל רוח או בקומה נצב, יען ידע בחכמת הרפואה אשר היא אחרית הטבע ומשפטה, כי סוף חכמת הטבע הוא האדם ותמונתו ובו תתחיל הרפואה מפני כי הוא נושאה. והבנתי זה ולקחתיו למשל ואמרתי: אלך אל היהודים הרופאים ואשאל מהם ואבקש מאת כבודם, יחמלו עלי וילמדוני מחכמתם בשכר מה או בחנם כי אזל הכסף מכלי והנה תם. והלכתי אחרי עקבותם ולא מצאתי בהם חסרון נרגש רק בחכמה ההיא לשתי הסבות הקדומות ושתים אחרות שהם ארבע. ואל תוסיף בהם מאלה לא תגרע והוא שרוב כלל אומתי המתעסק[ים] במלאכת הרפואה אין בדעתם להגיע עד תכליתה, גם כי יוכלו לעיין בה לא ירצו להטריח בזה שכלם כי פוערים פיהם במאמרם: אין זאת החכמה, חכמה כלל, אבל תחבולה וקול המולה להוציא כל איש ממנה המחיה ויהי להם למשל וילחשו בלחשם לאיזהו רופא חכם השואל ממון רב ולא בחנם ירפא והאיש ההוא, רופא אומן יקרא אשר בשקריו והבליו היותו יודע, לפעמים יראה היותו מזה בן מזה. וכמה רופאים רואים אנחנו הנעדרי הבינה אצרו אוצרות זהב וכסף מבלי בחינה ומהם עמדו תמיד אחרי הספרים ואליהם ההשקפה ולא השיגו ממון אפ[ילו] פרוטה. זאת ועוד אחרת לא יעיינו

[d11] Song of Sol. 2:2.
[d12] BT *Baba Meziʿa* 38b.
[d13] BT *Yebamoth* 16a.
[d14] Ezek. 1:24.

medical books, but in their leisure time they drink and lie together in the flesh and do other unworthy acts, such as reading books of fables, fantasies, and vanities. Not one of them wishes to be learned in the field of medicine so as to avoid entering Gehenna.

When I realized all this, I said to myself: there are no learned and expert men in our region. And I went in search of wise Christians so that they should guide me in such matters and so that they should show me the way, and so that they should show me / old and new volumes. Among them I saw the works of the learned physician Gordon, who was outstanding on the majority of subjects, both in theoretical study and in practical matters, and who achieved great fame. His works proliferated and his prestige increased more than that of his brethren. Some of his works have come down to us, such as the *Shoshan ha-refuʾah* [*Lilium medicine*] and the *Haqdamat ha-yediʿah* [*Tractatus de prognosticis*]; but the translations of these works are very defective, a shaky ladder. The Jews who translated [the *Lilium*] in these lands / gained access to it by means of the vernacular; they expressed the Latin in Romance, adding that not every Latin word may be translated in the vernacular tongue, and then they expressed it in the sacred language. In spite of that, the greater part of this book is understandable to us, with the exception of some points which I myself have hastened to correct and improve as was necessary so that the reader should be able to read it with ease; the same I have done with the book *Haqdamat ha-yediʿah,* the translator of which paid hardly any attention to the real meaning of the words. Seeking among their books, I found two / new books, "two golden pipes,"[d15] exemplary, excellent and worthy, which the people of our nation do not know. They are the books by the learned Gérard de Solo and by the master Jean de Tournemire, of whose [existence] I had known for ten years, but which I had been unable to acquire, neither in Montpellier, even though it was their place of origin, nor in Avignon, nor in other important places, since there were but very few [copies], and since the learned men of Montpellier / anathematize and excommunicate anybody who should sell to those who are not Christians. In order to acquire them, I invested all the funds that I was able [to spare], without reflecting on the consequences. And the books reached my hands this year, which is the year ninety-four according to the Christian calendar [1394]. The truth is that I paid double the price for them, owing to the yearning and desire that I felt for them. I saw their excellence, and that they explained things and answered matters in a suitable way. He who acts with them is as if he were grasping a column; / he will fear nothing, not even ten thousand physicians who might come with proofs and disputes, for they are pure flour. No men of their equal can be found in living memory. I believe that they did not fall behind and that they chose the best [aspects] of medicine.

Behold, thus, that I begin the book of Gérard, based on Book 9 of the *Book of Almansor* [by al-Rāzī, or Rhazes], short in length but great in quality, stronger than a rock. It provides suitable and opportune answers. / Its art is a safe art. It provides reasonable judgment on all things, which should be praised. Nothing is left out and nothing is forgotten. Therefore, the decision to translate it was taken calmly. When God wishes that I should finish it, I shall undertake Tournemire's book; in his time he was at the head of all the scholars of Montpellier, who were placed beneath him. I saw him with my own eyes and I spoke to him. He was a man who was pleasant to talk to. His behavior was not like that of the other scholars of his generation, who scorned those Jews who practiced the art of medicine, / for he guided them as far as he was able. May his soul rest in the treasure where the souls of the pious among gentile people live![d16] There is no book that is comparable to it for the beauty of its science. It speaks of the limbs and of the faculties, and of the illnesses that occur in them. It asks and answers, it explains and clarifies. He teaches like a father to a son, true and proper words, which are pleasing and agreeable to whoever listens to them.

I took the decision to translate these books, not for myself, but for the people / of my nation, both those who live alongside me today and those who will come after me, and who do not know the language of the Christians at all. When they

בספרי הרפואה, רק בעתות הפנאי בעברם עליהם בעתות השתיה והמשגל והדברים אשר להם גנאי בקראם על ספר מספרי המשלים, וההזיות וההבלים. אין איש מהם רוצה להיות ברפואה חכם למען לא יכנס בגיהנם.

ובהרגישי את כל זה אמרתי: אין נבון וחכם באיקלימנו זה. הלכתי אחרי עקבות החכמים הנוצרים והיישירוני בדברים והראוני הדרכים וגלו אלי הספרים חדשים גם ישנים. וראיתי ביניהם דברי החכם הרופא גורדו אשר ברוב דבריו תשובתו בצד הפליג לעשות בעיון ובמלאכה ולכתר שם טוב זכה רבו ספריו; וגדלו יקרותיו נתעלה על כל אחיו. והנה הגיעו אלינו קצת ספריו והוא שושן הרפואה והקדמת הידיעה. אמנם הגיע לנו בהעתקה מאד חלושה, סולם רעוע. הנה כי היהודים אשר העתיקוהו בארצות האלה לא השיגוהו רק באמצעות הלעוזות לעזו הלטין והוסיפו בטענות כי אין כל מלה אשר בלטין תוכל להיות לעוזה ובלשון הקדש להשיבה, אמנם רוב הספר ההוא על כל זה מובן אצלנו, ואם לא במקומות מה אשר טרחתי אני להגיהו ולתקנו כהלכתו למען ירוץ קורא בו וכן עשיתי בספר הקדמת הידיעה אשר המעתיקו באמתות הלשונות לא שעה. ובחפשי אמתחות ספריהם מצאתי שני ספרים חדשים לשני צנתרות הזהב ומשלים, מה מאוד הם טובים וראויים אשר מבני אומתי נעדרים. המה ספר החכם גיראבט דישולא וספר החכם מאישטרי יואן די טורנאמירא אשר זה עשר שנים שמעתי [ש]ומעם ולא יכולתי להשיגם לא בהר ואם הוא המקום אשר ממנו חוצבו, ולא באויניון ולא ביתר המקומות הטובים כי הנה במציאות מעטים, מצורף למה שחכמי ההר היו מחרימים ומנדים כל מי שימכרם לזולת הנוצרים, והוצאתי בהשגתם ממונות כפי כחי. ולא הרגשתי במי ומי והגיעו לידי בזאת השנה שהיא שנת תשעים וארבעה למספר הנוצרים לחשבונם, וחי האמת קניתים בכפלים משיווים לחשקי בהם ובתאותי ורצוני כם. וראיתי הפלגת טובם מראים פנים לכל הדברים ומשיבים כהלכה לכל הענינים והפועל עמהם שיעמור נשען בעמוד ובצר לא יירא מדבר ומרבבות עדת הרופאים אם יבואו אליו בנסיונות ובויכוחים להיות סולת נקייה לא קדם כמותם בזכירה. ואחשוב כי לא יתאחרו והיותר טוב מהרפואה בחרו.

והנה מתחיל אני בספר גיראבט הבנוי על הספר התשיעי מהאלמנצור אשר מעט הכמות ורב האיכות, חזק מצור, משיב כראוי ומגיד כהלכה ומלאכתו מלאכה בטוחה, ונותן טעם לכל דבריו טעם לשבח, לא נעלם ממנו דבר ולא נשכח ולכן שקטה ההסכמה להעתקתו. וכאשר יגזר השם בהשלמתו אתחיל אחריו ספר טורנו מירה אשר היה בימיו על כל חכמי ההר לראש והם עמדו תחתיו; ראיתיו בעניני ודברתי עמו, חסיד היה בדברו, לא היה חקו כחוק חכמי דורו לבזות היהודים אשר במלאכת הרפואה מתעסקים יען היה מישירם בכחו. בצרור חיי חסידי האומות תהיה צרורה נפשו, וספר אחד לא דמה אליו ביופי חכמתו. דבר באיברים וכחותיהם והחליים המתהוים בהם, שואל ומשיב, מברר ומלבן כאב המלמד את הבן חרש אמרים נכוחים וישרים ימתקו ויערבו לשומעים.

והנה עלה על רוחי להעתיק הס[פרים] ההם לא לעצמי אבל לזולתי מהעם, אשר עמי היום, ואשר יבואו אחרי הבלתי יודעים מאומה בלשונם כי

[d15] Zech. 4:12.
[d16] See 1 Sam. 25:29.

examine it and read it, they will see the perfection, the beauty, and the order of these books, they will bless me because of them and they will remember me for having been the reason why they should find them and the reason why they are able to compare themselves with the physicians in proofs and arguments, and this is a second life.

I believe that the fact that these books talk about things Christian is without significance unless [Jewish readers] take great pleasure in drinking wine, eating, drinking, and taking part in [Christian festivities], for, in that case, these translations will bring them no profit whatsoever; / it will be as if they had never been made and the yearning of their hearts will vanish. To tell the truth, if they read them many times, they will obtain different advantages, and they will feel calm and safe and will sleep peacefully in their beds. They will not fear him who attacks them in order to beat them with the stick of medicine, since they will be able to fight back without fear of the multitude, even if they are excommunicated. They will be able to put aside and put away all their other medical books, and should these two books be prohibited / they will be able to count on my explanations.[d17]

Thus, the aforementioned book of Gérard de Solo is Book 9 of the *Book of Almansor* [*Practica super nono Almansoris*] divided into the same parts and chapters as al-Rāzī divided his work. If this author [Gérard] does not point this out at the beginning of the book, as all authors of books are accustomed to do, it is because he trusted that everybody would understand that. I have prepared an index to these chapters, from the first to the last, so that everybody can find / what he wishes whenever he wants and so that he does not mix his thoughts or stray from the point. I have also thought to add in some chapters questions and answers following the disputes that I have found recorded, scattered here and there, some attributed to this same learned author, others to another eminent and authoritative scholar; others I drew up as well as I was able to when I could find nothing suitable that discussed the problem of that chapter in order to sharpen the intelligence and debate it and understand it in a suitable fashion. /

In the case of each question that is not from the book you will find at the beginning ALYH [*Amar Leon Yosef Ha-ma*^{c}*tiq* = Here speaks Leon Joseph, the translator], which are the initials of my name, so that you may know it is an addition. If you find any doubtful expression, do not reproach me or censure me in your hearts until you have checked it in another book, if God, in His mercy, has allowed you to learn the language of the Christians, or until you have consulted a learned physician. For the copy that I have translated contained errors, even though I have checked it twice / or thrice, [comparing it] with other books, and "all of them have been woven into the same cloth,"[d18] that is to say, it seems that they are all of the same origin, that all of them come from the same place. In those passages that turned out to be doubtful, there will be [the sign of] a small hand stretched out above them or some other sign at the side to indicate to whoever should be studying it that these passages have not passed unnoticed and that he can check them as well.

And to the community of physicians I say: Brothers, when you read the prologue of the author and see that he joins in his entreaty his king and his God and that / from one he obtains three and those different,[d19] I shall submit that I translated word for word, and do not get annoyed nor rail against me since you will have no other reasons for complaint after the prologue. My intention is that the book should reach you without suffering omissions or mistakes, so that you can understand it all and so that you can obtain benefits from it and sing its praises. If you do not wish to read the prologue, begin to study at the beginning of the book. I did not wish to remove any of its contents, rather / I wanted to add something to it.

I shall write [the name of] compound medicines in the Latin language, after having translated them into our language, with the help of God, so that those who are starting to practice the art of medicine can do so without effort or weariness. They will feel learned and intelligent, veterans in the art and perfect, even though they are but beginners. Without ever having seen the leading figure of the [medical] art, they will not be scorned by those crowned [with glory]. They will have no

בעברם עליהם וקראו ויראו שלמותם ויופי סידורם יברכוני בגללם ויזכרוני בלב[ם] להיותי סבת חיותם ושיוכלו עמוד נגד הרופאים בנסיונות ובויכוחים ואלה חיי שניים ידעתי כי עם אלה הספרים דבריהם נוצרים לאין אם לא ימשכו את בשרם ביין לאכול ולשתות ולחוג חגות כי אז לא יועילו להם ההעתקות, יען יהיו להם כמו שלא הועתקו וממורשי לבותם נתקו. אמנם אם יקראו בהם פעמים רבות יוציאו מהם תועלות מתחלפות ויעמדו בהשקט ובבטחה וישנו במטתם במנוחה. לא יפחדו מקול נוגש בשבט הרפואה יכם כי יוכלו ללחום מלחמותיהם לא ייראו מהמון אף כי יהיו מחורמים וכל שאר ספרי מלאכת הרפואה יוכלו להסתיר ולהעלים ועם שני אלה אם יחרימו תחרים ומפני זה בירותי בספרם.

והנה הספר הזה הנקר[א] גיראבט דישולא הוא הספר התשיעי מספר האלמנצור נחלק לאותם החלקים והפרקים אשר חלק ראזי את ספרו, ואם לא זכרם החכם הזה בתחילת ספרו כחק כל מחבר ספר מהספרים הנה סמך על המבינים. וערכתי אני הפרקים ההם זה מראש ועד סופו למצוא כל איש דבר חפצו כאשר ירצה ולא יבלבל מחשבתו ולא יטה. גם אמרתי: להוסיף בקצת פרקים שאלות ותשובות על צד הויכוחים מצאתים כתובים הנה והנה מפוזרים יוחסו קצתם אל החכם המחבר או לחכם אחר מטיב ומאשר וקצתם אחדש אני כפי יכלתי, כאשר לא אמצא איש עתי יתוכח בעיני הפרק ההוא לחדד השכל, ולפלפל ולדעת הפרק על אמתתו.

והנה תמצא בכל שאלה אשר לא תהיה בספר עצמו כתובה כתיבה בראשו אליה", והוא שמין שמי בראשי אותיות, למען תדע כי הן נוספות ואם תמצא לשונות מה מספקות אל תאשימני בלבך ואל תבזני בנפשך, עד שתדקדקו סבפר אחר, אם האל חננך לדעת לשונם או שאל לרופא חכם. כי הספר אשר ממנו העתקתי בו טעיות ואם דקדקתי עם ספרים אחרים שנים או ג" פעמים וכלהו מחתינהו בהדא מחתא נראה שכולם ממחצב אחד חוצבו וממקום אחד יצאו. והנה במקומות אשר יפול בו הספק ידו נטויה עליו או סימן אחר שבה כמו אל צדו להעיר לב המעיין ולהודיעו כי לא נעלמו מעיני ותוכל לדקדקו אחרי. ואת עדת הרופאים, אחי, כאשר תקראו בפתיחת המחבר ותראו אותו קושר מתפלל במלכו ובאלוהיו ולמעלה יפנה מאחד משלש ושונה ואני העתקתיו מלה במלה, אל תדברו עלי חרה ואל תלינו עלי תלונה, כי לא ישאר אליכם תרעומת אחר ההקדמה, כי דעתי רצויה יגיע לכם הספר בלי השמטה וחסרון יפול בו, למען תשיגוהו כולו ותוכלו לחתור מדבריו ולהשיב על מהלליו. ואם לא תרצו לקרות פתיחתות, תחילו לעין בתחלת ספרו ולא רציתי לחסר דבר ממה שדיו תחת רציתי להוסיף בו והנה אכתוב כל הרפואות מורכבות בלשון לטין אחר העתיקי אותם בלשוננו, בגבורת השם למען אועיל למתחילים להתעסק במלאכה יוכלו לסדר בלי עמל ויגיעה. יראו עצמם חכמים ונבונים, זקני המלאכה, ושלמים גם כי יהיו מתחילים. לא ראו מאורות במלאכה כל הימים, לא יבזו אותם העטרים ולא יצטרכו לעיין בספר שמות הסמים אם ידע הרפואות על

[d17] The meaning of this passage is unclear in Hebrew, and it is difficult to translate.
[d18] BT *Berakoth* 24a.
[d19] An allusion to Gérard de Solo's invocation of the Trinity in the proemium to his *Practica*.

need to consult any other book of medicine provided they know the remedies / by heart, just as is written: "[God] will keep your foot from being caught";[d20] they will be considered important physicians, which is what I hope to achieve.

God knows what my heart desires. I ask Him to help me and to guide me in my translation and to give me strength to bring my task to conclusion and to translate the other work as well. And that He should show me the wonders of His Torah, and that He should send us His Messiah. Amen.

APPENDIX E

Prologue to the translation by Abraham ben Meshullam ben Solomon Abigdor of Bernard Alberti's *Introductorium in practicam pro proiectis*[e1]

Abraham ben Meshullam ben Solomon Abigdor says: When I was young my desires were those of a young man, and equally my thoughts and my urges; not that I wished to study the art of medicine because of a yearning for knowledge of the science, but rather just the name itself was enough for me, / so that I would be called Master and earn those undeserved profits as is customary nowadays among the majority of the men who are engaged in this art, especially those of our people.

When I grew up, and reached the grade of manhood, my desires were those of a man, and equally my thoughts and my urges. I decided to study and to go deeply into this science from every side; and I wished to do so in order to attain true knowledge, not for anything / subject to destruction and corruption. Thus I went up to the mountain, to Montpellier, the renowned city, to hear the science of medicine from the mouths of Christian doctors and scholars, and there I found numerous books and useful commentaries on the fundamental principles of that science, and if the Lord should prolong my life, I shall translate some of them. I found useful books, which lead us straight to the art [of medicine], and from among them I specially chose this one called *Mabo ba-melakhah* [*Introduction to the Art*], which is a very useful guide / for anyone who wants to devote himself to this art with confidence and rectitude. The questions of which this book treats are all explained very clearly, as are the remedies that it includes, and that according to the time in which we live, the climates and the temperaments. [With its help,] the physician will be able to apply them with surety. I have translated it from the Christian language to that of our people, at the request of some of my friends and colleagues.

May the Lord protect me from all errors and make me worthy of translating this [book], as well as other books, / and may He prolong my days and the days of those who translate books of medicine, which are great things [?], and the days of all brothers of Israel [?].[e2] Amen.

The author says: This book, called *Introduction to the Art,* was written for the sake of those who have been instructed in the science of medicine but have not yet been trained in its use. It is founded on the first chapter of Book 4 of Avicenna['s *Canon*] and was composed by the distinguished scholar Bernard Alberti, a prominent figure in the honorable academy that is in the city of Montpellier, / at the request of his friends and pupils. These are the contents of his words: At your request, my friends, who have toiled and labored with me in the study of this science, the science of medicine, I decided to write for you a useful though small book concerning the art of medicines. I shall follow the path of the first chapter of Book 4 of Avicenna. I shall arrange, in an orderly way, the remedies that in my opinion are well known, efficient, and proven. I pray that this book / may not be trivial in your eyes, since I deem it to be of great utility. . . .

[d20] Prov. 3:26.

[e1] The Hebrew text (MS Halberstam 406, fol. 74) was edited by Moritz Steinschneider, "Medizinische Handschriften im Besitz des Herrn Halberstam," *Magazin für die Wissenschaft des Judentum,*

פה ככתוב וישמר רגל מלכד. ויחזיק[והו] לרופא חשוב וזאת היא כונתי. והאל הוא היודע מה הנכסף בלבי וממנו אשאל יהיה כעזרי ויישירני בהעתקתי, ויתן לי יכולת להשלים מלאכתי ולהעתיקו הספר האחר עמו ויראני נפלאות תורתו וישלח לנו את משיחו אמן סלה.

APPENDIX E

הקדמה לאברהם בן משולם אביגדור

אמר אברהם בן משולם בן שלמה (בן) אביגדור בהיותי נער (היו) תשוקותי תשוקות נער, ומחשבותי מחשבות נער, ותאותי תאות נער, וחשקתי ללמוד מלאכת הרפואה לא מפני כוסף ידיעת החכמה, אך הספיק לי בשם לבד כדי שאקרא רב, ארויח הרווחים ההם המגונים כמו שהוא היום מנהג כולל ברוב האנשים המתעסקים במלאכה הזאת ובפרט (וכל שכן ב) מבני אומתנו. וכאשר גדלתי והגעתי למדרגת האנשים היו תשקותי תשוקות איש ומחשבותי מחשבות איש ותאותי תאות איש ונתתי אל (את) לבי לדרוש ולתור ולחקור בזאת החכמה מכל צד לחשקתי בה מצד ידיעת האמת לא לתכלית כלה ונפסד, ואעלה ההר"ה הוא העיר ההוללה מונפשליר לשמוע חכמת הרפואה מפי נבוני הנוצרים וחכמיהם (מפי חכמי הנוצרים ונבוניהם) ומצאתי שם ספרים רבים וביאורים מועילים (בשרשי החכמה הזאת ואם יאריך השם ימי אעתיק מהם קצת. וספרים מועילים) מיישירים במלאכה ומכללם בחרתי בייחוד (ביארתי) זה הספר הנקרא מבוא במלאכה מועיל ומיישיר מאוד למי שירצה להתנהג במלאכה הזאת באמונה וביושר, והענינים אשר יכללם הספר הזה כולם מבוארים וגלוים והרפואות הנכללות בו כפי העת אשר אנחנו בו (והענינים) והאיקלימים והמזגים, יוכל הרופא להרגילם בבטחון. ולבקשת קצת אוהבי וחברי העתקתים מלשון ארומי אל לשון בני עמי. האל ישמרני מכל שגיאה ויזכני להעתיקו ולהעתיק ספרים אחרים ויאריך ימי וימי (מעתיקי רפואות דברים כבירים עם) כל ישראל חברים (אמן).

(אמר המחבר) זה הספר נקרא מבוא במלאכה חובר בעבור המשכילים בחכמת הרפואה ועדין לא הורגלו בשמושה ונבנה יסודו על האופן הראשון מהספר הרביעי (מאבן סיני) וחברו החכם המעולה ברנרט (ברנט) אלביריט האחד המיוחד בישיבה הנכבדת אשר בעיר מונפשל"ייר לבקשת אוהביו ותלמידיו וכה (וחביריו וזה) היו (sic) תורף דבריו, לבקשתכם ידידי אשר עמלתם ויגעתם עמי בלמוד החכמה הזאת (חכמת הרפואות) ראיתי לחבר לכם ספר קטן ומועיל במלאכת הרפואות אדרוך בו דרך האופן הראשון מהספר הרביעי מא"ס אתקן בו הרפואות הידועות המועילות (אשר ראויות) המורגלות לפי דעתי ואני משתחוה (!) אליכם שלא יהיה זה הספר נקל בעיניכם, כי הוא רב התועלת בעיני. ואם ימצא איש (על צד הקנאה) יורה חיצי סכלותו נגדי ראוי לכם לעמוד נגדו בכל מאמצי כחכם אחר שרציתי לעמוס עלי זה המשא הכבד בעבורכם ולתועלתכם.

1883, *10*:157–168, on p. 165. We have left the text as Steinschneider had it, including the use of parentheses for brackets.

[e2] The passage is difficult to decipher and translate.

V

Changes in the *Regimina sanitatis*
The Role of the Jewish Physicians

While working on public health in the fourteenth-century Crown of Aragon, I analyzed a medical literary genre called in Latin *regimen sanitatis,* health and its preservation.[1] I soon realized (1) that the factors that influenced medicine in late medieval Spanish kingdoms were also connected to changes in this kind of medical writing;[2] (2) that economic and ideological factors had an influence on the kind of readership of this genre that evolved during the fourteenth century (originally directed only to wealthy individuals, i.e. members of royalty and/or of civil or ecclesiastical nobility, the genre came to be extended to the population in general, especially the new urban social groups); and (3) that the use of the *regimina* by the most significant Christian physicians to express their thoughts and practical advice on the plague of 1348, and the subsequent acceptance of that advice by contemporary society,[3] could be another factor explaining the expanding audience of this medical literary genre.

Guy Beaujouan has pointed to four factors that affected the development of science in Spain in the late Middle Ages: the Muslim presence, the outstanding role played by the Jews, the precocious maturity of the peninsular languages, and the weakness of Spanish universities.[4] These four factors were also operative in the field of medicine, both as science and as practice; for medicine *qua* science these factors acted on what we might term the dynamics of the assimilation, the elaboration and the transmission of medical ideas. Specifically, they acted upon the text, for this was the vehicle for the transmission of science; and in the medical field this extended from what we today call medical sciences (anatomy and physiology) to theoretical and general therapeutics, passing through the complete range of pathology.

The complexities of medical practice, though intricately interwoven with the world of medical science, present another order of problems. These complexities include the practical dimensions in which the medical act was performed, the doctor's training and his performance as a professional, and the description of specific healing techniques. Furthermore, we must not lose sight of the fact that all this was carried out in a complex web involving the obvious interplay of scientific, economic, political, philosophical, religious, and other elements. An important part of this web, again, was composed of the four factors indicated by Beaujouan.

It is possible to observe in the late thirteenth century and during the fourteenth century an ideological change in the concept of health as perceived by laymen: health became a public good (*publica utilitas*), with implications for medicine but also with political repercussions and practical consequences for the everyday life of people. Municipalities, especially strong in the Crown of Aragon, took the lead in a new sanitary policy, dealing with, among other things, the control of foods (especially meat and fish), the cleaning of streets, the removal of garbage, disputes over pollution of the air (from irritating smoke) or of drinking-water (from liquids oozing out of olive-oil mills), the cultivation of rice fields in marshes, and the control of sanitary officers. Again, an important part of these measures was influenced by the four factors mentioned above.[5]

At the same time, however, health remained a private concern that was felt by the new urban groups (merchants, craftsmen, professionals, stockholders, in a word the *cives* or citizens of the late medieval Mediterranean cities). One of the educators of the new bourgeoisie at Valencia, the Franciscan Francesc Eiximenis (ca. 1327-1408), stressed this new concern – "love health in order that with your healthy body ... could you serve God with all your senses"[6] – and physicians shared this new emphasis.

Very recently, Jon Arrizabalaga, working on the perceptions and reactions that the so-called Black Death raised among Latin Mediterranean practitioners during the years 1348 and 1349, has demonstrated that the writings in which these physicians expressed their theoretical concerns and practical advice on the plague "represented the beginning of a new medical literary genre – that of the plague *regimina*",[7] and that the most relevant works of this genre written by the fourteenth-century learned physicians (e.g. Jacme d'Agramont, Gentile da Foligno, and the Paris masters) were addressed to the members of the bourgeoisie or to political authorities who were governing the municipalities or broader territories. All the sanitary measures put into practice by European communities against the pestilence after 1348 were closely interrelated with those suggested by learned physicians in their *regimina*.[8] But we must not forget that a probable reason why university physicians used this literary genre to address the laymen during the plague of 1348 is that the genre was already in normal circulation among the urban bourgeoisie. In this sense the successful application of plague *regimina* – a kind of writing that appeared for the first time in Europe in 1348-49 – reinforced the expansion of the medical literary genre.

This paper deals with a specific collection of medical techniques and their theoretical background, and with some of the problems derived from their application. These techniques covered both the preservation of health and the healing of the sick: the *regimina sanitatis.* I shall not attempt to analyze in depth this complex medical literary genre,[9] only to expose a conceptual change, as well as related practical consequences of it during the fourteenth century, and also the role played by Jewish physicians in this change.

The diffusion of the *Isagoge* of Iohannitius – one of the writings contained in the *Articella* – throughout the twelfth and thirteenth centuries[10] introduced into European learned circles its famous threefold organization of medicine's subject matter into naturals (things forming a part of living beings, such as elements, humours, qualities, and complexions), the contranaturals (things inimical to life and health, such as disease, causes of disease, and symptoms), and the nonnaturals (a set of things necessary for life and affecting the condition of the body).[11] The nonnaturals were organized under six headings: (1) air (and environment), (2) motion and rest, (3) food and drink, (4) sleep and waking, (5) evacuation and repletion (including sexuality), and (6) affections of the soul.[12] Nonnatural things are activities that are not essential for life, as are naturals, nor intrinsically pathological, like the contranaturals.[13] They are characterized by a high degree of choice on the part of the individual. "They are factors that operatively determine health or disease, depending on the circumstances of their use or abuse, to which human beings are unavoidably exposed in the course of daily life".[14] In fact, a substantial part of the causal and therapeutic system of medieval pathology was based on them, while at the same time all of the preventive doctrine for the preservation of health was built on them. The line between what was normal and what was pathological lay in the correct or incorrect, quantitative and/or qualitative management of each of these "six nonnatural things" on the part of the physician, with the active participation of the client. The latter may or may not have been ill, but he or she always needed to maintain a suitable standard of health. By means of this set of "things", medieval Galenism endeavoured to regulate human life from the standpoint of medicine. The management of this set of things was called *regimen,* and it was a task of the medieval physician. *Regimen* also provided a way to understand from the medical viewpoint the role of health, as both a public and a private value.

The "six nonnatural things" provided the skeleton for the kind of medical writing directly concerned with health and its preservation: the *regimina sanitatis.*[15] This type of writing was directed to those people for whom control over their lives according to the teachings of medicine could be accepted as a way of life. In other words, they were written for rich people (civil or ecclesiastical nobility or royalty). The *regimina sanitatis* were original creations of medieval medicine. One of the leading examples was the *Regimen sanitatis* written in 1306-07 by Arnald of Villanova for Jaume II, king of Aragon.[16] During the fourteenth century there was a change in the users of the *regimina:* the members of the urban bourgeoisie became the new consumers, and a relatively large market for the genre began to grow.

One of the most recent conclusions in our present research on Jewish practitioners in the western Mediterranean countries – especially Provence, Languedoc, and the Crown of Aragon – is that the fourteenth-century Latin scholastic system of medical learning had so developed as to establish itself as a model to be imitated and a resource to be exploited, at least in the eyes of a minority of Jewish practitioners: the so-called rationalist physicians and/or natural philosophers. One of the more highly appreciated products of scholastic medicine was precisely the *regimina sanitatis,* among both Christians and Jews. At least two rationalist Jews translated Arnald's *Regimen sanitatis* into Hebrew: Israel ben Josef Caslari in 1327, and Joseph bar Jehuda ha-Sefardi during the second half of the fourteenth century.[17]

Israel ben Josef Caslari, in the prologue to his translation of Arnald's *Regimen sanitatis,* introduced some very suggestive reflections on methodological problems of a theoretical nature; at the same time these comments also had considerable practical repercussions. Unfortunately, the extent of these reflections is not great and they lack a certain precision, in part because of difficulties in understanding the Hebrew text.[18] Be that as it may, they demonstrate the theoretical concern of such Jewish authors, while also offering us certain keys to an understanding of the reasons for the popularity of medical writings oriented as much towards the conservation of health as towards the cure of illnesses; they also tell us of the problems caused by their application.

The doctrinal basis on which writings concerned with the conservation of health and the cure of illness rested was the doctrine of the qualities hot, cold, dry, moist,[19] which allowed medieval medicine, whether Islamic, Jewish, or Christian, to produce a sophisticated elaboration of the "six nonnatural things". Special attention was given to the chapter on "food" – the basic source of energy. The writings on food and drink eventually became independent chapters and gained particular importance as a medical genre on their own.

Although a mathematical method of evaluating the qualities in substance had been developed in the Islamic world and was familiar to the physicians of the University of Montpellier, who applied it to the qualities of medicinal compositions in accordance with the doctrine of degree,[20] this method does not seem to have been applied to the doctrine of the qualities of nutritional substances. These continued to be known "by way of analogy (*derekh ha-hagasah*)".[21] Although the roots of the use of analogy, both in the more speculative aspects of medicine (those more directly related to natural philosophy) and in diagnosis itself, can be traced to Hippocratic writings, it was Galen who introduced it to the medical world.[22]

The diffusion of Galen's works in the Latin West provided the necessary doctrinal support for the use of analogy in the reasoning applied to medicine.[23] A writer such as Arnald of Villanova, like the other scholastic physicians, habitually used analogy as a legitimate procedure in order to discuss reality, when the latter is hidden from the senses and therefore inaccessible to medical observation. He did so, for example, when he wanted to establish the mechanism that produced fever – an obvious increase in temperature – inside the heart, the place where, according to Galenism, such an increase takes place. For this purpose he compared the cardiac chamber to a baker's oven and transferred a series of empirically verifiable consequences by way of analogy to the internal mechanism of temperature increase in fevers, not verifiable by use of the senses.[24] This must have been the method used to determine the character of the qualities of foodstuffs or nutritional substances (how dry, damp, or cold they were, among other points). These were natural principles for a scholastic physician and for the Jewish translator Israel ben Josef Caslari, who was completely familiar with scholastic terminology. Knowledge of these principles, only possible by means of the "way of analogy", was provided by natural philosophy and its intellectual tools, such as syllogism.[25]

However, this was not enough to establish an adequate diet for the conservation of health and for curing illnesses. The physician also had to unite his knowledge to the qualities that define the somatic characteristics (the constitution or temperament, *complexio / temperamentum*) of the individual whose health had to be protected, and in addition, he had to know the socio-physical surroundings in which the patient lived; in other words, what the terminology of the period in question called "climate" (the first of the "nonnatural things"), which was also defined by the doctrine of qualities. This is the reason for the latter's importance, if one wished to make the "art of medicine" (*melakhat ha-refu'ah*) an activity linked with the field of science (natural philosophy) (*hokhmat ha refu'ah*).[26] This was the principal argument employed in medical schools in order to maintain an exposition and clarification of the "natural principles" such as is contained, for example, in the first book of Avicenna's *Canon.*[27] Let us remember that this work was widely distributed also among medieval Jewish physicians.[28]

For all of these reasons, it is obvious that there were serious difficulties in the practical application of these works in order to extend their benefits to the population in general. These difficulties arose from the exact manner in which they were conceived (knowledge of the qualities of foodstuffs, of the constitution or temperament of the individual, and of the "climate" – i.e. socio-physical conditions of life). In the Christian, Islamic, and Jewish worlds, the *regimina* were conceived for particular individuals or groups living in special circumstances, for example Maimonides' *regimen* advising al-Adil, son of Saladin and sultan of Egypt.[29] This individuation provoked a proliferation of texts as a result of the need to adapt each diet to each individual case. It was as if, in the words of Israel ben Josef Caslari, "it could almost be said that every man needs a text written for himself".[30] The proliferation of texts was limited, since this type of prescription was only available to really wealthy individuals, and also only to those who carried out an activity compatible with the application of medicine as a way of life. "For this reason kings and magnates are accustomed to ask their doctors to write a text for them with the diet they should follow".[31] To this one must add the slowness of the process and the not particularly spectacular, indeed sometimes hazardous, nature of the results. This was especially true if these results were compared with the more spectacular and expeditious curative processes derived from the application of drugs, whose effectiveness only changed slightly, if at all, when applied to another individual.[32]

All this was closely related to an economic problem within the profession. The slow, hazardous nature of a diet (a thing that was always considered from the long-term point of view) could not compete with curative medicine, which produced rapid results that allowed physicians to increase the number of their patients, and, thereby, their income. Bernard de Gordon was able to see this clearly when he stated (1307-08): "Nowadays physicians do not take care to know the *regimen sanitatis* in their daily practice, because in their opinion there is no profit in it. On the other hand, they are very concerned about curing diseases, especially fevers".[33]

To these difficulties were added those derived from a way of life deeply rooted in religious rules and conditioned by them, as was the case for the Jewish community, with its meticulously detailed set of regulations that affected diet. We should remember the text of the Catalan rabbi Ishaq bar Seset Perfet, in which he makes specific reference to Jewish physicians who prescribed *regimina* inspired by Christian canons:

> We must not treat the laws and precepts of our Torah as do the students of medicine and the natural sciences. For if we believed – the Lord deliver us! – what they believe, what they assert in their deceitful teachings, the Torah did not come from of High. Likewise, if you interpreted the laws on unclean foods as do the physicians, you would receive a fat reward from the butchers ....[34]

This raises one immediate question: why, then, did Israel ben Josef Caslari and Josef bar Jehuda ha-Sefardi translate Arnald of Villanova's *Regimen sanitatis?* It is evident that the translators took all this into account from the moment they felt obliged to justify their work. But these same circumstances allow us to penetrate a little further into the complex world that we are analyzing.

The first reason that Israel ben Josef Caslari gives is of a technical nature: the work was written by an author – Arnald of Villanova (ob. 1311) – who was active in Languedoc and the Mediterranean region immediately to the south (Catalonia, Valencia); he was, moreover, in the service of a king who frequented the same lands. This was the same region in which the translator lived. Both "the nutritional substances that conserve the health" and "the climate" in which the readers of the Hebrew translation moved would be the same as the ones Arnald had in mind when he wrote his treatise a few years earlier.[35] Joseph bar Jehuda ha-Sefardi was to make the same point, "(because) he (Arnald) knew the natural things of these lands and their temperament (i.e. climate)".[36] This would have been true even if they had been thinking of Jewish clients, which they were not; however, this possibility should not be excluded. The Hebrew translation seems to have been aimed at those Jewish physicians with clients among the Christians "in whose lands we live".[37] This was the second reason adduced by Israel ben Josef Caslari. As will be seen, it had, furthermore, a pragmatic facet: the adaptation of the medical knowledge of the Jewish professionals to Christian customs, something that was particularly opportune, as it was a question of prescriptions that aimed to regulate the client's whole life. The third reason why Arnald's *Regimen sanitatis* was translated was the prestige that this Christian writer still enjoyed a generation after his death, among Jews and Christians alike, at least in the region between Avignon and Barcelona. "Great scholar", "brilliant physician", "prophet" were all expressions applied to Arnald by our translators, demonstrating that prestige.[38]

To these reasons, a fourth should be added, based on the evolution that this genre of medical literature, originally so personalized in nature, underwent. In the course of the fourteenth century a new form of medical literature was diffused, based on scientific knowledge of foodstuffs. An attempt was made to apply to a wider public what at the beginning of the fourteenth century was intended for particular individuals belonging to royalty or to the upper-level civil or ecclesiastical hierarchy. There was an attempt to convert the *regimina* themselves, like that of Arnald prepared for an individual, into more or less abstract treatises, suitable for application to patients who had little in common with the person for whom the work was originally written. There can be no doubt that this change in a medical genre whose roots were deeply set in a feudal society was due to the deep parallel changes that were taking place in Mediterranean society in the course of the fourteenth century. Thus it is not surprising that copies of Arnald's *Regimen* could be found in the libraries of merchants, members of the liberal professions, or church members.[39] This happened not only in the Christian world, but also in the Jewish and Islamic worlds. In the Islamic sphere, the appearance of writings "On foodstuffs" (*al-kalām ʿalā-l-aghdhiya*) can be found at the end of the fourteenth century in the kingdom of Granada. The author of one of these treatises (Abu Bakr Abd al-Aziz al-Arbuli from Almeira) gives us the key to this evolution: "foodstuffs are the principal cause of health, since if they are employed as they should be, a man's health is maintained and the damage that bodies may have suffered is repaired".[40]

An identical position can be seen in the work of the Toledan Jew who wrote the treatise *Book of Regal Castilian Medicine* (*Kitāb al-ṭibb al-qasṭalī al-mulūkī*), written in the first third of the fourteenth century.[41] In the Christian medical world, without going outside Arnald's *Regimen sanitatis,* we might think of the rich Latin manuscript tradition of this work, of which there are more than sixty surviving fourteenth- and fifteenth-century manuscripts, not counting its Catalan version.[42]

The way in which Jews perceived their relationship with Christians, both physicians and laymen, in other words the people whom they lived alongside and treated, is of interest in order to understand one aspect of the sociology of the practising Jewish physician in his contact with Christians during the period and in the area under consideration. It would appear that the habitual interaction in social and professional contacts between Christian physicians and their Jewish counterparts was no longer one of equals, but had become more distant.[43] In this context, we cannot pass over without comment Arnald of Villanova's recommendations to Frederick of Sicily, a brother of Jaume II, in which he insisted that the monarch should include clearly discriminatory measures against Jewish physicians in his dealings with his Christian clients in his "Constitution" (*Constitutiones*) of 1310.[44] We should recall the exceptional tone that

Leon Yosef de Carcassone, a Jewish rationalist physician who lived in Languedoc and Perpignan (at the time belonging to the Crown of Aragon), used for his contemporary Jean of Tournamire (fl. 1380), a professor at Montpellier, with whom he had personal contact: "I saw him with my own eyes and spoke to him. He was a man who was pleasant to talk to. His behaviour was not like that of the other scholars of his generation who scorned those Jews who practised the art of medicine".[45]

It is not difficult to see in the behaviour of these "other scholars" a problem of rivalry between practitioners in the same professional market. The Jews, in the opinion of Leon Yosef, also were scorned when they dealt with Christians who were not physicians. The same Leon, in the prologue to his Hebrew translation of Gerard de Solo's *Practica super nono Almansoris* (1394-1402), tells us:

> When I lived among the Christians, I was of an inferior condition in their eyes, for there is none of our nation who is honoured in their eyes, except he who is a physician and who cures them of their ills; in such a case, he sits at the table of kings and stays upright before them, be he modest or of high standard, owing to his knowledge of medical science.[46]

As a result of my work during the last ten years with Michael R. McVaugh, in the rich medieval archives of the Spanish lands that belonged to the old Crown of Aragon, we have verified that Jewish physicians and surgeons practised in a variable percentage among Christians, even after the pogrom of 1391. They attended the Jewish and the Christian population, and Christian practitioners also attended Jewish people. It was not unusual for a Christian and a Jewish doctor both to visit the same problematic patient.[47] In big cities such as Barcelona or Valencia (25,000-35,000 inhabitants), and in medium-sized or small towns (10,000-800 inhabitants), the presence of Jewish practitioners (*fisici, cirurgici*) practising medicine as a liberal profession, and/or by contract (of one to five years) with municipalities was normal. Despite ecclesiastical and civil prohibitions, all Christian social groups were attended by Jewish practitioners, who shared the medical practice – and also the technical contents of scholastic medicine – with their Christian colleagues.[48] We have to remember that, at least in some cases, the acceptance of scholastic medicine by the Jewish practitioners was not free of troubles within their own communities.[49] Thus it is not difficult to imagine the role played by the Jewish physicians in the change of the *regimina sanitatis* that took place, at least in the Mediterranean countries, during the fourteenth century.

Notes

1. An article, "Public Health and Medicine in the Fourteenth-Century Crown of Aragon", is in preparation.
2. See L. García-Ballester, "Medical Science in Thirteenth-Century Castile: Problems and Prospects", *Bulletin of the History of Medicine* 61 (1987) 183-202.
3. J. Arrizabalaga, "University Medical Practitioners Faced with the Black Death (1348-49) in the Latin Mediterranean Europe: Perceptions and Reactions", in *Practitioners and Medical Practice in the Latin Mediterranean, 1100-1350,* ed. L. García-Ballester, R.K. French, A. Cunningham, and J. Arrizabalaga (Cambridge, forthcoming).
4. G. Beaujouan, *La Science en Espagne aux XIVᵉ et XVᵉ siècles* (Paris 1967), p. 7.
5. See n. 1 above, and L. García-Ballester, *La medicina a la València medieval* (Valencia 1988), pp. 101-07; L. García-Ballester, M.R. McVaugh, and A. Rubio-Vela, *Medical Licensing and Learning in Fourteenth-Century Valencia,* Transactions of the American Philosophical Society 79, pt 6 (Philadelphia 1989).
6. F. Eiximenis, *Liber de virtutibus et peccatis, sive Ars maior praedicationis* (1385); see Martí de Barcelona, "Fra Francesc Eiximenis", *Estudis Franciscans* 22 (1928) 437-500 at 478.
7. See n. 3 above.
8. Ibid.
9. See H. Schipperges, *Lebendige Heilkunde* (Olten–Freiburg i. Br. 1962). At the present time, Pedro Gil-Sotres (University of La Laguna, Spain) is working on the rise and development of this medical genre in 13th- and 14th-century Latin medicine.
10. D. Jacquart, "A l'aube de la renaissance médicale des XIᵉ-XIIᵉ siècles: L'*Isagoge Johannitii* et son traducteur", *Bibliothèque de l'Ecole des chartes* 144 (1986) 209-40.
11. "Medicina dividitur in duas partes, scil. in theoricam et practicam, quarum theorica dividitur in tria, i. in contemplationem rerum naturalium et non naturalium et earum, quae sunt contra naturam, ex quibus sanitatis, aegritudinis et neutralitatis scientia procedit"; ed. G. Maurach, "Johannicius, *Isagoge ad Techne Galieni*", *[Sudhoffs] Archiv für Geschichte der Medizin* 62 (1978) 148-74 at 151, based on 13th- and 14th-century Latin MSS.
12. A marginal note of two Latin MSS – Metz, Cod. lat. 1256 (12th c.), fol. 1ff., and London, Wellcome Hist. Med. Libr. 82 (13th c.), fol. 1ff. – used by G. Maurach in his *Isagoge* edition, says: "Non naturalia sunt VI: aer, exercitium, optium, cibus et potus, somnus et vigilia, repletio et inanitio, accidentia anime"; "Johannicius", p. 157, n. 26.
13. L. García-Ballester, "On the Origin of the 'Six Nonnatural Things' in Galen", in *IV. internationales Galen-Symposium, Berlin, 18-20 September 1989,* forthcoming.

14. L.J. Rather, "The 'Six Things Non-Natural': A Note on the Origins and Fate of a Doctrine and a Phrase", *Clio medica* 3 (1968) 337-47 at 337.
15. Bernard de Gordon in his *Regimen sanitatis* says: "regimen sanitatis consistit in debita applicacione sex rerum non naturalium", *De conservatione* 4: *Regimen Sanitatis,* Vatican MS. Pal. lat. 1174, fol. 72v. Cited by L.E. Demaitre, *Doctor Bernard de Gordon: Professor and Practitioner,* Studies and Texts 51 (Toronto 1980), p. 69, n. 166.
16. *Arnaldi de Villanova opera* ... (Lyon 1504), fols 160r-172v. A critical edition by A. Trías, *Regimen sanitatis ad regem Aragonum,* is in preparation and will be vol. 10 in the series Arnaldi de Villanova opera medica omnia, ed. L. García-Ballester, M.R. McVaugh, and J.A. Paniagua (Barcelona 1974-).
17. L. García-Ballester, L. Ferre, and E. Feliu, "Jewish Appreciation of Fourteenth-Century Scholastic Medicine", *Osiris* 6 (1990), in press.
18. For a better understanding of this paper see our article just cited, "Jewish Appreciation", Appendix A, where we reproduce the English version of the prologue, published for the first time, together with the Hebrew text.
19. P.-G. Ottosson, *Scholastic Medicine and Philosophy: A Study of Commentaries on Galen's "Tegni" (ca. 1300-1450)* (Uppsala 1982). See the interesting distinction introduced by Danielle Jacquart between *complexio,* linked with the doctrine of qualities, and *temperamentum,* based on humoral theory: "De *crasis* a *complexio:* Note sur le vocabulaire du tempérament en latin médiéval", in *Textes médicaux latins antiques,* ed. G. Sabbah (St. Etienne 1984), pp. 71-76.
20. M.R. McVaugh, "Arnald of Villanova and Bradwardine's Law", *Isis* 58 (1967) 56-64; "Quantified Medical Theory and Practice at Fourteenth-Century Montpellier", *Bulletin of the History of Medicine* 43 (1969) 397-413; see also his edition, *Arnaldi de Villanova aphorismi de gradibus,* Arnaldi ... opera medica omnia 2 (Granada and Barcelona 1975), Introduction, pp. 1-136, esp. 75-122.
21. García-Ballester et al., "Jewish Appreciation", Appendix A, ll. 6-11.
22. L. García-Ballester, "Galen as a Medical Practitioner: Problems in Diagnosis", in *Galen: Problems and Prospects,* ed. V. Nutton (London 1981), pp. 13-46, esp. 36-38.
23. A medical work, very well known by learned physicians, in which Galen used the analogy as a normal heuristic procedure applied to everyday medical practice was *De locis affectis* (= *De interioribus*; e.g. to explain the mechanism of convulsions, 3.8:VIII 171-72 K, or how to apply causal discoveries in autopsies on animals to human sickness, 5.2:VIII 303-04 K).
24. *Commentum supra tractatum Galieni de malicia complexionis diverse,* ed. L. García-Ballester and E. Sánchez-Salor, Arnaldi ... opera medica omnia 15 (Barcelona 1985), p. 271, ll. 23-31.
25. García-Ballester et al., "Jewish Appreciation", Appendix A, ll. 7-9.
26. Ibid., Appendix A, ll. 2, 9, 30-33.
27. N. Siraisi, *Avicenna in Renaissance Italy: The Canon and Medical Teaching in Italian Universities after 1500* (Princeton 1987), pp. 221ff.

28. García-Ballester et al., "Jewish Appreciation".
29. S. Munter, ed., *Moshe ben Maimon (Maimonides), Regimen sanitatis ... Hebrew Translation of R. Moshe ibn Tibbon ...* (Jerusalem 1957), pp. x-xi.
30. García-Ballester et al., "Jewish Appreciation", Appendix A, ll. 60-61.
31. Ibid., Appendix A, ll. 61-63.
32. Ibid., Appendix A, ll. 47-50.
33. "... medici nostri temporis non curant scire regimen sanitatis quia videtur eis quod non sit *ibi* lucrum sed in curacione morborum et potissime febrium sunt bene solliciti", *De conservatione* 4: *Regimen sanitatis* 17, cited by Demaitre, *Doctor Bernard*, pp. 35, 69-70. The emphasis is mine.
34. Cited by Y. Baer, *Historia de los judíos en la España cristiana*, enlarged Spanish translation from Hebrew by J.L. Lacave, 2 vols (Madrid 1982), I, 364.
35. García-Ballester et al., "Jewish Appreciation", Appendix A, ll. 44-45, 68-70.
36. Ibid., Appendix B, ll. 8-9.
37. Ibid., Appendix A, l. 73 and Appendix B, l. 28.
38. Ibid.
39. See J.M. Madurell Marimón and J. Rubió y Balaguer, *Documentos para la historia de la imprenta y librería en Barcelona (1474-1553)* (Barcelona 1955), pp. 23-29, 43-45; Marimón, "Documents culturals medievals (1307-1485)", *Boletin de la Real Academia de buenas letras de Barcelona* 38 (1979-82) 301-473 at 339-41.
40. A. Díaz García, "Un tratado nazarí sobre alimentos: *Al-Kalam Ala-l-Aqdiya* de al-Arbuli. Edición, traducción, y estudio, con glosarios (I)", *Cuadernos de estudios medievales* (Granada) 6-7 (1978-79) 5-91 at 9.
41. Madrid, Biblioteca nacíonal, MS. Arabic, DCI, fols 1r-38v. The work is still unpublished. We are preparing a critical edition, with Spanish translation and commentaries, in collaboration with Concepción Vázquez (University of Salamanca) and Pedro Gil (University of La Laguna).
42. L. García-Ballester, M.R. McVaugh, and J.A. Paniagua, "Catálogo de incipits de los manuscritos médicos latinos atribuídos a Arnau de Vilanova" (Barcelona 1974-), typewritten copy.
43. We must not forget that normally when a Jewish physician was contracted by municipalities to give care to the population, he received only half the salary paid to a Christian physician with the same professional duties. The economic discrimination was a kind of institutional scorn. M.R. McVaugh and I are preparing a book on Jews and medicine in the 14th-century Crown of Aragon.
44. Arnald of Villanova wrote to the king: "Order, (Sir), that any Jew, as long as he professes his faith, does not dare to do medical practice with any Christian"; repr. M. Menéndez-Pelayo, *Historia de los heterodoxos españoles*, 8 vols, (Madrid 1963 [1st edn 1880]), vol. VIII: Apéndice I: Documentos, p. 276; see P. Diepgen, *Arnald of Villanova als Politiker und Laientheologe* (Berlin and Leipzig 1909), p. 89. Frederick of Sicily in his *Constitutiones* followed Arnald's advice; see H. Finke, *Acta Aragonensia*, 2 vols (Berlin and Leipzig 1908), I, 698.

45. See García-Ballester et al., "Jewish Appreciation", Appendix D.
46. Ibid.
47. As an example, we can mention a medical collaboration between the Christian doctor Anthonius de Campelles (fl. 1362) and the Jewish physician Samuel Adday (fl. 1362 in Puigcerdà, a small town in the Pyrenean valley of Cerdanya, where he practised as municipal physician; fl. 1363 in Perpignan). Their patient was Bertran Font, a Christian who finally died (Arxiu históric comarcal de Puigcerdà, Prot. Notarials, Joan Torrelles, lib. extraneorum, 1361-62, fol. 45v, 1362 March 18). The collaboration was not only between physicians, but also between barbers and surgeons: e.g. one Francisca, a Christian girl wounded in the head, was healed at the same time by the Christian barber Bartholomeus Spades and the Jewish surgeon Boniach Abram (both fl. in Puigcerdà in 1371) (Arxiu ..., Bernat Blanch, lib. firmitatis, 1370-71, fol. 95, 1371 October 10).
48. Christian people visited the houses of Jewish physicians in the Jewish quarter to receive medical assistance; this was the case, among others, of the Master Vital Rouen, who was a great success in his medical practice in Barcelona (Arxiu de la Corona d'Aragón, Cancillería, reg. 211, fol. 337v, 1315 June 17), and of the Jewish physician Ferrarius Cresques from Majorca (Arxiu del Regne de Majorca, Apellacions, 1355, fol. 54v, 1355 June 12). We deal with this topic in the book announced in n. 43 above.
49. García-Ballester et al., "Jewish Appreciation".

VI

Dietetic and Pharmacological Therapy: A Dilemma Among Fourteenth-Century Jewish Practitioners in the Montpellier Area

In the late thirteenth century, and during the fourtheenth century, health became a public value (*publica utilitas*), with medical implications. At the same time, health continued to be a private concern that was taken up by the new urban groups (merchants, craftsmen, professionals, rentiers, in a word the *cives* or citizens of the late medieval Mediterranean).[1] One of the educators of the new bourgeoisie at Valencia, the Franciscan Francesc Eiximenis (c. 1327-1408), points out the new value, *ama sanitatem, ut cum tuo corpore, quod erit sanum ... servias Deo per sentire et imaginari.*[2] (Love health, that with your healthy body you may serve God in mind and thought.) Physicians shared this new emphasis.

This paper deals with the problems derived from the application of a technique that covered both preservation of health and healing of the sick: the *regimina sanitatis*, regimes for health. My concern in this paper is, on the one hand, to expose the change in the users of the *regimina* outlined by physicians and surgeons for the nobility and royalty, on the other to analyse some of the problems which emerged from its therapeutical application and from the preference by physicians for the use of the most expeditious means possible (medicines instead of *regimen*) and, finally, the rôle played by Jewish physicians in these developments.[3]

One of the most recent conclusions of our work on Jewish practitioners in the Western Mediterranean is that the fourteenth-century Latin system of medical learning had so developed as to establish itself, in the eyes of Jewish practitioners, as a model to be imitated and a resource to be exploited. One of the more appreciated products of scholastic medicine — which had its own Jewish medical tradition — was precisely the *regimina sanitatis*, as both a technique and a literary genre. Two rationalist Jews translated into Hebrew Arnald of Villanova's *Regimen sanitatis*: Israel ben Joseph Caslari (1327), and Joseph ben Judah ha-Sefardi (*fl.* probably last decade of the fourteenth century); the first from Latin, the second from its Catalan version.[4]

I

The diffusion of the *Isagoge* of Joannitius — one of the writings contained in the *Articella* — throughout the twelfth and thirteenth centuries[5] introduced into European learned circles its famous three-fold organization of medicine's subject-matter into natural (things that are a part of living beings, such as elements, humours, qualities and complexions: *res naturales*), the contra-natural (things inimical to life and health, such as disease, causes of disease and symptoms: *res praeter naturam*), and the non-natural (things necessary for life and affecting the condition of the body: *res non naturales*). The last were organized into six groups: (1) air, environment or climate, (2) food and drink, (3) sleep and waking, (4) motion and rest, (5) evacuation and repletion, (6) motions or affections of the soul. Non-natural things are activities which are more or less optional, but not essential for life, as are the natural, or intrinsically pathological, as are the contra-natural.[6] "They are factors that operatively determine health or disease, depending on the circumstances of their use or abuse, to which human beings are unavoidably exposed in the course of daily life."[7] The management of this set of things was called *regimen*, and it was a task to be undertaken by the medieval physician. It provided a way of understanding from the medical viewpoint the rôle of health as both a public and a private concern.

The "six non-natural things" provided the conceptual frame for this kind of medical writing directly concerned with health and its preservation, and used also as a therapeutical technique: the *regimina sanitatis*.[8] Such medical writings were directed to those for whom medicine could be accepted as a way of life; in other words, for the rich (the civil or ecclesiastical nobility or royalty). Medieval learned physicians and surgeons were convinced that nobility and royalty had a peculiar bodily complexion. These biological characteristics came into existence at the very moment of conception and were hereditary — hence the individual way in which these groups of patients had to be treated both in sickness and in health. They could be detected only by a physician and they differentiated those who belonged by birth to the rank of the nobility from those who did not. The latter all shared a common nature. Thus their treatment or the norms for preserving their health did not require the same degree of individual attention as demanded by the nobility and the royal family. These arguments, from the viewpoint of biomedicine, stressed the social differences within Christian feudal society, which was served by Jewish and Christian physicians and surgeons.[9] The *regimina sanitatis* were an original creation of medieval medicine. One of its most important examples was the *Regimen sanitatis* written (1306-07) by Arnald of Villanova for Jaume II, king of the Crown of Aragon.[10] During the fourteenth century there was a change in the users of the *regimina*. The members of the urban bourgeoisie became the new consumers, the new audience; a relatively large market was growing up for this medical genre. We could say that this new market not only opened new economical resources to medical practitioners, but was the manifestation of deeper social changes.

Israel ben Joseph Caslari, in the prologue to his translation of Arnald of Villanova's *Regimen sanitatis*, introduced some very suggestive reflections of theoretical and methodological problems; at the same time, his comments also had considerable practical repercussions.[11] Unfortunately, their extent is not great and they are lacking in a certain precision, in part because of the difficulties involved in understanding the Hebrew text. Be that as it may, they demonstrate the theoretical concern of such Jewish authors, while also offering us certain keys to an understanding of the reasons for the popularity enjoyed by certain medical writings of a strictly therapeutic nature, concerned with the immediate cure of particular illnesses by means of medicines, as opposed to less drastic dietetic procedures, and oriented as much towards the conservation of health as towards the cure of illnesses themselves.

The doctrinal basis on which these writings rested was the doctrine of the qualities which allowed medieval medicine, whether Islamic, Jewish or Christian, to produce a sophisticated elaboration of the "six non-natural things". Special attention was given to the chapter on "foods" — the basic source that provided man with energy — which eventually became independent and gained particular importance as a medical literary genre by itself.[12] Natural philosophy provided to learned physicians the intellectual means to determine the character of the qualities of foodstuffs or nutritional substances (e.g. how dry, damp, hot, or cold they were). These were natural principles for a scholastic physician and for the Jewish translator Israel ben Joseph Caslari, who was totally familiar with Galenic terminology.

However, this was not enough to establish an adequate diet for the conservation of health and for curing illnesses. The physician also had to unite his knowledge of this to the qualities which defined the somatic characteristics (the constitution or temperament, *complexio*) of the individual whose health had to be protected. In addition, he had to know the very socio-physical surroundings in which the patient lived; in other words, what the terminology of the period in question called "climate" (the first of the "non-natural things"), which was also defined by the doctrine of qualities. This is the reason for the latter's importance, if one wished to make the "art of medicine" (*melakhat ha-refu'ah*) an activity linked with the field of science (natural philosophy) (*hokhmat ha-refu'ah*). This was the principal argument employed in medical teaching in order to maintain the validity of Book I of Avicenna's *Canon*, which was entirely devoted to an exposition and clarification of the "natural principles" (*res naturales*).[13]

For all these reasons, it is obvious that there were serious difficulties in the practical application of these works in order to extend their benefits to the population in general. These difficulties arose from the exact manner in which they were conceived (knowledge of the qualities of foodstuffs, of the consitution or temperament of the individual, and of the "climate" — i.e. socio-physical conditions of life). The *regimina sanitatis*, as we have already said, at least in the Christian world, were written for particular individuals. This individuation provoked a proliferation of texts as a result of the need to adapt each diet to each individual case. What is more, "each man would need a treatise written for him alone".[14] The proliferation of texts was limited since this type of prescription was available only to individuals of substance and nobility, and, among these, only to those who carried out an activity compatible with the conversion of medicine into a way of life. "For this reason only kings and magnates have the habit of asking their physicians to write a text on the diet they should follow".[15] To this one must add the slowness of the process and the not particularly spectacular, indeed hazardous, nature of the results. This was especially true if these results were compared with more spectacular and expeditious curative processes derived from the application of drugs "whose effectiveness only changes slightly, if at all, when we applied them to another individual".[16] The effectiveness of drugs or medicines derives from its own virtue, not from external circumstances; its effectiveness — in accordance with a medieval practitioner — does not change whoever they are applied to.

All this was closely related to an economic problem. The slow, hazardous nature of a diet (a thing which was always considered from the long-term point of view) could not compete with curative medicine in producing rapid results which allowed physicians to increase the number of their patients, and thereby their income. Bernard of Gordon saw this clearly when he stated in 1307-1308 that:

> Nowadays physicians do not use knowingly *regimen sanitatis* in their daily practice. The reason is because in their opinion they do not obtain any profit with it. On the other hand, they are very concerned about curing diseases, especially fevers.[17]

To these difficulties were added those derived from a way of life deeply rooted in and conditioned by religious norms, as was the case of the Jewish community with its meticulously detailed set of dietary regulations. We should remember the text of the Catalan rabbi Isaac ben Sheshet Perfet, in which he made specific reference to Jewish physicians who prescribed *regimina* inspired by Christian canons: "We should not judge the laws and commandments of our Torah according to the views of the scientists and physicians ... One who interpreted the laws relating to forbidden foods according to the ruler of the physicians would be richly rewarded by the butchers".[18]

We shall now consider here the reasons why Israel ben Joseph Caslari and Joseph be Juhad ha-Sefardi translated Arnald of Villanova's *Regimen sanitatis*.[19] As we have seen, in the course of the fourteenth century, the *regimina sanitatis*, originally so personalized in nature, underwent an evolution in their customers. Moreover, a new form of medical literature was diffused, based on scientific knowledge of foodstuffs.[20] An attempt was made to apply to a wider public what at the beginning of the fourteenth century was intended for particular individuals belonging to the royalty or civil or ecclesiastical nobility. There was an attempt to convert the *regimina* themselves, like that of Arnald prepared for an individual with a name and surname, into more or less abstract treatises, suitable for application to patients who had little in common with the person for whom the work was originally written. There can be no doubt that this change in a medical genre whose roots were deeply set in a feudal society was due to the deep parallel changes which were taking place in Mediterranean society in the course of the fourteenth century. Thus, it is not surprising that copies of Arnald's *Regimen* could be found in the libraries of merchants, members of the liberal professions or clerics.[21]

II

Alongside the use of foodstuffs and the complex world of the "six non-natural things" around which the *regimina sanitatis* were constructed, we have the world of medicines. In contrast to the difficulties of both a practical and doctrinal nature brought about by the use of *regimina* (the rationalistic approach to the qualities), medicines offered a more attractive alternative. And this was true from both a practical and doctrinale point of view.

a) Practical reasons

Let us not forget that the use of *regimina* did not mean that the physician completely dispensed with medicines as useful elements for maintaining health. The incorporation of medicines was not against the structure of the *regimina*. The use of medicines was also contemplated by the physician, within the system of the *regimen* especially when the diet was intended for a person who suffered from a particular illness or illnesses. This was, for instance, the case of Arnald's *Regimen*, drawn up for Jaume II, who suffered from haemorrhoids. Medicines were used in this case as reinforcements or complements.

We have already pointed out the economic reasons which would induce the physician to prefer a drastic medicinal treatment to a *regimen*. In such a situation, drastic medicinal treatment was seen to be opposed to dietetic treatment. This attitude formed part of the medical greed and picaresque behaviour denounced in the same period by Ramon Llull in his sermons (1313).[22] Leaving aside this weighty reason, shrewdly noted by Bernard of Gordon, there can be no doubt that physicians themselves were aware of the difficulties and the inconvenience that were involved in strictly following the thousand and one details which had to be observed for the complete effectiveness of dietetic treatment. The transgression of the diet on the part of the patient must have been fairly frequent. Thus there arose the desirability of incorporating medicinal therapeutic measures, and even surgical ones if necessary, in order to help to put the system imposed by the physician into action and to make it more efficacious.[23]

The chapter of the *Regimen* in which Arnald describes the use of medicines is the last one (chapter 18). All the previous chapters are dedicated to the systematic exposition of the "six non-natural things" (chapters 1 to 7) and to food, in other words the energy-supplying system (chapters 8 to 17). In spite of that, the Jewish translator gave special importance to the medicinal content of the eighteenth chapter, which contains "the medicines and remedies aimed at restoring health."

Bernard of Gordon's words emphasize that, already by the early fourteenth century, physicians were demonstrating a clear inclination towards curing illnesses by the most expeditious means possible; his words suggest a preference for the use of medicines. This demonstrates a clear predominance of the more pragmatic aspects of medicine over less aggressive procedures (the *regimina*), which were somewhat problematic in their effectiveness, because of the hazardous nature of their application. The employment of a drastic therapy, based on quite a large body of drugs, was guaranteed by several centuries of experience (trial and error) and by the medical authorities who had used and recommended them. They included, among others, the famous books of recipes or collections of *experimenta* which, anonymously or under the name of a famous physician, circulated in the medieval period and which enjoyed great popularity. We have to think of the prestige achieved by the fifth book of Avicenna's *Canon* (*Antidotarium*),[24] in fact a handy guide to treatment,[25] or in the pressure for Henri de Mondeville to complete the *antidotarium* (book five) of his treatise on surgery.[26]

To this should be added two fundamental elements: the physician's desire for profit (clearly diagnosed, as we have seen, by Bernard of Gordon and Ramon Llull, among others), and the fondness for polypharmacy among both the sick and physicians. Polypharmacy was not unrelated to the well-tilled commercial world of the apothecaries, who, by the fourteenth century, had strong commercial interests. The proof of this lies not only in the surviving prescriptions, but also in the great development of apothecaries and the extraordinarily wealth and variety of their stock of medicines, in both large and small centres of population.[27] The affection for a medical literature whose contents could be immediately applied to the patient (collections of clinical cases, *exempla*, aphorisms, prescriptions or *antidotaria*) is clear among fourteenth-century doctors, whether they were Christians, Jews or Moslems — what has been called the *via pragmatica*. It should not be forgotten that among the university physicians of Montpellier around the turn of the thirteenth to the fourteenth century, there was a certain insistence that medicine should never lose sight of its practical use (*utilitas*), and that this would only be achieved through the definite application of remedies or the conservation of health.[28] It should also be remembered that this concept — the *utilitas* (*to'elet*) — was the most commonly invoked by our Jewish translators to justify their work.[29]

A very deep pragmatism led some Jewish religious leaders in the fourteenth century to acknowledge the therapeutic value of all kinds of charms and other magical practices. However, the importance placed by Jewish tradition upon the saving of a life, in both the physical and moral sense of salvation, led some rabbis to acknowledge the therapeutic value not only of substances with the powers to cure specific illnesses, but also of all kinds of charms, incantations, and amulets.[30] What justified this acceptance was the possible efficacy (*utilitas*) of their use, as determined by trial and error. A mixture of empiricism and magic thus provided the basis for a range of therapeutic practices that, to judge from certain rabbinical texts (by Salomon ben Adret and Jacob ben Asher, among others), were very popular within Jewish society, including its intellectual minority, as has been pointed out by Eleazar Gutwirth.[31] They need not have been sanctioned by the Torah or mentioned in medical treatises. The use of things which possess curative properties as a seal engraved with the figure of a lion, formed part of a world of beliefs shared by medieval people, as much Jews as Christians.[32] Maimonides' opposition to the acceptance of such magical practices was not widely shared within late-medieval Jewish society.[33] In relation to our topic, it is interesting to note that the curative power resided in the thing, the word, the talisman; it was not the result of an individualized therapeutic procedure, as in the case of a *regimen sanitatis*. This ensured that such therapeutic measures could be extended to all people, whatever their social position and wherever they might dwell. Moreover, they were measured in perfect accord with the world of everyday beliefs, for they involved things that had no need of reason or natural philosophy (the province of the intellectual minority) in order to be understood.

b) Doctrinal reasons

There are also important differences, according to our Jewish translators, from a doctrinal point of view, between the world of "nutritional substances" or foodstuffs and that of "remedies aimed at restoring health" in order to cure illnesses. As we shall see, this point of view was not without practical repercussions. The former, according to our Jewish translators, are only "known by natural philosophy"; the latter, on the other hand, are known "by experimental reasoning". In the opinion of Israel ben Joseph Caslari, this technique demonstrates that:

> the effectiveness of medicines does not change (whoever they are applied to). We

> know, for example, that scammony purges the yellow bile, just as the ancients established, and it does not seem that anyone has ever taken scammony without something akin to the nature of saffron (i.e. of yellow colour) appearing on his body. Each of the learned experts in medicine tries to check for himself, not through others, the action of medicines, and each one writes a book about what he has proved, as happens with the science of the stars ... as is explained in the *Almagest*.[34]

However, what can be understood by "experimental reasoning" (*ha'iyun ha-nisavoni*), which is applied "to those things that come from the field of experimental science (*ha-hokmah ha-nisayonit*)"? Joseph Caslari centred his discussion on the field of therapy and, in particular, on non-alternative remedies, that is to say those which cure an illness by means of their virtues or the specific power they possess. He did not consider at all the alternative medicines that the doctor used when he wanted to modify the relation between the different qualities which defined the state of the patient (his *complexio*). Neither did he deal at all with the theoretical problem of the rôle of experimentation inmedicine, nor with that of the relationship between theory and practice, which can be considered as the moment when the physician tests his doctrinal baggage as a whole or when the latter must be adapted to the specific case.[35]

Caslari's allusions to the action of scammony and to the *Almagest* help us to establish the coordinates around which he was moving. The example of the purgative action of scammony is particularly significant. Experimental science must be that form based on experiments such as the one involving this medicine, whose singularity is provided by direct experience, something which cannot be rationally foreseen, but which can be relied on once the cause-and-effect relationship has been established by authors and by personal experience. "The word did not carry its modern sense in the Middle Ages ... These *experimenta* (experiments) obviously witness to the ongoing practical activities of physicians, and to their apparent success in treating a variety of medical problems".[36] It was not by chance that the Jew in question referred to the example of scammony. It was the experiment recorded by Galen in his work *On the natural faculties*[37] and later used by Avicenna to establish the conditions that must exist in induction and experiment (*tajriba*).[38] It was also the singular experiment cited by Robert Grosseteste when he wanted to explain the process of a type of inductive reasoning which we could well call "experimental reasoning" in accordance with Joseph Caslari's terminology.[39] The almost regular effect of medicines, both simple and compound in the form of prescriptions (*recepta*) is something that can be personally checked or verified and, in fact, we do so when we give a patient a prescription. The latter's effectiveness could only confirm the value of the experiment (*experimentum*) of the author from whose works it was taken and would legitimize the experimental reasoning (*ha-'iyun na-nisayoni*) applied. Medical authorities took great care to record these experiments in writing (in collections of prescriptions or *experimenta*) in which the *virtus specifica* or "hidden nature" (*teva' ne'elam*) of medicines is made evident.[40]

The allusion to the *Almagest* is less explicit and, for that reason, more difficult to define with precision. However, because of the context in which the reference is included, there can be no doubt that Joseph Caslari was alluding to the possibility that the astronomer has to check personally, with the necessary instruments, the observations carried out on definite stars by previous writers and to add his own evidence. Ptolemy said in the *Almagest*:

> The configurations observed in Hipparchus' time are seen to be absolutely identical now too ... This can be seen by anyone who is willing to make an inspection of the matter and examine, in the spirit of the love of truth, whether present phenomena agree with those recorded for Hipparchus' time ... We conducted this type of investigation by means of the instrument which we constructed previously for the observations of individual moon-sun distances ... So we thought it appropriate, in making our observations and records of each of the above fixed stars, and of the others too, to give their position, as observed in our time, in terms of longitude and latitude ...[41]

We know that rationalist Jewish scholars were familiar with the *Almagest.* Samuel ben Judah of Marseille's training in natural philosophy, begun in Salon under the supervision of Sen (don) Astruc de Noves (the same master under whom Qalonymos ben Qalonymos had studied a little earlier) commenced with this book "which occupied an important place in the cycle of philosophic studies".[42] This work, or alternatively Averroes' compendium, was in the library of the Jewish physician Jahuda (Leon) Mosconi in Majorca (1375).[43]

It is thus possible to establish some general norms which we know were to be followed with only slight variations in the application of these medicines. The usefulness (*utilitas, to'elet*) of remedies therefore lies in the almost invariable nature of their action and in the possibility of their being experimented with by everyone in their daily practice. In this way, the physician is able to remove the drawback of the individual character of the sick (derived from their personal *complexio*) and the inevitable peculiarities derived from the geographical differences in which the sick themselves live.

III

Everything we have seen so far required a considerable body of knowledge of Galenism on the part of Jewish doctors. It is legitimate to ask where Israel ben Joseph Caslari had acquired this familiarity.

The different stages in the diffusion of Galen's works in the Latin West (especially among intellectual physicians of the Western Mediterranean) in the thirteenth and fourteenth centuries are reasonably well known.[44] The same cannot be said of the Jewish world of the same region at the same date. In spite of that, it can be affirmed that by the end of the first third of the fourteenth century, such writings as the *De pulsibus ad tyrones* (*ad Theucrum*) [On pulses for beginners] and the collection known in the Latin world as *De morbo et accidenti* [On disease and its incidents], together with fifteen other Galenic treatises that formed the important Alexandrian nucleus of Galen's works, had been translated into Hebrew.[45] Likewise, *De malicia complexionis diverse* (= *de inequali intemperie*) [On bad temperament], a brief but important work within the new Galenism of the early fourteenth century, commented on by Arnald of Villanova,[46] was translated into Hebrew by David ben Abraham Caslari (1280-1337) (probably from the Latin version which was circulating in Montpellier).[47] All this Galenic corpus was translated into Hebrew in the first two decades of the fourteenth century. Of the translator of the Alexandrian nucleus (Simson ben Salomo) no more is known than that he was a contemporary of Qalonymus ben Qalonymus and that he finished his work in 1322.[48]

Another problem is that of the diffusion of all this medical literature among the Jewish physicians, many of whom had lost their training in Arabic language, from the point of view of both time and space. A physician such as Josef ben Abraham ibn Waqar from Toledo (*fl.* 1340-1355), who owned a substantial library, made Averroes his principal source of biologial information;[49] the same can be stated of Leon ben Moses Mosconi (1328-pre 1375), of whose library we possess a detailed inventory (Majorca, 1375), and in which the Galenic corpus is irrelevant.[50] The medical libraries of the Aragonese Jewish physicians Mosse Aventida (Monzón) and Astruch Rimoth (Fraga) (both *fl.* 1381) focused their medical information on, in the first place, Avicenna (*Canon*), followed by Albucasis (*Book on surgery* and *Abbreviamentum*), Serapion (*Practica*), Averroes (probably his commentaries on Aristotle's *libri phisicorum*) and Galen (commentaries on the Hippocratic *Aphorisms*). The copies of Avicenna's *Canon* and Serapion's *Practica* were written in Latin.[51] The Jewish author of the only medical treatise that has been preserved written in Arabic in the first third of the fourteenth century in Castile (probably in Toledo) — the *Kitab al-tibb al-qastali al-maluki*, or *Book of Royal Castilian medicine* — nourished his Galenism from the Galenic *corpus* written in Arabic and from Arabic authors such as Razes (*al-Hawi*) and Avicenna (*al-Qanun*); to all appearances he did not use medical works written in Hebrew. Probably the survival of Arabic among the minority of Jewish medical scholars seems to have acted as a limiting factor for their knowledge of Galen's works, at least till the middle years of the fourteenth century.[52]

Very little is known about this question. This prevents us from drawing any conclusions about the importance that the diffusion of the "new Galen" in Hebrew might have had among the Jewish minority that was aware of this form of literature (if indeed this is what happened). Nor is it clear that what we are emphasizing among certain Jewish figures of the Western Mediterranean is more than a reflection of the impact of the "new Galen" on the Christian intellectual circles with which they were in touch (e.g. this is what Steinschneider suggests for the medical sources of the Catalan Jewish physician Moses Narboni (died 1362), who spent his life in Perpignan and Valencia, but who also travelled to the Jewish communities of Castile (Toledo and Soria), and was one of the principal commentators on Averroes' writings on natural philosophy).[53] What does seem to be true is that Avicenna's *Canon*, at least by the second half of the fourteenth century — a period in which western Jewish physicians were no longer in contact with the Arabic language — figures as the principal source of medical information for intellectually ambitious Spanish and Provençal Jewish physicians, with the consequent risks caused by the defective Hebrew versions.[54]

REFERENCES

1. L. García-Ballester, *La medicina a la València medieval*, València, Institució Valenciana d'Estudis Investigació, 1988, pp. 101-107; L. Garcia-Ballester, M.R. McVaugh, and A. Rubio-Vela, *Medical Licensing and Learning in Fourteenth-Century Valencia*, Philadelphia, The American Philosophical Society, 1989 (*Transactions of the American Philosophical Society*, vol. 79, Part 6).

2. F. Eiximenis, *Liber de virtutibus et peccatis sive Ars maior praedicationis* (1335), edited by Martí de Barcelona, "Fra Francesc Eiximenis", *Estudis Franciscans*, 1928, 22: 437-500, on p. 478.

3. The first part of the present paper is summarized from L. García-Ballester, "Changes in the *regimina sanitatis*: the Rôle of the Jewish Physicians", in: Sheila Campbell, (ed.), *Health, Disease and Healing in Medieval Culture*, Toronto, St. Martin's Press, 1990, in press.

4. L. García-Ballester, L. Ferre, and E. Feliu, "Jewish Appreciation of Fourteenth-Century Scholastic Medicine", *Osiris*, 1990, 6: in press.

5. D. Jacquart, "A l'aube de la renaissance médicale des XIe-XIIe siècles: L'*Isagoge Johannitii* et son traducteur", *Bibliothèque de l'Ecole des Chartes*, 1986, 144: 209-240.

6. See L. García-Ballester, "On the Origins of the 'Six Non-Natural Things' in Galen", in: Jutta Kollesch (ed.) *Galen und das hellenistische Erbe*, Wiesbaden, F. Steiner, 1991, in press.

7. L.J. Rather, "The 'Six Things Non-Natural': A Note on the Origins and Fate of a Doctrine and a Phrase", *Clio Medica*, 1968, 3: 337-347, on p. 337.

8. Bernard of Gordon in his *Regimen sanitatis* says: "regimen sanitatis consistit in debita applicatione sex rerum non naturalium", cited by L.E. Demaitre, *Doctor Bernard of Gordon: Professor and Practitioner*, Toronto, Pontifical Institute of Mediaeval Studies, 1980, p. 69, n. 166.

9. This doctrine was exposed by the Jewish author of the medical treatise, *K. al-tibb al-qastali al-maluki* (*Book of Royal Castilian Medicine*), written probably in Toledo, near 1312; it was also explained by his contemporary, the Christian surgeon Henri de

Mondeville, in his long introduction to the second book of his treatise on surgery, see L. García-Ballester and Concepción Vázquez de Benito, "Los médicos judíos castellanos del siglo XIV y el galenismo árabe: el *Kitab al-tibb al-qastali al-maluki* (Libro de medicina castellana regia), *c.* 1312", *Asclepio*, 1990, 42: 119-147.

10. *Arnaldi de Villanova Opera* ... Lyon, 1504, fols. 79ᵛ-84ᵛ. Critical edition is preparing by Ana Trias, *Regimen sanitatis ad regem Aragonum* (Vol. X, in *Arnaldi de Villanova Opera Medica Omnia*, Barcelona, University of Barcelona Press, 1974-).

11. The Hebrew text, with its English translation, has been published in García-Ballester, Ferre and Feliu, op. cit., note 4 above, appendix B.

12. See the work *On foodstuffs*, written by the Muslim physician Abu Bakr Abd al-Aziz al-Arbuli from Almeria (Kingdom of Granada), edited and translated into Spanish by A. Díaz Gracía, "Un tratado nazarí sobre alimentos: *Al-Kalam Ala-l-Agdiya* de Al-Arbuli", *Cuadernos de Estudios Medievales* (Granada), 1978-79, 6-7: 5-91; and the wearisome insistence on this topic by the Jewish author of the *K. al-tibb al-qastali*, note 9 above.

13. Nancy Siraisi, *Avicenna in Renaissance Italy. The Canon and Medical Teaching in Italian Universities after 1500*, Princeton, Princeton University Press, 1987, pp. 221ff. This work was widely distributed also amongst medieval Jewish physicians, see L. García-Ballester, *et al.*, *Osiris* (1990).

14. Appendix A, see note 4.

15. *Ibidem.*

16. *Ibidem.* 17. *Regimen sanitatis*, 17, cited by L. Demaitre, *Doctor Bernard de Gordon*, pp. 35, n. 187, and 69-70, n. 169.

18. Cited by Ytzhak Baer, *A history of the Jews in Christian Spain*, 2 vols., Philadelphia, The Jewish Publication Society of America, 1978, II, p. 75. A similar assertion was made by Jacob ben Sheshet Gerundi (*c.* 1250 in the polemic on Maimonidism): "In their madness they (the rationalists) follow the science of the Greeks ... It is illicit to learn something from the Gentiles", cited by G. Vajda, *Recherches sur la philosophie et la kabbala dans la pensée juive du Moyen Age*, Paris, Mouton & Co., 1962, pp. 357-358.

19. These reasons were explained in detail in García-Ballester, note 3 above.

20. See note 12.

21. See L. García-Ballester, "Tres bibliotecas médicas en la Valencia del siglo XV", *Asclepio*, 1966-67, 18-19: 383-405.

22. "Medicus avarus, qui de facili posset curare infirmum, differt infirmitatem, ut possit ab infirmo multos denarios extorquere; et lucratur multos denarios, et ponit aegrum in casu mortis atque periculo", *Liber de virtutibus et peccatis*, ed. F. Rodríguez Reboiras and A. Soria Flores, in *Raimundi Lulli Opera Latina*, vol. XV, Turnhout, Brepols, 1987, p. 143. 65-68.

23. Arnald bore this in mind: "Sed quia frequenter a debito regimine declinantur, ideo convenit ut hii, qui per naturam sunt proni ad talem vexacionem (in the case of the king of Aragon, to haemorrhoids, but they could be other ailments), sciant quibus remediis in actu passionis potuerunt se iuvare", *Arnaldi de Villanova Opera* ... Lyon, 1504, fol. 79ᵛ-84ᵛ, on fol. 84ʳ.

24. Specially useful for physicians was the second part of Avicenna's *Antidotarium*, dealing with medicines arranged according to diseases.

25. An anonymous Spanish Jewish physician (*fl.* first third of the fourteenth century) gave this opinion on Avicenna and his *Canon*: "Avicenna consolidates the art of medicine with the book *al-Qanun*, something which no other author has managed to achieve until now <...>. His antidotary (*agrabadhin*) contains marvellous texts which are the fruit of his experience", see García-Ballester and Vázquez de Benito, op. cit., note 9.

26. E. Nicaise (ed. and transl.), *Chirurgie de Maître Henri de Mondeville ...* Traduction française avec des notes ..., Paris, F. Alcan, 1893, pp. xxvi-xxvii.

27. As a result of my work during the last years on practical medicine in the fourteenth-century Crown of Aragon (North-east Spain) with Michael R. McVaugh in the rich medieval archives of the Spanish lands, we have verified in big cities such as Barcelona or Valencia (25.000-35.000 inhabitants), and in medium size or small towns (5.000-800 inhabitants) the presence of apothecaries with their stores well supplied with drugs.

28. Cardinalis (d. *c.* 1290), master in the Faculty of Medicine of Montpellier in 1240, distinguished — as did Avicenna in his *Canon* — between "*philosophi, qui causas et rerum essencias investigant*, and the "*medicus, (quod) plus attendit utilitatem quam veritatem*", Commentary to *Ysagoge*, MS Kues 222, fol. 40va.

29. About the presence of practical considerations in fourteenth-century Arabic science and medicine, see A.I. Sabra, "The appropriation and subsequent naturalization of Greek science in medieval Islam: a preliminary statement", *Hist Sci*, 1987, 25: 223-243, on pp. 235-36. On the so called "via pragmatica" in medical circles of late medieval Paris, Eduard Seidler, *Die Heilkunde des ausgehenden Mittelalters in Paris*, Wiesbaden, Franz Steiner Verlag, 1967, pp. 110 onwards.

30. Ron Barkai, "L'ús dels salms en la màgia jueva de l'edat mitjana i el Renaixement: el llibre *Shimush tehil.lim*", in *La Càbala*, Barcelona, Fundació Caixa de Pensions, 1989, pp. 17-57 (in Hebrew, Catalan transl. by E. Feliu).

31. Eleazar Gutwirth, "Casta, classe i màgia: bruixes i amulets entre els jueus espanyols del segle XV", in *La Càbala*, Barcelona, Fundació Caixa de Pensions, 1989, pp. 85-99 (in Hebrew, Catalan transl. by E. Feliu).

32. Mosse ben Nahman of Gerona used a seal engraved with the figure of a lion as a remedy, see Barkai, op. cit., note 30 above, pp. 30, n. 54. Arnau de Villanova used this kind of seal, who was mentioned at least in two of his works (*Speculum medicine* and *De parte operativa*), see Juan A. Paniagua, *El Maestro Arnau de Villanova, médico*, Valencia, Universidad de Valencia, 1969, p. 71, also Lynn Thorndike, *A history of magic and experimental science*, vol. 2, New York, Columbia University Press, 1923, pp. 857-58. About the possibility of a relationship between Jewish and Christian authors on this topic in Montpellier area, see Joseph Shatzmiller, "Contacts et échanges entre savants juifs et chrétiens à Montpellier vers 1300", in M.-H. Vicaire, and B. Blumenkranz (eds.), *Juifs et judaïsme de Languedoc, XIIIe siècle-début XIVe siècle*, Toulouse, Edouard Privat, 1977, pp. 337-344.

33. See the above mentioned articles by Barkai, Gutwirth and Shatzmiller.

34. Appendix B, see note 4 above.

35. About the discussions on all these theoretical problems in academic medical circles of Montpellier, and their areas of influence, during the fourteenth century, see, Michael McVaugh, "The development of medieval pharmaceutical theory", in L.

García-Ballester, M. McVaugh and J.A. Paniagua (eds.), *Arnaldi de Villanova Opera Medica Omnia*, vol. II: *Aphorismi de gradibus*, ed. by M. McVaugh, Barcelona, Universidad de Barcelona, 1975, pp. 1-136.

36. Michael McVaugh, "Two Montpellier recipe collections", in N.G. Siraisi and L. Dumaitre (eds.), *Science, medicine and the university: 1200-1550*, part II, *Manuscripta*, 1976, 20: 175-180, on pp. 178-9.

37. *De naturalibus facultatibus*, I 13: II 42-44K (English translation by A.J. Brock, Loeb class. lib. num. 71, pp. 67-71).

38. "In Arabic works of peripatetic and Galenic ancestry the most commonly used word to convey the meaning of experience is *tajriba*, which in these works corresponds to *empeiria*", A.I. Sabra, "The astronomical origin of Ibn al-Haytham's concept of experiment", *Actes XIIe Congrès International d'Histoire des Sciences, Paris 1968*, Tome IIIA, *Science et Philosophie*, Paris, Albert Blanchard, pp. 133-136, on p. 133. See, Mathias Schramm, "Aristotelianism: basis and obstacle to scientific progress in the Middle Ages", *Hist. Sci.*, 1963, 2: 91-113, on p. 105. The work of Avicenna corresponds to his *Kitab al-Burhan* (I, 9), ed. A.E., Cairo, 1956, pp. 93-98, see Schramm, p. 112, note 35.

39. On Grosseteste's experiment, see A.C. Crombie, *From Augustine to Galileo*, 2nd ed., 2 vols., London, Heinemann, II, pp. 24ss.

40. On these kind of collections, see McVaugh, note 36 above.

41. *Almagest*, ed. and transl. by G.J. Toomer, New York, F. Springer, 1984, lib. VII, pp. 321-33; 328-29, and 339.

42. Lawrence V. Berman, "Greek into Hebrew: Samuel ben Judah of Marseilles, fourteenth-century philosopher and translator", in A. Allmann (ed.), *Jewish medieval and renaissance studies*, Cambridge, Mass., Harvard University Press, 1967, pp. 289-320. The owner, a scholar Jew said: "It is the book (the *Almagest*) which I first studied in my youth", Berman, pp. 297-8. On the complex process of Almagest's translation into Hebrew, see Moritz Steinschneider, *Die hebraeischen Übersetzungen des Mittelalters und die Juden als Dolmetscher*, Berlin, 1893, p. 547 (Repr. Graz, 1956). Samuel ben Judah of Marseilles explained his personal participation in these processes, see Berman, appendix D, pp. 313-15.

43. Moritz Steinschneider, E. Aguiló, I. Levi and N. Kayserling, "Inventari de la heretat i llibreria del metge jueu Jahuda o Lleo Mosconi", *Bol. Soc. Arq. Lulliana*, 1903, 10: 80-91 and 140-151.

44. See Nancy G. Siraisi, *Taddeo Alderotti and his pupils. Two generations of Italian medical learning*, Princeton, Princeton University Press, 1981. Luis García-Ballester, "Arnau de Villanova (*c.* 1240-1311) y la reforma de los estudios médicos en Montpellier (1309): el Hipócrates latino y la introducción del nuevo Galeno", *Dynamis*, 1982, 2: 97-158. Marie-Thérèse d'Alverny, "Piëtro d'Abano traducteur de Galien", *Medioevo*, 1985, 11: 19-64.

45. Steinschneider, op. cit., note 45 above, pp. 654-55.

46. Luis García-Ballester, Introduction to *Commentum super tractatum Galieni de malicia complexionis diverse,* ed. by L. García-Ballester and E. Sánchez Salor, in García-Ballester, McVaugh and Panigua, op. cit., note 38 above, pp. 13-36 and 73-137.

47. Steinschneider, op. cit., note 45 above, p. 653.

48. Steinschneider, op. cit., note 45 above, p. 654.

49. Georges Vajda, "Joseph ben Abraham Ibn Waqar et sa tentative de concilation de la philosophie et de la réligion", in *Recherches sur la philosophie et la kabbale dans la pensée juive du Moyen Age*, Paris, Mouton & Co., 1962, pp. 115-297, on p. 128. Joseph ben Abraham Ibn Waqar, who lived in Toledo in the first part of the fourteenth century, was a trilingual scholar (Arabic and Hebrew and Spanish). From the contents of a medical work written in Arabic by an anonymous Jewish physician, probably from Toledo, and a contemporary of Ibn Waqar, we know that learned Jewish physicians living in Castile in the first third of the fourteenth century had a accurate knowledge of the Galenic *corpus* written in Arabic, a circumstance that apparently did not take place in North-east Spain (Crown of Aragon) in the second part of the century. See, García-Ballester, Ferre and Feliu, op. cit., note 4 above.

50. Steinschneider *et al.*, op. cit., note 46 above.

51. Archive of the Crown of Aragon (Barcelona), Cancilleria, reg. 819, fol. 151. See, Antoni Rubió y Lluch, *Documents per l'historia de la cultura catalana mig-eval*, vol. II, Barcelona, Institut d'Estudis Catalans, 1921, pp. 246-47.

52. García-Ballester, Ferre and Feliu, op. cit., note 4 above.

53. Steinschneider, op. cit., note 45 above, pp. 311-12.

54. García-Ballester, Ferre and Feliu, op. cit., note 4 above.

VII

A marginal learned medical world: Jewish, Muslim and Christian medical practitioners, and the use of Arabic medical sources in late medieval Spain

The Christian conquest of Muslim-ruled areas in that part of the Iberian peninsula within the confines of present-day Spain did not mean that the Arabic language disappeared from those areas. From the late eleventh century onwards the frontiers of Castile included such important cities as Toledo (from 1085 onwards); during the course of the thirteenth century the Guadalquivir valley was incorporated (with the conquest of Cordoba, 1236, and Seville, 1248), as was the Kingdom of Murcia (1243 onwards); the Muslim Kingdom of Granada was not conquered until 1492. For their part, the Christians of the Crown of Aragon, in the eastern coastal area of the Iberian peninsula, conquered the Kingdom of Valencia, as far as the frontier with Murcia, in 1237–40. All these cities and regions contained a population whose everyday language of communication was Arabic, and who, to a great extent, remained settled in the area after the conquest. Furthermore, Arabic maintained its role as a language of scholarly communication and as the vehicle which allowed continued access to medical sources of unquestionable theoretical and practical value.[1]

[1] On the small number of medical works written in or translated into Arabic, which were translated into Latin, see Danielle Jacquart and Françoise Micheau, *La médecine arabe et l'occident médiéval* (Paris, 1990), pp. 230–43. On the role played by knowledge of the Arabic language in the medical training of the Jewish and Muslim physicians practising in medieval Spanish kingdoms, see L. García-Ballester, 'Medical science in thirteenth-century Castile: problems and prospects', *Bulletin of the History of Medicine*, 61 (1987), 183–202, and L. García-Ballester, Lola Ferre, and Eduard Feliu, 'Jewish appreciation of fourteenth-century scholastic medicine in the Western Mediterranean', in McVaugh and Siraisi (eds.), *Renaissance medical learning* (*Osiris*, 2nd series, 6 (1990), 85–117). The conclusion reached by L. P. Harvey after the analysis of two medical consultations, the one in 1492 and the other in 1501, between Christian patients and Muslim practitioners, one of them, a woman, about the situation of Arabic medicine among Muslim practitioners living under the new

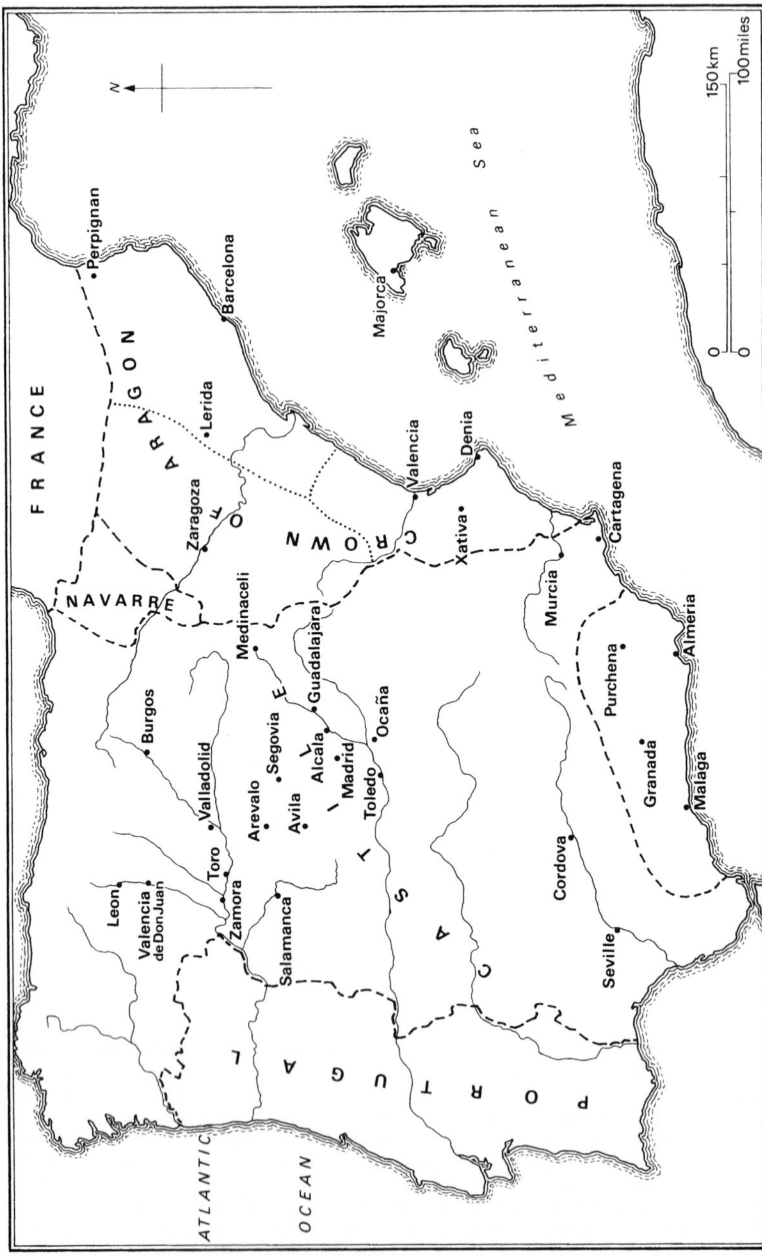

The Iberian peninsula in the thirteenth, fourteenth and fifteenth centuries.

During the last few years, various experts on Arabic culture in medieval and Renaissance Spain have discovered, described and studied surviving manuscripts of all kinds written in Arabic that were used by members of the three religious groups (Christians, Muslims and Jews) that lived alongside each other in the Christian kingdoms of Spain between the eleventh and sixteenth centuries. The most recent and most complete of all these works is that produced by P. S. van Koningsveld.[2] He describes 105 manuscript codices. Twenty-four of them contain a total of sixty-five medical works with various texts by Hippocrates, Galen, Dioscorides, Avicenna, Rhazes, Maimonides, Averroes and other lesser authors. All the manuscripts with medical contents were copied between *c.* 1150 and 1480. This is fundamentally the material upon which this chapter, which continues and brings up to date other earlier contributions on the same subject,[3] is based.

The present chapter is divided into three parts. In the first we shall describe the uses these manuscripts were put to by physicians of the three religious groups (Christians, Muslims and Jews) that lived alongside one another in the peninsular Kingdoms of Castile and the Crown of Aragon from the twelfth to the fifteenth centuries and who are recorded as having made use of the Arabic language to establish the foundations of their medical knowledge. In the second part, we shall offer a general panorama, based on an analysis of the evidence of reading and transmission present in the manuscripts themselves. This analysis demonstrates the continued use of (Greek and Arabic) medical sources written in Arabic, which contributed to the development of the medieval Galenism of these physicians (who were most commonly of Jewish origin, although the other two groups should not be forgotten). If our analysis is basically restricted to Castile, this is due to the fact that all the *surviving* Arabic medical manuscripts which circulated in Spanish Christian lands come from this Kingdom, with the exception of two (one from Barcelona, the other from Valencia, both of which were cities of the Crown of Aragon). The close relationship existing between the population of the lands of Castile and the

Christian conquerors is highly illustrative of the situation: 'Granada [we could say also Valencia or Murcia] was a place where the culture of the conqueror was for a time challenged by the continuing reality of the culture of the conquered': see 'In Granada under the Catholic monarchs: a call from a doctor and another from a *curandera*', in *The age of the Catholic monarchs, 1474–1516, Literary studies in memory of Keith Whinnom* (Liverpool, 1989), pp. 71–5.

2 P. S. van Koningsveld, 'Andalusian-Arabic manuscripts from Christian Spain: a comparative, intercultural, approach', *Israel Oriental Studies*, 12 (1992), 75–110; van Koningsveld, 'Andalusian-Arabic manuscripts from medieval Christian Spain: some supplementary notes', in *Festgabe für H.-R. Singer* (Frankfurt a. M., 1991), pp. 811–23. I have used the typescript version of both papers by courtesy of the author.

3 The first attempt to use this approach on the medieval medical manuscripts written in Arabic and preserved in Western libraries, especially El Escorial and Biblioteca Nacional of Madrid, was made by L. García-Ballester, *Historia social de la medicina en la España de los siglos XIII al XVI* (Madrid, 1976), pp. 31–42.

people of the Crown of Aragon has meant that it is advisable to make reference to events that took place in the Crown of Aragon, when it is relevant. The third part will be dedicated to the analysis of the intellectual characteristics of the only medical work written in Arabic in the first third of fourteenth-century Castile to survive to the present day. This is the *Kitab al-tibb al-qastali al-maluki* (Book of regal Castilian medicine), an important systematic medical treatise, written by an anonymous Jew from Toledo (*fl.* 1295–1312).[4] It will enable us to consider in great depth the role played by the rationalist Jewish minority in the maintenance and growth of the medical literature that circulated among the Jewish minority in Castile. In addition, as will be seen, this medical literature acted as a support for a particular approach to professional practice. Thus, the medical activity of certain physicians – to be more precise Jewish practitioners – was not limited to mere empiricism, nor to the blind application of prescriptions repeated from generation to generation; it was, in fact, the manifestation in practice of theoretical knowledge, transmitted and developed in accordance with an 'open' system, distinct from that of the Latin scholastic university world.[5]

I

Three population groups continued to use Arabic as a language of communication in Christian Spain: Muslims, Jews and Christians, both those of Arabic culture (Mozarabs) and those formed in Latin culture. The survival of the Arabic language among these different groups was not uniform; the time and other circumstances of a social and intellectual nature influenced the survival of Arabic among them to a greater or lesser extent.

Christians

One of the most interesting peculiarities of the new area conquered by Christians from the north – especially in the case of Toledo, but also of other cities – was the presence in them of communities of Christians of Arabic culture, who had lived as a minority in what had hitherto been Muslim territories, and who, after the conquest, remained alongside their brothers-in-religion of Latin culture. They received the name *Mozarabs*.[6]

[4] L. García-Ballester, and Concepción Vázquez de Benito, 'Los médicos judíos del siglo XIV y el galenismo árabe: el *Kitab al-tibb al-qastali al-maluki* (Libro de medicina castellana regia), *c.* 1312', *Asclepio*, 42 (1990), 119–47.

[5] On the relationship between both systems of medical training in western Mediterranean countries, see García-Ballester, Ferre and Feliu, 'Jewish appreciation'.

[6] On *Mozarabs* and medicine, see F. Girón-Irueste, 'Los médicos mozárabes y el proceso de constitución de la medicina árabe en Al-andalus, siglos VIII–X', *Asclepio*, 30–1 (1978–9), 209–22, which, in my opinion, over-emphasizes the role of *Mozarabs* in this process. See also Jacquart and Micheau, *La médecine arabe*, pp. 134–53, and P. S. van Koningsveld, *The*

The strength of Latin culture and the continuing uneasiness of the Church at the presence of Christians of Arabic culture, whether they were Christians of long standing or recent converts, meant that Mozarabic culture underwent a rapid process of decline, already apparent in the early thirteenth century.[7] Even though it is possible to identify documents composed in Arabic by members of this Christian minority in the early fourteenth century, all available indications point to this language rarely being used from the second half of the thirteenth century onwards by those individuals among them who practised medicine. None of the surviving medical manuscripts in Arabic that have come down to us, and which are known to have circulated in Christian lands, were copied by or belonged to a member of the Mozarabic community.[8]

Christian physicians trained in Latin culture were not averse to using Arabic medical manuscripts. Throughout the thirteenth century, and even at the beginning of the fourteenth century, nobody among the Christian intellectual minority of Europe doubted that an effective way to gain access to medical learning was still through a knowledge of Arabic.[9] Moreover, Christian scholars were aware that there existed valuable medical works unknown to scholastic medical circles because they had not been translated into Latin. Very few Christian university physicians were capable of handling these Arabic sources directly. Moreover, Arabic medical manuscripts do not seem to have been particularly abundant in the late thirteenth century and the first decades of the fourteenth century, to judge from the available information. However, the Arabic medical manuscripts that were in existence in Christian lands were highly regarded, and were used habitually by Christian physicians and scholars, either in Latin translation, or, by those few with sufficient knowledge of Arabic, in the original.

One of the few Christian physicians of this period who is known to have had a knowledge of Arabic was Arnau de Vilanova (*c.* 1240–1311), who spent part of his life in those areas of the Crown of Aragon where the majority of the population – for example in the Kingdom of Valencia –

Latin Arabic glossary of the Leiden University Library. A contribution to the study of Mozarabic manuscripts and literature (Leiden, 1977).

7 This mistrust of the Spanish Catholic Church, and the relationship of this phenomenon with the medicine practised by the appropriate minority, have been studied within the context of the so-called 'Moriscos' or new Christians compulsorily converted from the Muslim religion at the beginning of sixteenth-century Spain: see L. García-Ballester, *Los moriscos y la medicina. Un capítulo de la medicina y la ciencia marginadas en la España del siglo XVI* (Barcelona, 1984).

8 Van Koningsveld, 'Andalusian-Arabic manuscripts from Christian Spain', pp. 29–30 of his typescript, and 'Andalusian-Arabic manuscripts from medieval Christian Spain', number xiv of the Appendix.

9 Roger Bacon's (d. 1294) opinion with regard to this is very well known. See J. S. Brewer (ed.), *Fr. Rogeri Bacon opera quaedam hactenus inedita* (London, 1859), vol. 1, *Compendium studii*, cap. 8, pp. 467–8, and 471–2.

spoke Arabic.[10] He is known to have translated at least three works of medicine from Arabic into Latin: *De tremore, iectigatione et spasmo* by Galen; *De viribus cordis* by Avicenna and *De simplicibus medicinis* by Abu Salt (1067–1134), a physician from Denia, Valencia.[11] He appears to have undertaken his translations in Barcelona, during the time of his first period in the service of the King of Aragon (1280s).[12] From his own writings we know that he also frequently used medical works in Arabic to discuss unclear passages in the Latin versions.[13] On his death, in the inventory of his library, which was located in the city of Valencia, there figure eight works 'in arabica lingua', two of which we know were certainly of medical content.[14] Evidence of Arabic texts similarly being either translated or used to check accuracy can be seen in the request that Guillelmus de Biterris directed (1302), via the king, to the Jews of Catalonia for the loan of 'certain books of medicine written in Arabic, which were necessary for him'. In this way he intended to increase the number of Latin medical manuscripts at, and to improve the quality of those already in the possession of, the recently created University of Lerida, where on the orders of the king, he was establishing a faculty of medicine.[15]

The Christian university doctors who did not know Arabic turned to those of their Christian pupils who came from lands where Arabic was a living language to translate for them the medical writings in which they were interested. Such was the case of Bernard de Gordon (fl. 1283–1308), a colleague of Arnau at the faculty of medicine in Montpellier, who asked Berenguer Eymerich of Valencia to translate the work entitled *De cibariis infirmorum*.[16]

[10] J. A. Paniagua, 'L'arabisme à Montpellier dans l'œuvre d'Arnau de Vilanova', *Comptes-rendus du XVIe Congrès International d'Histoire de la Médecine*. (Montpellier, 1958), pp. 163–9; L. García-Ballester, 'Arnau de Vilanova (*c*. 1240–1311) y la reforma de los estudios médicos en Montpellier (1309): el Hipócrates latino y la introducción del nuevo Galeno', *Dynamis*, 2 (1982), 97–158, at 141–5.

[11] The three translations are being published in *Arnaldi de Villanova opera medica omnia* (AVOMO hereafter) (Barcelona, 1975–), see M. R. McVaugh (ed.), *Translatio libri Galieni de rigore et tremore et iectigatione et spasmo* (Barcelona, 1981), AVOMO, vol. XVI.

[12] McVaugh, *Translatio*, pp. 30–7.

[13] '... nec est imputandum errori transferentis, quia in omnibus libris arabum, quos invenire potuimus, sic invenimus contineri; nec similiter imputandum est defectui vocabulorum in illa lingua, quod ad notificandum dolorem secundo modo acceptum scimus in ea copiosos esse sermones', *Commentum supra tractatum Galieni de malicia complexionis diverse*, ed. by L. García-Ballester and E. Sánchez Salor (Barcelona, 1985), AVOMO, vol. XV, p. 192, lines 15–20.

[14] R. Chabas, 'Inventario de los libros, ropas y demás efectos de Arnaldo de Vilanova', *Boletín de la Real Academia de la Historia*, 9 (1903), 189–203, nos. 48, 65, 76, 93, 115, 150, 173 and 183; at least nos. 76 and 173 are medical works.

[15] Archive of the Crown of Aragon (hereafter ACA) in Barcelona, C., reg. 299, fol. 52v, 2 September 1352, published in A. Rubió y Lluch, *Documents per l'història de la cultura catalana mig-eval* (Barcelona, 1921), pp. 13–14, doc. 16.

[16] Probably a part of the 28th book of Albucasis' (az-Zaharawi) *Tasrif*, which circulated in Latin with the title of *Liber servitoris*, and where the author shows how to prepare medical prescriptions. Berenguer Eymerich's translation has never been edited: see

Another place where Christian scholars used Arabic manuscripts was in the recently conquered territory of Murcia, which became part of the Kingdom of Castile. There, the context was different from that which has been seen in the Crown of Aragon. In Murcia the active scholars were members of the mendicant orders (Dominicans and Franciscans) and Italian scholars, who showed enough intellectual curiosity about natural and medical sciences contained in Arabic manuscripts to maintain a limited programme of translation and study. These regions were unique in bordering territories of Arabic culture (the Muslim Kingdom of Granada, North Africa), as well as the Mediterranean Sea, which meant that after the Christian conquest an intense commercial and cultural interchange was quickly established with meridional regions of Europe (Italy, among others) and with the nearest Arabic countries.[17]

The first translations from Arabic to Latin in these territories were made by the Franciscan Pedro Gallego (*c.* 1200–67), who was named first Bishop of Cartagena (Murcia) in 1250. During the seventeen years of his bishopric he completed translations of four works of natural philosophy with implications for medicine: an abridgement (with personal touches) of the *Liber de animalibus* (from *Historia animalium*, Books 1–9) of Aristotle; an abridgement of Averroes' compendium to the *De partibus animalium* (from *Historia animalium*, Books 1–2, chapter 2) of Aristotle; and a text on *Oeconomia* (*in regitiva domus*), probably based on the pseudo-Galenic work. He also wrote a *Summa astronomica*, in which he appears to summarize the treatise of Al-Fargani, *Elementa astronomica*.[18]

The second place in Murcia where medical works were translated was the school of Arabic and Hebrew languages ('Studium Arabicum et Hebraicum') founded by the Dominicans in 1266 for missionary and apologetic purposes. This school was similar to others created in the thirteenth century in territories on the frontiers of Christendom ('Germania', 'Hungaria', 'Hispania'). For reasons unknown to us, Rufinus Alexandrinus (from Alessandria in Italy, to the north of Genoa) arrived in Murcia to learn Arabic. He was taught the language there by a Dominican, Dominicus Marrochinus.[19] With the latter's help he translated at least two works: the first was an ophthalmic work, which he finished in 1271;[20] the second was a group of works collected in a manual like those used in teaching medicine, and entitled in Latin *Liber questionum medicinalium discentibus in medicina*, attributed to 'Huneyn filius Ysaac medici qui latine dicitur

L. García-Ballester, *La medicina a la València medieval* (Valencia, 1988), p. 92, n. 163. These kinds of work were much appreciated by medical practitioners: see Jacquart and Micheau, *La médecine arabe*, p. 210.

17 See, García-Ballester, 'Medical science in thirteenth-century Castile', p. 199.

18 Ibid., pp. 199–200.

19 Ibid., p. 200.

20 Berne, Bürgerbibliothek, MS 216, fols. 1ra–43vb. This copy dates from 1279 (fol. 43vb).

Johannicius'.[21] This second item is an authentic student textbook. That this Arabic-language students' manual should have been current in Murcia between the years of 1270 and 1280 is of great interest, and tells us of the presence and circulation among the Muslim population of a medical literature elaborated and prepared for didactic purposes.[22]

After the treaty of Alcaraz (1243), the Muslim Kingdom of Murcia was subjected to Castile, although it maintained a certain degree of autonomy (language, religion, land ownership, even the Muslim monarch himself remained until the early 1260s). Around 1257 the Christians started seriously to contravene the terms of the settlement, and an increasing exodus of Muslim inhabitants in the direction of the neighbouring Kingdom of Granada can be detected; in 1264 a rebellion broke out among the Muslim inhabitants of Murcia.[23] From that moment onwards, the situation of tolerance that had previously existed disappeared. It is known from Arabic sources that the Muslim scholar and physician, Abu Bakr M. ibn Ahmad al-Riquti, remained in Murcia after the advent of the Christians, at least until 1272. During these years he resisted pressure from King Alfonso X of Castile to convert to Christianity, unlike other Muslim scholars of Murcia such as Bernard the Arab. Bernard translated a treatise on a kind of astrolabe (*azafea*) by Al-Zarqali (Azarquiel) from Arabic to Castilian with the collaboration of the Jew don Abraham in Burgos in 1278. Until recently, the presence of al-Riquti has been associated, although without any documentary support, with the translating activity of Pedro Gallego, and also with the existence of a possible *Madrasa* or school of Islamic studies, which may have functioned in Murcia during those years in which this Muslim scholar remained in this land. This last point springs from the well-known evidence of Ibn al-Khatib, in which he affirms that 'the tyrant-king of the Christians knew [his scholarship], and built for him, after he had conquered Murcia, a *Madrasa* in which he could teach Muslims, Christians and Jews and [where] he continued to be held in esteem by him [i.e. the king]'.[24] Nevertheless, there is no documentary

[21] Erfurt, Staatsbibliothek Amploniana MS, F 271, fols. 11ra–25rb. In the copy (fol. 18vb) there is a mention of 'Huneyn filius Ysaac medici qui latine dicitur Johannicius'. See also M. Steinschneider, *Die hebräischen Übersetzungen des Mittelalters, und die Juden als Dolmetscher* (Berlin, 1893), pp. 710–11. It could be the variant *Kitab al-masa 'il fi t-tibb* of Hunain ibn Ishaq's introduction to medicine: see Jacquart and Micheau, *La médecine arabe*, pp. 46–7.

[22] Another problem is why this translation did not become diffused through Latin Europe. The Murcia translation has been preserved only in the above-mentioned manuscript.

[23] J. Torres Fontes, 'El obispado de Cartagena en el siglo XIII', *Hispania*, 13 (1953), 339–580.

[24] Ibn Al-Khatib, *Al-Ihata fi akjbar Gharnata*, ed. by M. A. 'Inan, 4 vols. (Cairo, c. 1975–7), vol. III, pp. 67–8. Van Koningsveld gives an English translation of the passage from al-Khatib: see his 'Andalusian-Arabic manuscripts from Christian Spain', pp. 9–10 of his typescript. The Muslim King of Granada, Yusuf surnamed 'Al-Faqih' (1272–1302) of the Banu Nasr family, took in al-Riquti and gave him facilities for teaching and practising medicine. On the Banu Nasr of Granada, see R. Arié, *L'Espagne musulmane au temps des Nasrides, 1232–1492* (Paris, 1973).

evidence to prove that this institution ever functioned. Van Koningsveld has recently brought to light new evidence, also from Arabic sources, unknown until now. It comes from Abu 'Ali al-Husain ibn Rashiq (*fl* 1275), who lived in Murcia after the Christian conquest. It is of great significance, firstly because it confirms the existence of scientific manuscripts in Arabic among the Muslim population that remained after the conquest. Secondly it provides information about the attraction exerted by the knowledge of natural and medical things contained in these manuscripts upon Christians. In addition, it enables us to appreciate how members of the enlightened Muslim minority perceived this situation. It thus complements what is known about Pedro Gallego and the *studium* founded by the Dominicans.

> I was in the city of Murcia – may God restore it! – during the days when its inhabitants were afflicted by the *dain* [i.e. by subjection to a non-Muslim ruler] ... At that time a group of their priests and monks had come to that city on behalf of the Tyrant-King of the Christians, in order to dedicate themselves – as they thought – to devotion and scientific study, eagerly stretching out their necks to look into the sciences of the Muslims and to translate them into their own language, for the sake of criticism – may God thwart their effort! They were especially fond of disputing with the Muslims and had a blameworthy intention in attracting weak minds.[25]

We have evidence about the existence in Murcia of Arabic manuscripts on natural philosophy a few years later, around 1325. But this evidence is no longer associated with the Muslim minority or with Christian scholars. Now the information comes from Jewish sources and the users were likewise Jews. We refer to Samuel ben Judah of Marseilles, who, on being expelled by the King of France, sought refuge, like so many other Jews, in the Christian Kingdoms of the Crown of Aragon and Castile. He went to Murcia (1324) where he traced the Arabic version of Alexander of Aphrodisias' *De anima*, which he translated into Hebrew.[26] In the fifteenth century – when Arabic had been abandoned by the scholars in favour of Latin, Greek or Romance languages – there appear two further Christian physicians from Valencia who knew Arabic and who handled scientific manuscripts in circulation there; they were Martín Villarroya (*fl.* 1414–21) and Juan de Bosnia (*fl.* 1456–84).[27] After that date we have to wait until 1540 to find Christian physicians in Valencia in possession of medical

[25] Muhammad Hajji (ed.), *Abu' l-'Abbas Ahmad ibn Yahya, Al-Mi'yār al-mu'rib wa-al-jāmi' al-mughrib 'an fatāwá 'ulamā Ifrīqīyah wa-al-Andalus wa-al-Maghrib*, 13 vols. (Rabat, 1981), vol. XI, p. 155. Quoted and translated into English by van Koningsveld, 'Andalusian-Arabic manuscripts from Christian Spain', p. 11 of his typescript.

[26] L. V. Berman, 'Greek into Hebrew: Samuel ben Judah of Marseilles, fourteenth century philosopher and translator', in A. Altmann (ed.), *Jewish medieval and Renaissance studies* (Cambridge, Mass., 1967), pp. 289–320, on pp. 317–18.

[27] See, García-Ballester, *Historia social de la medicina*, pp. 72–3.

manuscripts in Arabic (Avicenna's *Qanun*) and with sufficient knowledge of this language to enable them to read such works.[28]

The Muslim minority

As regards the Muslims that remained in Christian lands after the conquest, the educated minority emigrated southwards, to those areas of the peninsula still in the hands of Muslims, or alternatively, to the areas occupied by present-day Morocco. In spite of this, attitudes towards the Arabic language and medical writings were not the same in the various parts of Spain in the later Middle Ages. The Muslim inhabitants of Castile soon lost all knowledge of Arabic, to the point that by the fifteenth century even the Koran had to be read to them in a Romance language, since Arabic was unintelligible to them.[29] After 1265, there is no evidence that any of the surviving medical manuscripts among those that circulated in Christian zones of Castile were copied by Muslim scribes. In the case of those surviving from before that date (between 1166 and 1265), which were copied by Muslims in either Castile or Catalonia, all the scribes were prisoners of war, who carried out their work for Jewish masters.[30] In spite of this we know that still in 1346 there were Muslims in Toledo with enough knowledge of Arabic to translate notarial documents written in Arabic into Castilian to be used by the king.[31] However, the only surviving manuscript with medical contents belonging to Castilian Muslims is of the fifteenth century and is partly in 'aljamiado' (Castilian in Arabic letters) and partly in Arabic. Empirical and magical elements are predominant in this work.[32]

The same did not occur in the lands of the Crown of Aragon, where there was a substantial Muslim population with a certain level of literacy, which we can establish with documentary evidence. As an example, it is possible to find in the notarial archive of Zaragoza (Aragon) many documents from the second part of the fourteenth century, related to business between Muslim people and Christians or Jews, which are signed in Arabic with the name of the Muslim participants.[33] There is fifteenth-century evidence

28 See, García-Ballester, *Los moriscos y la medicina*, pp. 24–8.

29 *Tratados de legislación musulmana* (Madrid, Real Academia de la Historia, 1853), pp. 7 and 248, quoted by A. Castro, *Sobre el nombre y el quién de los españoles* (Madrid, 1973), p. 276.

30 See, van Koningsveld, 'Andalusian-Arabic manuscripts from Christian Spain', p. 21 of his typescript.

31 See, F. Fita, 'Marjadraque, según el fuero de Toledo', *Boletin de la Real Academia de la Historia*, 7 (1885), 360–94, document no. 5, pp. 371–6, where are given the names of two 'mudéjares' (Muslims) – don Mahomad Xaraffi and his son don Hamete – who translated into Spanish for the king some documents written in Arabic, which were stored in the archive of Toledo Cathedral.

32 J. Albarracín Navarro and J. Martíinez Ruiz, *Medicina, farmacopea y magia en el 'Misceláneo de Salomón'. Texto árabe, traducción y glosas aljamiadas, estudio y glosario* (Granada, 1987).

33 Notarial Archive of Zaragoza (ANZ hereafter), Pedro López de Anso, 22 February 1361, fol. 27; the document is signed by Abrayim Avenjucez, mayor of the Muslim community of Azuara, a little town near Zaragoza; a witness of the document is Muça de Jamez, a

from both Aragon and Valencia that members of the Muslim minority maintained contact with the medical sources of their own culture expressed in Arabic. We are referring to – as far as Aragon is concerned – the existence of regular medical studies in the *Madrasa* of Zaragoza, where in 1447 and 1495 it can be demonstrated that medicine was being taught together with its foundations in natural philosophy; Avicenna's *Qanun* and the same author's *Uryuza fi-l-tibb*, among others, were being used as the standard texts for this purpose.

These significant pieces of information are derived from the contents of both a colophon of an Arabic manuscript copied in 1447 (19 June 851) 'in the Madrasa built by the Muslims of the city of Zaragoza', and a letter written by a Muslim student of medicine to his master, Abu 'Abd Allah M. al-Gazi, *alfaquí* of Belchite (Aragon) from Zaragoza in 1494. The documents were published in Arabic by Ribera.[34] The fact that the letter had not been translated into a western language was probably the reason why it was not taken into consideration until 1975, the year in which it was translated into Spanish and its contents analysed.[35] The letter has two parts, both of which are important for our purposes. In the first, the student, whose name was Muhammad al-Qurasi, promised his master, among other things, that he would not forget to send him a copy of some commentaries on writings of Al-Yasiti (d. 1189), in all probability the well-known Malikite theologian who was so influential among Spanish Muslims.[36] In the second part, he informs his master about his medical studies:

> As regards your request that I should send you the commentaries on the writings of al-Yaziri ... I do not have the copies of the commentaries with me, except a few insignificant fragments ... However ... when Muhammad b. Yusuf comes, I shall ask him for these commentaries so as to make a copy of them and to be able to send them to you ... And if I have other business to attend to, I shall abandon it in order to be at your immediate service ...
>
> Concerning your kind enquiries about my situation and the way of teaching for the goal that I am pursuing [i.e. to be a physician], I inform you that I am in perfect health, thanks to God, and that I have just read the commentary on Avicenna's *Uryuza*, and that, with the will of God, I shall start to read the first book of the *Canon*. I shall have to work day and night to achieve my goal, because the above-mentioned work deals with the general aspects of medicine, which are: knowledge of the limits of medical science; the mixture of the humours; the elements; the nature of bodies; the science of the necessary things, such as meals,

Muslim barber from Zaragoza. ANZ, Rodrigo López Castillón, 23 February 1363, *s.f.*; the document is signed both by Moçat de Marquna and Ali de Marquna, boilermakers from Huesca, who were contracted to repair the bathtub of the king.

34 J. Ribera, 'La enseñanza entre los musulmanes españoles', in *Disertaciones y opúsculos* (Madrid, 1928), vol. 1, pp. 229–359; colophon and letter are on pp. 351–4.

35 See the Spanish translation in García-Ballester, *Historia social de la medicina*, pp. 68–9 (letter) and p. 71, n. 171 (colophon).

36 See, W. Hoenerbach, *Spanisch-islamische Urkunden aus der Zeit der Nasriden und Moriscos* (Bonn, 1965), p. xxxiii.

drink, sleep, wakefulness, movement and rest; knowledge of illness and its causes; and many other things which I shall not detail. All this forms but some of the subtleties of this science, which also takes into account logic and philosophy. And all this can only be accomplished by means of effort and application.[37]

We have to emphasize the significance of the presence of the Malikite theological tradition within the context of the only surviving document in fifteenth-century Spain in order to understand medical teaching among the Muslim minority in Aragon.[38] Van Koningsveld, after analysing the manuscripts that are known to have belonged to members of the Muslim or Morisco minority, emphasizes the leading social and intellectual role of religious institutions (mosques) and leaders (*alfaquies*) among the Muslim minority living in Spanish Christian lands.[39]

In this context, we believe it to be acceptable to connect what has just been mentioned on the subject of the teaching of medicine among the Muslim minority in Aragon with recently discovered evidence. This has been provided by van Koningsveld and relates to the copying, in Valencia in 1480, and subsequent circulation of a medical work by ibn Rushd, the *Mansuma fi-l-tibb*, a medical poem (like the *Uryuza*) used in teaching.[40] Together with these points we should also mention the presence, also in the Kingdom of Valencia, of an *alfaquí* (*fl.* 1450–6) from Paterna, a small town with a largely Muslim population near the city of Valencia. This *alfaquí* brought from Cairo a manuscript describing the *Sexagenarium*, the Latin name for the instrument used by Egyptian astronomers, which, by means of the graphic application of trigonometrical formulae, in accordance with Ptolemaic science, provides equations for the centre of the earth and the theory of the planets.[41]

These data from Aragon (1447 and 1495) and Valencia (1450 and 1480), all concentrated in the central and final years of the fifteenth century, have a further common feature in that all of them can be found in Spanish Muslim sources. The plentiful Christian documentation preserved in the archives says nothing of these matters, yet, in contrast, it provides numerous examples that point to the lack of cultural (and medical) integration which Muslim communities experienced in Christian lands. Unfortunately, it is impossible to go beyond what has already been said, in view of the paucity of sources we are faced with. Moreover, we lack similar data for the thirteenth and fourteenth centuries. Nevertheless, by the sixteenth century, scarcely two generations after 1495, two significant developments should provide food for thought. In the first place, the Muslim tradition of

[37] Arabic text in Ribera, 'La enseñanza', vol. 1, pp. 352–4.

[38] See García-Ballester, *Historia social de la medicina*, pp. 50–3 and 69.

[39] Van Koningsveld, 'Andalusian-Arabic manuscripts from Christian Spain'.

[40] Ibid., Appendix 1, no. 70; see P. K. Hitti, *Descriptive catalog of the Garrett Collection in the Princeton University Library* (Princeton, 1938), p. 343.

[41] E. Poulle, 'Théorie des planètes et trigonométrie au XVè siècle, d'après un équatoire inédit, le sexagenarium', *Journal des Savants*, 3 (1966), 129–61.

medical teaching had been completely forgotten by the old Christian society of Aragon when they thought of creating a new faculty of medicine in Zaragoza (1584); and, secondly, the descendants of Muhammad al-Qurasi, who proclaimed that 'medical science . . . can only be achieved by means of effort and application', were only able to write their medical works, fundamentally based on magic, in 'aljamiado' (the text of Spanish written in Arabic characters).[42]

Everything seems to indicate that in the period between the thirteenth and fifteenth centuries, and at a faster rate in Castile than in the Crown of Aragon, a series of factors led the Muslim minority in Christian lands towards a state of progressive cultural disintegration, with consequent repercussions on the form of medicine which they practised, which drifted towards empirical and magical forms as the dominant style of medical activity. Among these factors we might mention: (1) The social and economic conditions in which they were obliged to live (in effect as serfs to Christian lords). (2) The possible influence of their own religious leaders, around whom the cultural and political life of Muslim communities revolved. These leaders were heavily influenced by Malikism, the dominant spiritual movement among the Spanish Muslim population, both in Castile and the Crown of Aragon, and this was not at all well disposed towards intellectual activity, such as natural philosophy. (3) The fact that it was impossible for them to enter centres of medical teaching (faculties of medicine and schools of surgery) which were accessible to Christians (we only have the exception of Zaragoza in the fifteenth century and in this particular case our reference is to a specifically Islamic institution). (4) The flight of the intellectual minority to nearby Muslim territories (Granada and Morocco), where members of the medical profession could practise freely. Although there is little definite evidence on this last point, we can cite two examples, first the already mentioned intellectual and physician Abu Bakr M. ibn Ahmad al-Riquti (*fl.* 1264–78) from Murcia, who went on to practise and teach medicine in courtly circles of the Muslim monarch of Granada, 'Al Muhammad b.M.b. Yusuf (1272–1302);[43] and second, that of Muhammad al-Safra (*c.* 1280–*c.* 1350), a surgeon from Crevillente (Valencia) who left for Granada (probably in 1318) and later Fez (1344),

[42] Nevertheless, I am in agreement with Harvey and with van Koningsveld about the fact that in Christian Spain there was a survival of Arabic culture (and *a fortiori* of Arabic medicine) from the thirteenth through to the sixteenth century, embodied first in the Muslim minority and finally in the Morisco minority: L. P. Harvey, 'The literary culture of the Moriscos, 1492–1609. A study based on the extant manuscripts in Arabic and Aljamia, 2 vols., Ph.D. thesis (University of Oxford, 1958); Harvey, 'The survival of Arabic culture in Spain after 1492', *Actes du 8me Congrès de l'Union Européenne des Arabisants et Islamisants, Aix-en-Provence, Septembre 1976* (Aix-en-Provence, 1978), pp. 85–8; van Koningsveld, 'Andalusian-Arabic manuscripts from Christian Spain', p. 20 of his typescript; see also García-Ballester, *Los moriscos y la medicina*, *passim*.

[43] See note 24 above.

where he died shortly afterwards.[44] All these four factors, at least, were present simultaneously and help to explain the progressive disintegration of the minority's intellectual and cultural life, which also affected the medicine they practised, in so far as the medicine practised by a social group is an integral part of its cultural identity.

Paradoxically, a factor that tended to assist this disintegration of medical culture was the pressure applied by Christian authorities via control of medical practitioners of non-university origins. This control was exerted through an examination which reproduced at a lower level the procedures of the Christian schools of medicine. It was in fact an indirect method of acculturing the scholastic medical model among those Muslim or Jewish practitioners who wished to open the circle of their medical practice wider to the Christian population. It is noteworthy that in the Kingdom of Valencia – whose Muslim population in many areas was not just the dominant, but also the only community – we have been able to find only four requests from Muslims for a medical licence in the whole of the fourteenth and fifteenth centuries (Hamet Hatequia in 1338, Maymó Abdochaxis in 1388, Cahat Azeit in 1434, and Abdalla Gasí in 1445).[45] Obviously, this number of licences bears no relation to the actual number of practitioners in the Muslim community. It is extremely difficult, of course, to know what kind of health care was available to the large numbers of Muslims in the Kingdom of Valencia, or who attended them; yet, in spite of a lack of documentation providing concrete details, everything seems to indicate that they were treated by healers from their own community who, with rare exceptions, did not practise among Christians or Jews. For instance, in the two hundred and fifty years between 1250 and 1500, we have not been able to trace a single document in which there appears a Muslim physician or surgeon contracted by a municipal council, either of a large or a small town, to exercise medicine or surgery among its inhabitants. Quite the opposite occurred in the case of Jewish physicians and surgeons, whose presence among the practitioners hired by Christian municipal councils was frequent. Muslim healers appear in Catalan or Valencian records only when a member of the Muslim community accepted the professional model of the Christian society and requested an examination; or, more often, when he was prosecuted for illegal medical practice. In these latter instances, our little data reveal in effect 'sub-profess-

[44] H.-P.-J. Renaud, 'Un chirurgien musulma du royaume de Grenade: Muhammad al-Safra', *Hesperis*, 20 (1935), 1–20; Arié, *L'Espagne musulmane*, p. 430; García-Ballester *Historia social de la medicina*, pp. 21–2.

[45] ACA, C., reg. 863, fol. 161r (Hamet Hatequia); Archive of the Kingdom of Valencia (ARV hereafter), Justicia Civil, 550, fols. 30r–31r (Maymó Abdochaxis); ARV, Real, 264, fol. 133 (Cahat Azeit), and ARV, Real, 51, fols. 111v–112 (Abdalla Gasi). On the first two, see L. García-Ballester, M. R. McVaugh, and A. Rubio-Vela, *Medical licensing and learning in fourteenth-century Valencia*, Transactions of the American Philosophical Society, 79, part 6, (Philadelphia, 1989), pp. 17, 25–6 and 98–101.

ionals' (quacks, both men and women), and show us how deeply medicine was affected by the broad cultural disintegration that afflicted the Valencian Muslims living under Christian rule.[46]

In connection with this last point, we should also mention the prestige that scholastic medicine, and its Christian professionals, acquired from the thirteenth century onwards among the members of the non-Christian religious groups. We have been able to demonstrate this point among the 'rationalist' minority of the Jewish community,[47] but, despite the scarcity of information, it is also known to have taken place among the scholarly members of the Muslim minority who, before they emigrated to Muslim-ruled areas, lived in lands conquered by the Christians. Such was the case of the above-mentioned surgeon Muhammad al-Safra. After his arrival in Fez (1344), he wrote his *K. al-Istiqsa wa al-ibram fi-cilay al-yiraha wa al-awram* (*On the treatment of wounds and tumours*), a surgical treatise in which he denounced the poor position of surgery among the Muslims, and emphasized his training in Valencia with the Christian surgeon 'magister Bernard'.[48] We can also confirm the view that Christian medicine was prestigious among the Muslims from evidence that has been gathered about the wish of the Muslim monarch of the Kingdom of Granada to be attended in his illness by Christian physicians (13 August 1378), in particular by the famous Majorcan surgeon, Pere ça Flor, surgeon to the King of the Crown of Aragon.[49] What can be confirmed in connection with the Muslim minority remaining in Christian areas is that during the period under consideration (the thirteenth to fifteenth centuries), there is no indication that any of its members wrote a medical work of any description.

The Jewish minority

Nothing seems to indicate, on the other hand, that the Jewish population followed the steps of the cultivated Muslim minority. On the contrary, some of them achieved a high level of penetration and influence even among the Christian ruling circles themselves.[50] Their medical practitioners (both physicians – *phisici* – and surgeons – *cirurgici*) can be traced in any Christian community during the fourteenth and fifteenth centuries, both in Castile and the Crown of Aragon. They were hired by the Christian municipal authorities for the medical attention of the community

[46] This is the hypothesis proposed by García-Ballester, McVaugh and Rubio-Vela, *Medical licensing and learning*, pp. 25–9.

[47] See García-Ballester, Ferre and Feliu, 'Jewish appreciation'.

[48] See note 44 above. I have not been able to identify this Christian master of surgeons.

[49] Archive of the Kingdom of Majorca (ARM hereafter), Gobernación, LR-30, fol. 187r, 19 July 1378. We give particular thanks to Manuel Becerra, who called our attention to this document.

[50] For a general view of the Jewish minority in medieval Spain, see Y. Baer, *A history of the Jews in Christian Spain*, 2 vols. (Philadelphia, 1978).

and shared this activity with Christian medical practitioners, in spite of ecclesiastical prohibitions to the contrary.[51]

Thus, Jewish physicians were held in high esteem by the members of Christian society. On the other hand, during the fourteenth century, part of the learned Jewish minorities was intellectually drawn towards Christian scholastic medicine. These physicians belonged to the so-called 'rationalists'. We may summarize intellectual activity in the heart of Jewish communities under three headings. Firstly, there were the rabbis, whose principal interests were oriented towards problems of the faith and Talmudic exegesis; secondly, the Cabalists, whose concern was with what we might call theosophic speculation; finally came the rationalists, who were interested in natural philosophy, and whose intellectual sphere was centred upon knowledge of nature.[52] The latter made the practice of their Jewish faith compatible with the rational study of nature (natural philosophy). Physicians who were members of this group made an effort not to reduce medicine to a mere application of remedies and routine practice but to make it an activity based on natural philosophy. As a result, this minority was also drawn by the intellectual attraction of natural philosophy and the medicine based on it, that is, of Latin scholasticism, which, from the late thirteenth century onwards, was able to offer practical and intellectually worthwhile responses to the specific medical problems (both of a theoretical and a practical nature) that contemporary Europe posed. For the first time there appeared in Europe new medical works in Latin, together with Latin translations (on natural philosophy and medicine) of classical writers (Aristotle, Galen), which were able to compete in quality with those works hitherto only available in Arabic. Jewish physicians belonging to rationalist groups tried to incorporate into their own culture, by means of translations into Hebrew, the new written intellectual product of the Latin medical scholasticism elaborated in the university circles of Montpellier throughout the fourteenth century. They considered it to be useful, both as a tool in medical practice and as an intellectual model to follow.[53]

As for the question that concerns us here – the survival of Arabic as a vehicle for scientific communication – it would seem that the behaviour of the Jewish minorities was not identical in Castile and in the Crown of Aragon. The Jewish communities of this second area (like those of Provence and other territories of the south of present-day France), or at least the rationalist minority, gradually forgot Arabic as the fourteenth century

51 L. García-Ballester and M. R. McVaugh are preparing a book on medicine and Jewish practitioners in the fourteenth-century Crown of Aragon.

52 Berman, 'Greek into Hebrew', pp. 289–90 and 293. On the division of Jewish medieval society into three rival social groups, see also the Hebrew grammar by Profiat Duran (Perpignan, 1340/5–1414), *Ma'ase Efod* (Vienna, 1865). We are grateful to Eduard Feliu (Barcelona) for this piece of information.

53 García-Ballester, Ferre and Feliu, 'Jewish appreciation'.

progressed, and as a result lost the ability to read medical manuscripts in Arabic, using instead Hebrew, Romance languages or Latin itself.[54]

In the case of Castile, the first clear evidence for the intellectual fascination that Latin scholastic natural philosophy exercised over the Jewish minority belongs to the last third of the fourteenth century.[55] This, however, did not mean that the Jewish minority abandoned contact with medical sources written in Arabic, and they continued to produce them in this language almost until their expulsion. We have proof of this in the Castilian communities of Toledo and Guadalajara. Even after their conversion to Christianity, some *conversos*, such as García de la Estrella b. Juan Gozalbez b. Gato (*fl.* 1420) of Toledo, continued to make use of Arabic to copy medical manuscripts written in that language.[56] This does not mean that they lived without any contact with the Christian medical works that were being produced. As we shall have occasion to see, there is evidence that in the early fourteenth century scholastic medical writings of the last third of the thirteenth century (in all probability Teodorico Borgognoni of Lucca's *Cirurgia*) were known to Castilian Jewish physicians, who argued about these works from a position of full intellectual equality.

The Jews were the only non-Christian socio-religious group in Castile that could count on a minority within their number who were interested in natural philosophy and in a form of medicine related to it, and who at the same time were actively practising medicine. This medical practice was not limited to members of their own communities, but also included the Christian population.[57] As will be seen below, their activity (as that of Christian practitioners) was basically itinerant, which provided them with detailed knowledge of Christian people and places. This knowledge was by no means irrelevant for their knowledge of medicine. In fact, as will also be seen at a later stage, some of them were able to integrate these new aspects derived from their itinerant practice of medicine into the doctrinal *corpus* of a demanding form of Galenism, written in Arabic, that was nourished by a wide range of medical sources by Greek and Arab authors.[58] Their interest in a medicine based on natural philosophy was rooted in their own

[54] Although they have not been conserved, it is known that medical manuscripts in Arabic circulated among the Jewish communities of Catalonia in the first decade of the fourteenth century: ibid.

[55] Steinschneider, *Die hebräischen Übersetzungen*, p. 210 (don Meir Alguadez ben Salomo, physician of Enrique III, King of Castile, 1390–1406).

[56] F. Guillén Robles, *Catálogo de los manuscritos árabes existentes en la Biblioteca Nacional de Madrid* (Madrid, 1889), no. 101–10, p. 248. See R. Kuhne, 'El Sirr Sina'at al-Tibb de Abu Bahr Muhammad b. Zakariyya' Al-Razi', *Al-Qantara*, 3 (1982), 347–414, at 352; P. Leon Tello, *Judíos de Toledo*, 2 vols. (Madrid, 1979), under Abengato.

[57] See note 51 above. Even the community of canons of Avila Cathedral (Castile) hired two Jewish physicians (R. Meyr and R. Yuçé Cohen), Spanish National Archive (AHN hereafter), Clero, lib. 816, fols. 37r, 50r, 167r, 179v and 218v (2 July 1460 to 19 February 1468); AHN, cod. 411–B, fols. 5v and 85v. I am grateful to Carlos Carrete (University of Salamanca) for these pieces of information.

[58] See the third part of this chapter.

intellectual rationalist tradition. In Castile, these rationalist Jewish physicians were able to preserve sufficient knowledge of the Arabic language to enable them not only to read these Arabic medical sources, but also to use Arabic as a means of written communication as late as the first third of the fourteenth century and even later. This demonstrates at least the following: in the first place that the circulation of medical manuscripts in Arabic was normal among members of Castilian Jewish communities; secondly, that there existed a public that was by no means indifferent to medical matters as part of natural learning; thirdly, that part of this public was made up by those who wished to learn the physician's craft and to take the first steps in medical learning; fourthly, that medical manuscripts were indeed copied and transmitted. We shall have occasion to see that some Castilian Jewish physicians, at least until the first half of the fourteenth century, maintained a degree of contact with medical science and did not limit themselves to being mere readers, copiers and/or transmitters of other authors' medical works: they also participated in the process of intellectual creation. We have direct evidence of this through a fascinating medical work written by a Jewish physician, probably of Toledo, in the first third of the fourteenth century.[59] However, as we shall have the opportunity to see, we can demonstrate the presence of medical manuscripts in Arabic at the heart of Castilian Jewish communities until the fifteenth century, almost until the same year as their expulsion from Spain (1492). Unfortunately we do not have evidence in the fourteenth-century Crown of Aragon of such medical intellectual creativity by a member of the Jewish community. This does not imply its total absence. We have evidence, for example, of the presence in the Jewish quarter of Xàtiva (Valencia) in 1347, prior to the Black Death, of either a school where medicine was taught, or a prestigious master in medical teaching.[60] Were any medical works produced by such masters? It remains unknown to us.

II

The socio-religious norms according to which the Jewish and Muslim minorities had to live in the later Middle Ages became increasingly strict in the course of the fifteenth century. One of the results of these conditions was the conversion of members of the Jewish and Muslim communities to Christianity, a process which did not at all aid the survival of manuscripts composed in Arabic. We should not forget that conversion to Christianity also meant encouraging a change in cultural model. As has already been noted, the Christians' cultural model was dominated by the Latin scholastic model. The same pressure from Latin culture (both direct and indirect) that

[59] See García-Ballester and Vázquez de Benito, 'Los médicos judíos castellanos del siglo XIV y el galenismo árabe'.

[60] I am very grateful to Michael McVaugh for this piece of information.

was felt by Christians of Arabic culture (*Mozarabs*) was also exerted on converts. Furthermore, Latin scholastic scientific and medical culture could rely on the strength of its own prestige. After the expulsion of the Jews and the conquest of the Kingdom of Granada (the last part of the Iberian peninsula with inhabitants of Arabic language and culture, who continued to live in their land after the conquest), both of which occurred in 1492, a political tendency to seek uniformity in language, religion and culture gained strength among Christian rulers. After the enforced conversions to Christianity of the early sixteenth century, the use of Arabic became identified with the old Muslim faith. The use of Arabic was soon to become an activity that might arouse political or religious suspicion. The Christian political and religious authorities, both within and outside the Inquisition, made the use of Arabic a political matter. The possession of texts in Arabic (let alone speaking it) became something rather suspicious and even dangerous.[61] These were all rather unfavourable circumstances for the conservation of manuscripts written in Arabic, even though they might contain medical and/or scientific material, both of which were subjects that Christian scholars and rulers were trying to preserve. In spite of all this, a considerable number of medical manuscripts in Arabic that were copied or circulated among these minorities of Christian Spain both in the Crown of Aragon and in Castile have been preserved, spread amongst various libraries. This must mean that many more have been lost, as has happened in the case of almost all those that are known for sure to have circulated in the Crown of Aragon until the first third, at least, of the fourteenth century.[62] Those that have been preserved allow us to analyse the phenomenon – unique in European Christian lands – of the actual use of medical manuscripts in Arabic in Christian areas by members of the three cultures then co-existing in Europe between the mid twelfth century and the last decade of the fifteenth century (see table on p. 372).

The medical manuscripts in Arabic that were copied or circulated in the kingdoms of the Iberian peninsula (Portugal has not been considered here) under Christian rule can be divided into three groups on the grounds of their origins:[63] (1) Those that were composed in the Muslim period and that survived after the Christian conquest. (2) Those that went from the Muslim areas of the peninsula (whether old or new copies) to the Christian

61 The Belgian humanist Nicolas Clénard found great difficulties in Seville (1539) in learning Arabic because Muslim people recently converted to Christianity refused to talk in Arabic in order not to show any signs of their old faith: see A. Roersch (ed.), *Correspondance de Nicolas Clénard*, 3 vols. (Brussels, 1940–1), vol. 1, pp. 151–2, nos. 34–49. For an analysis of the medical contents of this correspondence and its relationship with the role played by Arabic language for recovering Greek medical sources in the European Renaissance, see L. García-Ballester, 'The circulation and use of manuscripts in Arabic in sixteenth-century Spain', *Journal for the History of Arabic Science*, 3 (1979), 183–99.

62 See note 54 above.

63 Van Koningsveld, 'Andalusian-Arabic manuscripts from Christian Spain', pp. 1–2 of his typescript.

Places and years in which medical manuscripts in Arabic were written, corrected or used in medieval Spanish kingdoms. The figures indicate the number of medical works

	Twelfth century								Thirteenth century													Fourteenth century														Fifteenth century										
	13	18	26	45	64	65	82	90	13	26	27	29	30	32	37	48	65	66	80	94	96	23	33	41	44	46	56	61	75	76	79	85	87	88	89	13	24	25	28	32	66	80	83	94	undated	Total
Alcala																				1	1													2	1											5
Almeria				1																																										1
Barcelona					4																						1																			5
Cordoba																									1			4																		5
Granada		1											1			1																				1										4
Guadalajara																							1										1					1	3	1	1					8
Malaga																																			1											1
Murcia																			3																											3
Ocaña																																						1							1	2
Purchena														1	1																															2
Seville				1															1																								1			3
Toledo	1		1		1	1	1	1	1	2	2	1					1	1		2		3		1		1			4	1	12	1	1				3									43
Valencia																																										1				1
Zaragoza																																												2		2

Sources: Catalogues from the libraries of El Escorial, BN Madrid, BN Paris, and Princeton (Garret Collection).
The two MSS from Zaragoza (1494) have not survived. Indirect description by J. Ribera, 'La enseñanza entre los musulmanes españoles' (see note 34 above).

areas of the north. There even seems to have existed a real market of copyists in the Muslim south (Kingdom of Granada) that accepted orders from people living in Christian regions. All the orders that are known are from Jews living in thirteenth–fourteenth-century Castile, a group which played an important part in scientific communication between Muslim and Christian Spain. We have to remember for instance the travels to Granada of the Jewish physician Yusuf ibn Waqqar of Toledo (*fl.* 1312–40), and his friendship with Ibn al-Khatib (1313–75), a Muslim medical writer at the royal court of Granada.[64] (3) Those copied in Christian lands. These make up the largest group. As has already been mentioned, some were copied by Muslim scribes who were prisoners of war. The majority, however, were copied by Jewish scribes and physicians for their own personal use, and they remained in the hands of Jewish families for several generations between the twelfth and the fourteenth centuries (for example, the Banu Susan family, Toledo), or fourteenth–fifteenth centuries (the Banu Waqqar family, Guadalajara–Toledo). All except two of the surviving medical manuscripts belonged to members of Jewish communities. These circumstances led van Koningsveld to state that 'the Jews . . . [were] the main heirs of the specifically secular, purely scientifical elements of the Arabic civilization in medieval Christian Spain'.[65] However, we must not forget the survival of Arabic medical culture amongst the practitioners and the people of the numerous Muslim minority of Christian Spain.

If we arrange the surviving medical manuscripts chronologically (see table), it can be observed that they range from 1113 until 1494. With the exception of information from Valencia, Zaragoza and Ocaña (all of fifteenth-century date), the rest of the evidence is concentrated in towns with large Jewish communities. The most active centres were Toledo and Guadalajara (fourteenth and fifteenth centuries). Of particular significance was the Jewish community of Toledo, where a substantial number of medieval manuscripts in Arabic were composed, copied or transmitted. The fact that Toledo was the leading western centre for the translation of medical and scientific works from Arabic to Latin between 1150 and 1300 was, I believe, not unrelated to this state of affairs. Moreover, members of the Jewish community had a decisive role in this process.[66]

It can also be seen from the table that from the 1390s onwards there appears to be an interruption in the copyists' activity and, therefore, clearly

[64] See M. M. Antuña, 'Una versión árabe compendiada de la "Historia de España" de Alfonso el Sabio', *Al-Andalus*, I (1933), 105–54, at 116 (Arabic text) and 129 (Spanish translation), where the *A'mal al'a'lam* by Ibn al-Khatib is edited. On the Waqqar family, see *Encyclopaedia Judaica* (Jerusalem, 1972), vol. VIII (1205–7), and Steinschneider, *Die hebräischen Übersetzungen*, pp. 598–9, and 921–2; on Ibn al-Khatib, see *Encyclopédie de l'Islam* (Leiden and Paris, 1971), vol. III, pp. 859–60.

[65] Van Koningsveld, 'Andalusian-Arabic manuscripts from Christian Spain', p. 28 of his typescript.

[66] On this process see Jacquart and Micheau, *La médecine arabe*, pp. 131ff.

in the case of Toledo a slowing down in the rhythm of transmission and circulation of medical literature in Arabic. In the first half of the fifteenth century this was restricted to the activity of the Banu Waqqar family. In the last part of the century we have only the Valencia manuscript and information from Zaragoza, both cases involving Muslim communities. This situation must have been a consequence of the clear crisis of co-existence between the dominant Christian group and the other two minorities in the late fourteenth century; this crisis was expressed in social terms in many cities, both in the Crown of Aragon and Castile, by a series of pogroms, which were repeated in the fifteenth century and culminated in the expulsion of those members of the Jewish minority who did not convert to Christianity.[67] Another factor which must have been influential in the almost total cessation of the copyists' activity was the gradual loss of knowledge of Arabic on the part of Jewish rationalist physicians, and its replacement by Hebrew, Latin or a Romance language.[68] Both factors – one of a social nature (the crisis of co-existence), the other of intellectual scope (the gradual disappearance of Arabic from the intellectual horizon) – might well explain the void observable between the fourteenth and fifteenth centuries.

If, instead of arranging the surviving medical manuscripts on a chronological basis, their contents are analysed, we find that the Hippocratic corpus is represented, but only by the *Aphorisms* and books from the *Epidemics* and *On prognostics*; that is to say, it is represented by books that were eminently didactic and clinical in character. On the other hand, the available material includes the most interesting of Galen's extensive medical output, ranging from his treatises on anatomy and physiology (*De usu partium*, and *De facultatibus naturalibus*) to his semiological writings (*De symptomatum differentiis*, *De differentiis febrium*), writings on pathology (*De locis affectis*, *De crisibus*, *De diebus criticis*, *De differentiis morborum*), on therapeutics and dietetics (*De compositione medicamentorum*, *De alimentorum facultatibus*), and on hygiene (*De sanitate tuenda*). One of the manuscripts contains, grouped together, the collection of Galen's most important medical (pathological and clinical) works, which in Latin scholastic medicine was to be known by the title of *De morbo et accidenti*, and was to be the nucleus of the important commentaries on general pathology in the freshest and most attractive scholastic writing during the transition from the thirteenth to the fourteenth century, especially in Montpellier.[69] Another manuscript contains Dioscorides' *Materia medica*, the most important source of Galenic therapeutics. Together with this impressive sample from

[67] Baer, *History of the Jews in Christian Spain*.

[68] See García-Ballester, Ferre and Feliu, 'Jewish appreciation'.

[69] See Fernando Salmón, 'La couleur dans les théories visuelles des cercles médicaux universitaires à la fin du XIIIè siècle', Colloque 'Maladies, médecines et sociétés' (Paris, May 1990, in press).

the Galenic corpus, works of the great masters of Jewish and Arabic medicine were also in circulation; the writings of Rhazes, Avicenna, Haly Abbas, Avenzoar and Maimonides were copied frequently and assiduously. It is interesting to note that the text used most often was the *Continens* (*al-Hawi*) of Rhazes, followed by the *Canon* of Avicenna.[70] While the *Canon* was not well received in Al-Andalus,[71] it was however popular among the Jewish minorities living in Christian Castile at least from the beginning of the fourteenth century;[72] in the Latin West;[73] and among the Jewish minorities of Provence and Catalonia.[74] Many of these writings had not been translated from Arabic into Latin in late twelfth-century Toledo, and some of them, by both Greeks (Galen) and Arabs (Rhazes, Avenzoar), would not appear in Latin until the 1270s or 1280s, when they contributed in a decisive way to the renovation of scholastic medicine in European university circles.[75] The presence and circulation of these works among Jewish communities in thirteenth-, fourteenth- and fifteenth-century Castile tells us of the vitality of medical practice among this minority, whose knowledge of Arabic guaranteed them access to the most authentic sources of a form of medicine based on natural philosophy.

Another example of the intellectual vitality of these Jewish physicians was the way they put this medical literature to use. Although the amount of evidence available is very restricted, the contents themselves of some of the surviving manuscripts demonstrate that these works were used for the teaching of medicine, for the production of medical works of a systematic nature, and in order to provide an intellectual and doctrinal basis for medical practice, at least for the most learned physicians. In the following section, we shall analyse the only surviving work, which can serve to illustrate the last two points mentioned.

Some of the extant manuscripts do not reproduce a medical work by a classical author, but tend to be of the nature of medical *florilegia*. These were Arabic manuscripts copied at Toledo in 1379 and at Guadalajara in

[70] For a critical description of these manuscripts in van Koningsveld's papers on Andalusian-Arabic manuscripts, see note 2 above. For a detailed description of the contents of manuscripts, see H. Derenbourg, 'Notes critiques sur les manuscrits arabes de la Bibliothèque Nationale de Madrid', in *Homenaje a don Francisco Codera* (Zaragoza, 1904), pp. 571–618; H. Derenbourg and H.-P.-J. Renaud, *Les manuscrits arabes de l'Escurial*, vol. II, fasc. 2: 'Médecine et histoire naturelle' (Paris, 1941).

[71] R. Arnaldez and A. Z. Iskandar, 'Ibn Rushd (Averroes)', in *Dictionary of Scientific Biography* (*DSB* hereafter), ed. C. C. Gillispie (New York, 1981), vol. XII, pp. 7b–8. The popularity of the *Hawi* of Rhazes is testified to by the great number of manuscript copies transmitted and written by Castilian Jewish physicians: see Derenbourg and Renaud, *Les manuscripts arabes*, nos. 806–18, *passim*.

[72] See the third part of this chapter.

[73] Nancy Siraisi, *Avicenna in Renaissance Italy. The 'Canon' and medical teaching in Italian universities after 1500* (Princeton, NJ, 1987), pp. 43–76; Jacquart and Micheau, *La médecine arabe*, pp. 79–85 and 167ff.

[74] García-Ballester, Ferre and Feliu, 'Jewish appreciation'.

[75] García-Ballester, 'Arnau de Vilanova y la reforma de los estudios médicos', pp. 119–45; Jacquart and Micheau, *La médecine arabe*, p. 176.

1387 and 1425 using clinical and dietetic texts by Hippocrates, Galen, Paul Aegineta, Rhazes, Maimonides, Mesue, Avenzoar and others. Their educational nature is obvious since they adopt the question-and-answer format.[76] Another of the manuscripts copied in Guadalajara in 1432 by a member of the Banu Waqqar family for his son appears to have a similar educational purpose; it contains extracts from Avicenna's *Canon*.[77] As will be seen shortly, the one surviving work of a systematic nature, written in the first third of the fourteenth century and copied in 1376, was also composed with a clear didactic intention. Some fragments of the late manuscripts have an astrological character, such as tables to establish the astrological profile of a patient.[78]

In this context, it is interesting to remember what has been noted concerning the existence of regular medical teaching in the Islamic *Madrasa* of Zaragoza in the fifteenth century. We do not know whether it was being undertaken in previous centuries. Neither do we know anything after the year 1494. Teaching activity is likely to have given rise to some form of medical writing. But we do not have any evidence for this either. However, the only medical manuscript that has come down to us from the Muslim minority of Valencia, a medical poem by Averroes, copied in 1480, was for didactic purposes.[79]

III

As has already been pointed out, the Jewish physicians of Castile – probably those belonging to the rationalist group – did not limit themselves to reading and handing down classical works, however important these may have been, but were also involved in a second and parallel task, the creation of new medical works. Only one has been preserved: the *Kitab al-tibb al-qastali al-maluki* (*Book of regal Castilian medicine*).[80] Its author, whose name has not been preserved, was a Jew, as he himself informs us (fol. 21r). The work was probably written at some time in the first two decades of the fourteenth century and in any case before 1348, for there is no mention whatsoever of the plague of that year in the analysis that the author makes in his ninth chapter of the unusual illnesses that affected Castile in a particularly virulent fashion during the period of his medical practice. From the evidence of the author we know him to have been physician to

[76] Derenbourg and Renaud, *Les manuscrits arabes*, no. 873,8 (Toledo, 1379), no. 873,11 (Guadalajara, 1387), and no. 870,1 (Guadalajara, 1425), pp. 83–4.

[77] Ibid., no. 870,4, pp. 77–8.

[78] Ibid., no. 873,1, p. 81. The astrological fragments are being studied by Margarita Castells (University of Barcelona).

[79] *Manzuma fi'l-tibb*, with glosses in Latin and Spanish: see note 40 above.

[80] On the description of the two surviving manuscripts, see García-Ballester and Vázquez de Benito, 'Los médicos judíos castellanos del siglo XIV y el galenismo árabe'. Our references are to the oldest copy, Madrid, Biblioteca Nacional, Arabic MS, no. 601, fols. 1r–38v.

Ferdinand IV, King of Castile (1295–1312) (fol. 19v). The constant advice about how the physician should behave in the presence of members of the nobility and royalty, abundant throughout the work, together with the recommendations he makes concerning the *regimina sanitatis* dedicated to such persons, is indicative of how familiar this physician was with courtly circles in Castile. We also know by the author's own admission that he wrote this work when he had reached a considerable age. In fact, throughout the work there appear references to how beneficial 'experience' can be in medical practice, as well as other remarks to the effect that the arguments adduced were 'what has been obtained during my lengthy experience' (fol. 26r). From the manner in which he constantly alludes to Toledo, he must have retired to that city after having practised for the greater part of his life in the lands of Castile. The constant references to Burgos, and to specific patients in that city, also lead one to consider that he may have been a physician there under contract to the town council.[81] Also apparent from his work is the itinerant nature of his medical practice, a particular characteristic of these Jewish physicians, who were hired by Christian town councils for periods of rarely more than five years, or, alternatively, who used to follow the court, or who went to wherever the king or nobles called for their services. His professional activity enabled him to get to know an extensive part of the Kingdoms of Leon and Castile. To be more precise, the cities of Leon, Valencia de Don Juan, Toro, Valladolid, Burgos, Segovia, Arevalo, Avila and Medinaceli, as well as Toledo and Seville to the south, are mentioned in the work (see map).

A description of the contents and structure of the work is the best way to penetrate the intellectual background and purposes of the author. The work consists of two clearly differentiated parts. The first is an introduction of the natural philosophical foundations of medicine and the activity of the physician, all of which tends to justify the purpose and suitability of the work (fols. 1–7v). It is divided into five brief sections: in the first, the concept of illness is expounded and the task of the physician within society is justified, everything connected with health and illness being claimed as the latter's rightful field of activity. The second section presents the conceptual foundation of the work as a whole. It is none other than the Aristotelian scheme of the four causes (material, formal, final and efficient). The author adapted to this what was known in the Latin West by the name of *res naturales* and *res non-naturales* (the naturals and the non-naturals). He makes obvious use of medical sources other than Johannitius' *Isagoge*, the translation of which into Latin and the subsequent diffusion of which was,

[81] We know the name of at least one of these Jewish physicians contracted by the municipality of Burgos in 1388 and in 1411, 'don Salomon el Leví': see Municipal Archive of Burgos, Libros de Actas, 30 April 1388 and 6 April 1411. See J. A. Bonachia Hernando, *El concejo de Burgos en la Baja Edad Media, 1345–1426* (Valladolid, 1978), pp. 118 and 188. I am very grateful to Carlos Carrete for this piece of information.

as is well known, the starting point for the medieval scheme of Latin Galenism (together with the *res praeter naturam*) from the twelfth century onwards.[82] The work in question does not devote a specific section to the group of things against nature formed by illness, its causes and its manifestations or signs (*res praeter naturam*), although they are present in the book. On the basis of Avicenna's *Canon*, with slight modifications,[83] this Castilian Jew distributed what he called 'natural causes' in the following way: material causes (elements, humours, spirits and limbs or organs), formal causes (complexion, qualities and virtues, including the natural, the vital and the animal), final cause (essential operations) and efficient causes. The last, denominated 'natural causes of health and illness' by the author, were grouped in the following six sections, according to their order of importance: air, food and drink, evacuation and repletion, motion and rest, sleep and wakefulness, and accidents of the soul.[84] If the physician is to use procedures consonant with nature, his intervention in health and illness has to be carried out through these six 'efficient causes'. However, the physician's activity is not limited to them; he may intervene in the processes of illness and health by means of procedures that are not at all natural, such as 'medication and manual operation [surgery]' (fol. 2v). In the third section, the author explains the reasons for focusing his work on the 'six natural [efficient] causes', without nevertheless thereby renouncing the use of medicines. On the other hand, he rejects surgery. He takes special care to emphasize that his work aims to be 'useful' (*intafa'*); it is for this reason that he decides not to develop at length the components that make up the other three causes (elements, humours, spirits, etc.), all of which are subjects more appropriate in a work of natural philosophy. The author made a particular effort to stress the physician's capacity to manipulate these six components, both for the preservation of health (what in the Latin West was to be known by the name of *regimina sanitatis*), and for the cure of illness, by means of the therapeutic use of diet. This last point was something on which the author placed great importance, preferring this technique to treatment involving medicines, whether simple or compound; however, he did not renounce medicinal treatment out of hand. From this point onwards, the author repeatedly insists on the importance of the air. The complex Galenic concept of 'climate' was in effect to be one of the principal axes around which the whole work revolved; on this the author based the comparative analysis that he carried out throughout the work, distin-

82 D. Jacquart, 'A l'aube de la renaissance médicale des XIe–XIIe siècles: L'*Isagoge Johannitii* et son traducteur', *Bibliothèque de l'École des Chartes*, 144 (1986), 209–40.

83 The work I describe here is a very interesting testimony to the diffusion and popularity of Avicenna's *Canon* amongst learned Jewish physicians of this time.

84 We have to remember the importance given by Rhazes to these 'non natural things', following the path opened up by Hunain ibn Ishaq: see Rhazes' *Introduction to medicine*, edited with Arabic text and Spanish translation by C. Vázquez de Benito, *Libro de la introducción al arte de la medicina o 'Isagoge'* (Salamanca, 1979).

guishing between different cities and regions of Castile (Burgos, Leon, Valladolid, Toro, Segovia, Avila among others), on the one hand, and what he calls Al-Andalus centred upon Toledo, on the other. The fourth, very brief, section is devoted to pointing out the importance of the curative action of nature through the 'natural causes', without there being any need for action on the part of the physician. In the fifth and final part the greater or lesser significance of the 'six natural [efficient] causes' is considered once again, the 'necessity' that man has of each one of them in order to maintain life being used as a comparative factor. The result of these deliberations is a hierarchy of these six groups, at the top of which is situated the air, followed by food and drink. Both – but more especially the first one – acted as a support for the four remaining ones. The author does not hide his interest in writings on food, a subject constantly present throughout the work.[85]

The second part is the longer (fols. 7v–38v). It consists of ten chapters, of very variable length, preceded by a section in which the different chapters are listed and a brief summary of each of them is presented. The work concludes with an appendix containing a collection of prescriptions (*agrabadin*) with compound medicines suitable for the people of Castile. This appendix has been lost. The contents of the different chapters are as follows: in the first (fols. 7v–13v) 'the illnesses in which the patient should abstain from consuming any sort of meat, and also the circumstances in which [the physician] allows the patients of the region [Castile] to eat it' are mentioned (fol. 7v). The second (fols. 13v–17v) 'deals with the illnesses in which patients in this region should refrain from consuming wine, and in which they need not; and also the various classes of wine and their characteristics, according to the different places' (fol. 13v). All the third chapter (fols. 17v–23r) is dedicated to 'the rules which should be observed when blood-letting, the [appropriate] quantity of blood to extract, and a list of the illnesses of this region in which it can or cannot be undertaken' (fols. 17v). The fourth chapter (fols. 23r–24r) 'deals with the application of cupping-glasses, scarification and leeches in Castile' (fol. 23r), special attention being devoted to the technique of scarification as applied to children and adolescents. The fifth chapter (fols. 24r–27r) is totally devoted to 'the prescription of purgatives in this region [Castile]' (fol. 24r). Chapter six (fols. 27r–v) deals with 'the norms concerning vomiting (that the physician should observe) in this region' (fol. 27r). Chapter seven (fol. 27v–31r) deals with baths. After a reminder of Galen's bio-energetic scheme (the three digestions that take place in the human body), with the consequent

85 This kind of medical literature became highly prestigious among Jewish physicians according to manuscripts listing books of foodstuffs, which have been preserved in El Escorial's Library: see Derenbourg and Renaud, *Les manuscrits arabes*, nos. 833,4 (1265), 871,2 (1336) and 873,2 (n.d.), pp. 42, 79 and 81.

problem of the elimination of waste matter, the author makes a more detailed analysis of the problem of baths in Castile, showing his preference for the 'dry bath' (sauna), the technique of which is described in detail. According to the author, this type of bath – one not without risks – was frequently used in Castile, and Christian physicians also demonstrated their preference for it. The eighth chapter (fols. 31r–34r) is devoted to the use of cold water 'both in a state of health and in illness', bearing in mind the complexional characteristics of the people of Castile, the climate of the region and its particular illnesses. For obvious reasons, this chapter is closely related to the second one, the one that deals with wine. The ninth chapter (fols. 34r–38r) has two clearly differentiated parts: the first is devoted to the conceptual foundations of such terms as 'putrefaction' (*al-'afuna*), 'pestilential air' (*al-hawa al-wubai*), 'celestial causes' (*al-sabab samawi*) among others, as well as the suitable means of treatment for certain unusual illnesses of sudden widespread appearance, in particular 'smallpox' (*yudari*); the author was witness to one outbreak of an especially virulent nature – 'that not even old people of sixty knew' (fol. 35r) – during his career. The author insists that all these illnesses are produced by natural causes (*al-amr al-tabi'i*). The second part is dedicated to explaining the mechanism of production of 'the specific illnesses of this region', that is to say, what we might call the standard pathology of Castile during the author's lifetime (*c.* 1270–*c.* 1340). The most frequent illnesses were 'nasal and chest catarrhs, consumption, lung ulcers, those illnesses that affect the tendons [painful and particularly common owing to the cold climate of the region], back pains [kidney stones and colics located in the intestinal zone] and the illnesses proper to each season' (fol. 35r). He ends the chapter with a digression on the therapeutic use of cauterization, especially indicated in chronic illnesses that exhibit pain (pains in joints, gout, tendon conditions). A technique of cauterization not described by the most frequently used authors, nor employed in Al-Andalus, is detailed – 'in my opinion it is a treatment characteristic of this region [Castile]' (38r). It consisted of provoking a wound by means of cauterization in one of the lower limbs, between the knee and the heel, which takes in both sides of the leg where the veins run; to keep the wound purulent use was made of a shackle of the same size as the wound provided with a hole through which the 'superfluous humour accumulated at the point of the chronic illness' is eliminated (fol. 37v). The tenth chapter (38r–v), the last in the work, is very brief. In it the author endeavoured to answer the problem of what therapeutic and preventive attitude the physician should adopt when faced with people who were born in regions other than Castile, but who had gone to live there. The book finishes with the following epilogue:

> This is the end of our book. May God help us. Praise be to Him. Those who believe in Him will be saved. This book was finished in Toledo – may God protect it. Praise be – on the tenth day of February in the year 1414 of the Christian Era

[= A.D.1376], by the hand of Musa b. Sasun [*sic*]. May God protect him! (fol. 38v).[86]

As has already been stated, the manuscript does not preserve the appendix containing compound medicines. We do not know whether the author never managed to draw it up, or if the exemplar for the surviving copy did not include it, or whether the copyist had no interest in it.

This is a work written in Arabic as a response to the particular intellectual, clinical and therapeutic problems of his times. It demonstrates that at the time when it was composed (*c.* 1312–40) and copied (Toledo, 1376) there existed a certain level of debate concerning medical problems within the Jewish community of Toledo, to which the author probably belonged. According to the evidence of the author, the atmosphere of intellectual discussion on medical and natural questions had also spread to other cities, both to the north (e.g. Burgos) and to the south (Seville); indeed, he indulged in a polemic with a physician among his contemporaries from the latter city – the Jew Abu Harun b. al-Lawi (fols. 20v–21r). Furthermore, the fact that reference is frequently made to specific works by Galen, Rhazes, Isaac Israeli and Avicenna as a matter of course, together with the polemic which he sustained on certain of the doctrinal points of Avicenna, indicates a personal knowledge of all these works; in addition, it indicates that they were accessible and familiar to those of his kind for whom the author wrote. The process of creating a new medical work, with explicitly clinical and therapeutic purposes – and thus aimed at informing others of the author's own medical experience – clearly shows the existence of points of common understanding between the author and his audience. These intellectual points were in the form of easily accessible references, a shared technical vocabulary and scientific methodology, in addition to a whole complex, elaborate common intellectual background which allowed the author and his readers to communicate with each other in an intelligible fashion. We should not forget that in order to achieve a reasonable degree of understanding, a thorough appreciation of all the methodological, terminological and biological arsenal that made up the doctrinal *corpus* of medieval Arabic natural philosophy was required. The summary that we have provided of the *K. al-tibb al-qastali* demonstrates in sufficient detail that both the author and his public were familiar with this *corpus*.[87] Above

[86] Musa ibn Sasun (or Susan), probably a member of the Banu Susan, a family of physicians of Toledo to whom belong some of the medical manuscripts which have been preserved. The first of them was written in 1182 in Toledo. The last famous member of this family associated with medical manuscripts was Mayir b. Ishaq b. Susan, physician and financial adviser of Alfonso X, King of Castile (1252–84): see van Koningsveld, 'Andalusian-Arabic manuscripts in Christian Spain', Appendix, no. 72.

[87] A good summary of Arabic medicine and its relationship with the natural philosophy used by physicians is given in the long introduction written by M. W. Dols, *Medieval Islamic medicine. Ibn Ridwan's treatise 'On the prevention of bodily ills in Egypt'* (Berkeley, 1984), pp. 1–42.

all else, the work reveals the existence of an intellectual atmosphere in which medical problems were of interest and discussed, a process for which the Arabic language was used.

The work which is being described adopts as its starting point a clinical problem that was apparent to any medieval physician who approached his medical career with a minimum of rigorousness. What were the causes of the clinical peculiarities of the sick in the various parts of Castile, whose diseases were on occasions different from the descriptions to be found in classical medical works, and how could they be explained? What could be done when the intellectual tools which were available to the physician (i.e. the works of the great physicians) were of no use in finding effective advice that enabled him to solve the particular cases that occurred in his everyday medical practice? The author provides an answer by resorting to two tools: rational analysis by means of the intellectual resources that contemporary natural philosophy and Galenism made available to him, and personal clinical experience, extraordinarily rich in his own case. For all these reasons, the *K. al-tibb al-qastali* cannot be considered to have been an isolated phenomenon, a matter of chance. It is evident that its existence and contents place before our eyes a chink that enables us to peek into a medical intellectual world that has been lost. Our image of this world is strengthened if we bear in mind the eminently educational nature of the text:

> Many times, on reflecting upon the works that the great authors composed concerning medical science, I found that their approach was limited, especially as regards the particular aspects of medicine that are connected with the maintenance of health and the cure of diseases in specific regions never alluded to by them in their books of medicine (fol. 1r).

> All the medical treatises that circulate nowadays among us – both the most famous and the more ordinary – were composed in regions and countries with very different customs to those of this region of Castile. Thus none of the peculiarities described in them can be applied in Castile. For this reason I have seen fit to draw up this work, which deals with the practical norms to take into account in the treatment of the diseases of this region. These norms differ from those listed in the treatises, especially with regard to the two kingdoms [he is referring to Leon and Castile] of this region (fols. 7r–v).

The author took great care to indicate directly or indirectly (through the references he used) which were the authors and works that normally circulated among the Jews of Castile. The most frequently cited author, both as regards the number of references and the number of works, is Galen. The following works are directly referred to: *De methodo medendi*, *Quod animi mores corporis temperamenta sequantur*, *De flebotomia*, *De compositione medicamentorum secundum locos*, *De sanitate tuenda*. The Galenic commentary to the Hippocratic treatise *Airs, waters, places*, which was translated from the Arabic into the Hebrew in the year 1299 by Solomon ha-Me'ati, is not explicitly quoted.[88] The texts of Hippocrates cited are the *Aphorismi* and *Epidemiarum libri*. As for Arabic authors, at the end of the first introductory part, the author says:

The most famous treatises of medicine existing today and known unto us [the Jews] are: the *Kitab al-Hawi fi-l-tibb* [*Continens*] of al-Razi, the *Kitab al-Qanun fi-l-tibb* [*Canon*] by ibn Sina, which follows in its particularities [the clinical part] the instructions of *al-Hawi*, the book of al-Mayusi [*Pantegni*] and that of Julaf al-Zahrawi [*Kitab al-Tasrif*], in addition to other habitual treatises (fol. 7r).[89]

Among these are mentioned *On the pains of the joints* and *On blood-letting* by Rhazes and the *Book of Foodstuffs* by Isaac Israeli.[90] He also includes works of natural philosophy, such as *al-Tahafut* (*The refutation*) by Abu Hamid al-Gazzali, and he summarizes the cosmological opinions of Al-Zarqali (Azarquiel), whom he describes as 'modern' (fol. 21v).[91] He also seems to make allusion to Ibn al-Kammad (fol. 21v).[92] He has a wide knowledge of Galen's works, which is especially evident when he demonstrates the authenticity of the Galenic text *De flebotomia* – probably based on the authority of Rhazes – the authorship of which had been placed in doubt by Abu Harun b. al-Lawi, the Jewish physician of Seville with whom he maintained a dispute (fols. 20v–21r).[93] Galen was for him the unquestionable medical authority. It is his work which is always chosen to settle conflicting views. This Jewish physician held the following opinion of him:

Galen displaced all other physicians both of Antiquity and those of modern times, like Asclepiades, Thessalus and others, in such a way that his teachings have remained beyond any doubt down to our days (fol. 15r).

Of Avicenna he states that:

It is he who consolidates the art of medicine with the book *al-Qanun*, something which no other author has managed to achieve until now ... His Agrabadin [*Antidotarium*, Book v of the *Canon*] contains marvellous texts which are the fruit of his experience (fol. 20v).

88 A. Wasserstein (ed.), *Galen's Commentary on the Hippocratic treatise* Airs, waters, places, *in the Hebrew translation of Solomon ha-Me'ati* (Jerusalem, 1982).

89 The *Kitab al-Tasrif*, as is known, consists of thirty books; only four were translated into Latin, and have the following names: *Liber theoricae necnon practicae* (Books 1 and 2: generalities and description of diseases *a capite ad calcem*), *Liber servitoris* (Book 28: in fact a treatise on pharmacy), and *Chirurgia* (Book 30: the most famous and influential Arabic treatise on surgery).

90 F. Sezgin, *Geschichte des arabischen Schrifttums*, vol. III (Leiden, 1970), pp. 287–8 (al-Razi), and p. 296 (Ishaq al-Isra'ili).

91 *DSB*, vol. XIV, pp. 592–5.

92 On Ibn al-Kammad (d. 1195), an astronomer who lived in Al-Andalus, see J. Vernet, 'Un tractat d'obstetricia astrològica', in *Estudios sobre historia de la ciencia medieval* (Barcelona and Bellaterra, 1979), pp. 273–300. I am grateful to Julio Samsó (University of Barcelona) for his help in acquiring this information.

93 The authorship of this work has been questioned by scholars of medieval Arabic writings: see Sezgin, *Geschichte*, pp. 115–16. On al-Razzi's references, see ibid.

This did not prevent him from disagreeing with him on those points that he considered to be unsuitable for application to patients in Castile, and even on matters of natural philosophy, as in the case of his disagreement about the components of the 'efficient natural causes' cited by Avicenna.

It is worth considering briefly the attitude that this Jewish physician adopted towards the Christian physicians that he had contact with during his medical career, and to whom he makes allusion on several occasions. Throughout the work, it is possible to detect a climate of constant critical contrast with what his Christian colleagues did and wrote. On one occasion, he explicitly refers to a Christian surgical treatise with the title in Arabic of *Balagtu-hu al-yabr al-yadid* (*On the new art of surgery*). He does so in connection with a debate on the therapeutic use of wine in the case of patients with wounds, 'according to the nature of each injured individual and the part of the body where the wound is to be found' (fol. 15r). In opposition to the attitude of those who took into account both sets of circumstances (which is the position defended by the author), there existed that of

> [some] Christian surgeons in favour of giving wine instead of water to those who are injured whether by blows or by wounds. They base their argument on what was written by a great Christian friar, who composed a book on the subject some sixty years ago, to which he gave the title *On the new art of surgery*. He believed that he had invented something new and different from what Galen had already put forward on this art of surgery. As a consequence of this book, two groups were formed among Christians surgeons: the ones who professed the new surgery; and those others who supported the ancient view, which is none other than Galen's medicine (fol. 15r).

He appears to be referring to the *Cyrurgia* of Teodorico Borgognoni, who was a Dominican friar (*c.* 1205–98).[94] From the evidence of Henri de Mondeville (1316), a disciple and fervent supporter of the new surgery, we know that the therapeutic procedures explained by this Dominican caused great debate among the Christian surgeons of Italy, Montpellier and Paris, and his supporters were described as 'modern'.[95]

Putting aside the dispute, and the version of it that is provided by this Castilian Jew, what is important to point out at this stage is his opinion of

[94] The date ('sixty years ago'), the debate (the giving of wine 'to those who are injured whether by blows or by wounds'), the social condition of the Christian author ('a great friar'), and the controversies following the spreading of the work are coincident with the circumstances surrounding Teodorico Borgognoni and his treatise on surgery. This treatise was translated twice into Catalan in the first decade of the fourteenth century, and it was very well known both by Jewish and Christian Catalonian physicians and surgeons of the time. I suspect that the treatise was also translated into Spanish at the end of the thirteenth or beginning of the fourteenth century. On Teodorico's opinion on the use of wine, see his *Chirurgia* (Venice, 1499), vol. I, p. 25. He based his therapy on the authority both of his teacher Ugo da Lucca and Galen himself (*De methodo medendi*, 8,3).

[95] Henri de Mondeville agreed with Teodorico. See E. Nicaise (ed. and trans.), *Chirurgie de maître Henri de Mondeville ... composée de 1306 à 1320* (Paris, 1893), pp. 187–8 and 284.

the new Christian medical literature. He was not full of admiration for the writings of the medical scholasticism of Montpellier, unlike his brothers in religion who were physicians in Provence or Catalonia in the second half of the fourteenth century.[96] On the contrary, the Jewish physician of Toledo, living in the last third of the thirteenth and first decades of the fourteenth centuries, disputed, on an equal footing, certain specific opinions sustained by Christian physicians, calling upon his training in natural philosophy and his knowledge of the Galenic *corpus* to which he had access in Arabic, something which his brothers in religion in Provence and Catalonia were unable to do as they had forgotten this language and because manuscripts in Arabic were scarce amongst them. On the other hand, neither is there any feeling of respect in the passages in which the author of the *K. al-tibb al-qastali* mentions his relationship with Christian colleagues in the case of specific patients. It was a relationship of professional equality, and even endowed with a certain superiority on his part. Expressions such as 'his opinion is erroneous' (fol. 32r), 'it is easy to refute them' (fol. 31v), 'do not pay attention to what is mentioned by non-Arabic-speaking practitioners' (fol. 31r) are not unusual when he mentions Christian physicians. He clashed with them, not only on clinical matters (differences of opinion in the case of a course of treatment, as in the above-mentioned situation), but also on others of a theoretical character, in which both parties put forward 'logical arguments taken from natural philosophy' (fol. 31r) to settle the questions raised (all of clinical origin), as, for instance, the suitability or unsuitability of using cold water on patients suffering from certain fevers.

The author was aware of the differences and even contradictions existing between the various authors mentioned (both ancient and modern) when it came to deciding upon a form of treatment. In a way similar to what happened in the already sophisticated Galenism of Latin scholasticism, he made an effort to find arguments that harmonized the conflicting opinions and endeavoured to explain the differences rationally. As regards the question of the amount of blood that should be let on each occasion, a subject that was widely debated in Jewish medical circles in Toledo, as we know from this work, the author was faced with serious differences between what was stated to be usual by Galen (six pounds!), what was practised by Rhazes (three pounds), and what his own common sense imposed on his practice of medicine (not more than a pound and a half). The reasoning used by this author allows us, to a certain extent, to come close to the type of arguments put forward in these discussions among Jewish rationalist physicians, about which we otherwise know hardly anything. It was in these discussions that the greater or lesser degree of training in natural philosophy of the participants was made evident. At the core of the argument was the cosmological question of whether the created

[96] See García-Ballester, Ferre and Feliu, 'Jewish appreciation'.

world was or was not variable. The author himself states: 'on reflecting upon this problem, I saw that it had to be considered in the context of natural philosophy [*'ilm al-falsafa*]' (fol. 21r). He adduces arguments from al-Gazzali, Ptolemy and Al-Zarqali (Azarquiel), among others, against 'those who maintain the theory that both the world and all that there is in it have suffered no changes from their original state' (fol. 21v). When he discovered that the above-mentioned quantities of blood were in the proportion of 1:2, he concluded as follows:

If we accept our arguments as valid, the question for which we could not find an answer is resolved. I refer to the quantity of blood to extract indicated by Galen and by al-Razi. According to our suppositions, in the time of Galen – let us remember that more than one thousand two hundred years have elapsed until the present time – people used to bleed the quantity of six pounds, in view of the size of their bodies and the vigorousness of their faculties or virtues. In contrast in the time of al-Razi – let us not forget that more than six hundred years have passed down to our days – the quantity of three pounds was bled. That is to say, half the amount that was let in Galen's time. However, since the time of al-Razi to our days exactly half the length of time from the period of Galen to that of al-Razi has gone by. For this reason, at present, the maximum quantity of blood that is let is exactly half that extracted in the time of al-Razi, approximately a pound and a half, a quantity similar to that which I have just mentioned that I let from a heavily built woman [22 ounces] (fol. 22r).

This reasoning indicates a certain concern for quantifying biological processes, but unfortunately, the author does not offer us any more data to enable us to develop such conjectures any further. The work is planned in a context of a debate – if I might say so – of a very academic nature, the structural framework for which makes use of the scheme of the 'six natural efficient causes' mentioned earlier, together with the elements that make up the other three causes (material, formal and final), all in an intimate functional relationship. These are of course the same as the scheme of the *res naturales, non naturales* and *praeter naturam*, so familiar to Latin medieval Galenism. The *K. al-tibb al-qastali* is in no way a rough, direct, word-by-word commentary on a text of a medical authority. It is an authentic systematic medical treatise which integrates the reality of the author's own clinical experience with this Aristotelian-Galenic scheme. The author introduces his clinical experience as a problematic factor – the different forms of behaviour of the sick and the healthy according to whether they live in the high, cold lands of Leon and Castile (Burgos, Avila, Segovia) or in the warmer, lower areas of Toledo and Seville. Together with this factor, the author puts forward the Galenic doctrine of the relative nature of the individual and climatic constitution as the key to the intellectual problem of the divergence between experiential knowledge and what is stated by medical authorities, who not only lived in other climates, but also – like Galen, Rhazes or Avicenna – several hundred years beforehand.

For example, the inhabitants of the region of Toledo forbid youths to drink wine until they reach the age of twenty; and neither do those with fever consume wine for several days. This is due to the fact that the air of the region of Toledo is very warm in comparison with that of the area of Burgos, apart from the fact that its wines are thicker and warmer than those of Burgos. In contrast, the inhabitants of Burgos agree with their children drinking wine, and some even give it to those who are suffering from fevers – provided they are not continuous or burning fevers. And this is because the air of Burgos is softer in comparison with that of Toledo, and as a result the wine is also thin and acid-tasting, so much so that it may be compared with the juice of the bitter pomegranate, as is easy to prove. If this is the difference existing in medical treatment caused by the different air of the two cities mentioned, between which there is only a difference in latitude of two degrees, how much greater will be the variation in treatment [between cities] whose difference in latitude is of five or ten degrees (fol. 7r).

The author of the *K. al-tibb al-qastali* did not aim to write an abstract treatise, but a work addressed to the practising physician – a 'useful' work – but without renouncing the intellectual equipment without which medicine is reduced to a simple handbook of prescriptions or to a catalogue of clinical casuistry. He placed great emphasis on this last point. All the steps that he mentions directed towards the maintenance of health or towards explaining the application of specific treatments are preceded by a brief physiological summary which gives a natural basis for the particular medical approach that he is considering. Recommendations like the following, with a touch of medical ethics, are not unusual:

The practising physician will apply this treatment [one associated with wine in the case of special patients] only after having acquired solid knowledge and when able to diagnose the disease well. He should not use it to challenge the merits of other physicians, and for this reason neither will he pretend to establish a precise diagnosis to gain fame (fol. 14r).

We have already mentioned the complex doctrinal background that the author presupposes in his potential readers, and the authors and medical works recommended. We are now going to turn to a discipline that has not yet been mentioned, but is present in the medical activity of this author: astrology. We have already alluded to the knowledge that he demonstrates of the works of Ptolemy and Al-Zarqali (Algazel). He also seems to have known the astrological work of Ibn al-Kammad. The clearest allusion to astrology appears in a digression in which he considers one of the questions that most concerned Castilian Jewish physicians: the amount of medicine necessary to achieve a certain measurable effect. This is closely connected with the concern for measuring biological phenomena mentioned before. The author resorts to a minor therapeutic experiment for this purpose. His account helps us to recognize the central role that astrology played in the practical medicine of his time.

As for the relation existing between the amount of medicine needed in this region [Castile] and what has to be given in warm regions, I can explain what I obtained in the course of my lengthy experience. I have frequently seen that the quantity of medicine required to evacuate any quantity of humour in this region has to be double what needs to be taken in Al-Andalus [Toledo] in order to evacuate the same amount of humour. In fact, a single drachm of finely powdered agaric evacuates five depositions of humour from any body in Toledo. The same quantity in Burgos does not produce this effect in a body of similar nature and build ... What I have just said does not rule out any individual from Burgos responding favourably, and the person from Toledo unfavourably. This is due to the fact that the natural disposition and complexion of people differ considerably and that is decisive. This is the norm in this matter. For this reason I pointed out that the following requirements should be met to check the strength of one or two grains of agaric: that the two individuals who are the object of study in both these regions should be similar in nature, complexion and in the abundance of humours. However, if we wish to be more demanding in this matter, we also have to make the position of the moon at the moment when the purgative is consumed a condition in order to be able to compare both individuals in the two regions. This is a natural circumstance that may or may not facilitate the action of the medicine. In effect, if, at the moment when the laxative is taken by the man in Toledo, looking towards the planets the moon is to be found in the astrological houses of earth and fire – in other words with all the circumstances required to diminish the strength of the medicine – its efficacy will be reduced. The humours even though they naturally tend towards it, will not respond to evacuation easily. In contrast, we will assist the response of the humours – even though the humours are not disposed [towards evacuation] – if the man from Burgos should consume the purgative when the moon is in a watery sign of the zodiac, other than Cancer, and with aspects towards Venus or Mercury, and both are also placed in the same sign of the zodiac (fol. 26r–v).

The *K. al-tibb al-qastali* had a clear didactic intention. The work is aimed at a hypothetical pupil to whom instructions and recommendations are given. As a result it provides us with the means to reconstruct the most personal parts of the system of medical instruction practised within Jewish quarters, the general lines of which are already known. We refer to what has been called the 'open' model, in contrast to the closed institutional model practised by the Christian university institutions, to which the Jews were forbidden access. According to the open model, he who possessed medical learning transmitted it or imparted it, following his own personal criteria and without being protected by any institution. Teaching activity in the open system reflected the master's interests and abilities rather than the university system.[97] This is apparent in the case of this author, who made an effort to place the pupil who was to practise in the lands of Castile face to face with continual practical examples and specific situations. As we have already seen, the work is not just a set of specific cases hurriedly put

[97] Ibid.

together, but is endowed with a logical structure and a certain standard of abstraction. This latter aspect was to enable the author to pass on his personal experience in a more efficient manner since it was set within the framework of the underlying doctrinal Galenism of his medical practice. He endeavoured to focus the pupil's attention, using the starting point of a specific problem which is likely to arise when the student comes to practise medicine. On other occasions, the pupil's attention is attracted by discussion of questions that were the subject of debate among the practitioners of his time. In this case, the teacher immediately follows with examples from his own experience. He then moves towards an ever-increasing level of abstraction. For example, when dealing with the therapeutic use of cold water with patients suffering from fever in Castile, once he has encouraged the pupil to consult Galen's works on the matter, he explains the seven conditions necessary to establish the individual treatment (this was the abstract level):

> First, that the humour causing the fever should not be either phlegm nor black bile. If it were yellow bile, this would have to be subtle and mature. Secondly, that the functions of the stomach should not be weakened nor should they be cold; this last circumstance rarely comes to pass in this region [i.e. Castile]. Thirdly, that the liver should perform its functions perfectly and should not be cold, which also rarely happens in this region since the internal organs of the inhabitants are usually found to be, in the majority of cases, healthy and they are warm, as we have already explained. Fourthly, that there should exist no inflammation nor pain in any intestine, nor subtle yellow bile, something that has to be taken into account in this land. Fifthly, that the patient should possess plenty of innate warmth and blood. Among the inhabitants of this region, those who belong to the nobility and royalty usually fulfil this condition, as we have already explained in the first chapter of this book. Sixthly, notice whether the feverish patient, when in a state of good health, was or was not in the habit of drinking cold water; this point may affect the consumption of cold water in this region. Seventhly, that the person affected by fever should not be an extremely thin person. When you know that these conditions are fulfilled, or are dominant, in the person suffering from fever, then you may let him drink cold water (fols. 31r–v and 32r).

After a series of theoretical considerations, he goes on to explain an individual case history (the case of an old man of seventy who was suffering from fever and severe back pains); the aim of this was to capture the attention of the pupil and lead him towards the specific field of medical practice: 'I mention this example so that you take it into account during treatment, and so that you know the norms of medicine as regards the consumption of cold water during sickness' (fol. 32v).

One aspect of the medical practice of the author of the *K. al-tibb al-qastali* that has been mentioned and which we should not omit is his relationship with noble and royal circles. The biological justification for the 'different' character of the physiology of those belonging to such high ranks was the basis on which rested the whole literary genre of what Christian physicians called *regimina sanitatis*. This genre reached its peak in such circles in the early fourteenth century. By means of these texts, physicians aspired to order the whole life of the addressee, both when he enjoyed good health and when he was sick, thereby hoping to convert medicine into a way of life for the individual in question.[98] These biological characteristics came into existence at the very moment of conception and were hereditary – hence the individual way in which patients had to be treated both in health and in sickness. They could only be detected by a physician, and they differentiated those who belonged by birth to the rank of the nobility from those who did not. The latter all shared a common nature. Thus, their treatment or the norms for preserving their health did not require the same degree of individual attention as demanded by the nobility and the royal family. These arguments, from the point of view of bio-medicine, stressed the social differences of Christian feudal society, which was served by the Jewish author of the work being described. These social characteristics were clearly reflected in the medical treatment provided (fols. 10r–11r). Such arguments were also developed by his Christian contemporary, the royal physician and surgeon Henri de Mondeville, when he describes the social and bio-medical elements that the practitioner has to bear in mind when starting to establish a relationship with his patient.[99]

CONCLUSIONS

Medieval medical Galenism found in the Arabic language an adequate and rigorous vehicle of scientific communication, which survived in south Europe during the late medieval centuries and the Renaissance; people trained in this language could have access to medical texts of scientific and practical value. Between the twelfth and the fifteenth centuries Arabic medical manuscripts circulated in the Christian Kingdoms of Castile and the Crown of Aragon. Although the majority have been lost, nevertheless a total of eighty-one medical works by Greek and Arabic authors, written in Arabic, that circulated in this period and in these regions, are available for study today, surviving in various repositories. The users were members of the three religious communities that co-existed in the Christian kingdoms of the Iberian peninsula during these centuries – Christians, Muslims and Jews. Within the Christian group we have to distinguish between those of Arabic culture (*Mozarabs*) and those of Latin culture. The former would appear to have ceased to make use of Arabic in the early thirteenth century,

[98] L. García-Ballester, 'Changes in the *regimina sanitatis*: the role of the Jewish practitioners', in S. Campbell (ed.), *Health, disease and healing in medieval culture* (Toronto, 1992).

[99] The biological and social characteristics on which medieval physicians, both Jews or Christians, grounded their socially differentiated treatment were systematized and described by Henri de Mondeville in the long introduction to the second book of his treatise on surgery: see Nicaise's edition of the *Chirurgie*, pp. 121–81.

whereas the latter continued to demonstrate interest in medical writings in Arabic down to the transition from the thirteenth to the fourteenth centuries. There is direct evidence that this is actually what happened in the Crown of Aragon and in Murcia. Interest in the employment of Arabic on the part of Latin Christians can again be detected at very localized centres in Valencia in the second half of the fifteenth century.

The only geographical areas where intellectual medical activity on the part of members of the Muslim minority requiring the use of Arabic medical manuscripts can be identified were in the south of Valencia (Crevillente) and Murcia (late thirteenth to early fourteenth centuries), together with Aragon and Valencia once again (last third of the fifteenth century). The evidence is scanty and that from the fifteenth century is particularly difficult to interpret. It is of interest to note that the latter information is derived from Muslim sources, which would appear to indicate that the culture of the Muslim communities was not as poorly integrated as might be suggested by the use of Christian documentary sources alone.

As far as the Jewish minority is concerned, both their own and Christian sources are unanimous in confirming the intense activity of Jewish practitioners – both in Castile and in the Crown of Aragon – which also involved the treatment of members of the Christian community. There is no available information as regards them practising their profession among the Muslim minority. Diachronic analysis of the surviving medical manuscripts in Arabic, as well as the study of the medical sources mentioned in the only surviving fourteenth-century medical work, written in Arabic by a Castilian Jewish physician (probably from Toledo) – the *K. al-tibb al-qastali al-maluki* (*c.* 1312) – demonstrate that the level of medical culture of certain Castilian Jewish rationalist physicians in the first third of the fourteenth century was equal to that of their contemporary Christian colleagues in universities. This learning was nourished by the *corpus* of Galen's medical works, by certain works of Hippocrates, and by the medical writings of Arabic and Jewish authors, written in Arabic. Works of natural philosophy of Aristotelian inspiration and of astrology are to be added to these. All this circulated among the Jewish communities of Castile during the whole period under study here, although the pace of movement declined substantially in the late fourteenth century. The survival of Arabic among the minority of Jewish medical scholars seems to have acted as a limiting factor for their level of scientific knowledge and their intellectual independence as regards Latin scholastic science and medicine.

Internal analysis of *K. al-tibb al-qastali* allows us to draw further conclusions. This work illustrates the author's concern for the application of doctrinal considerations to particular problems and, on urgent occasions, to everyday medical practice. Throughout the work, the author presents himself as a physician who practised for the greater part of his life in the area of Castile now known as the autonomous region of Castile-Leon (see map). There is a predominance of clinical problems and others concerning the maintenance of health of the highest ranking members of society (the nobility and royalty), circles which were well known to the author. He took particular care to emphasize prudence in the application of remedies (e.g. blood-letting) and also to point out the need to study the clients belonging to such ranks of society individually.

Although the author made use of surgery, and had no reservations about employing medicines, of both simple and compound nature, the text reveals that he is also convinced of the benefits that the physician's use of the natural agents that regulate the functions of the body, ranging from the air to the movements of the soul, can have for the client – whether he be sick or healthy. He considered that the physician's study of these external agents (among which astrological factors are also included) should be accompanied by knowledge of the individual 'complexion' of each patient. Thus the physician must be in possession of detailed knowledge of both the region in which he works and of the natural resources of the region. The patient is not an abstract entity disconnected from his environment, but a part of a microcosm incorporating a complex series of natural factors (the word 'natural' should be emphasized) that must be familiar to the physician for him to evaluate them correctly. The diagnosis-prognosis will effectively consist of this. The physician's actions – both in order to maintain health, and also to recover it if lost – will make sense only after this process of evaluation; this process tries to integrate the microcosm–macrocosm relationship at an individual level, by resorting to astrological techniques. This relationship is a consistent factor in the work under study and makes up the core of the natural factors mentioned above.

The author does not reject the study of the great treatises, nor the constant consultation of medical authorities. Three stand out among these: in the first place, Galen, to whose writings he resorted in order to settle conflicting points in medical disputes, whether of a practical or a theoretical nature; in the second place, Rhazes' *Hawi*; in the third place, Avicenna's *Canon*. The intellectual leadership of the last author was for him indisputable, in spite of minor points of disagreement. Avicenna thus appears as the most suitable and lucid interpreter of the Galenic *corpus*. Concerning this point, we can point to the earlier and more direct evidence for Avicenna's prestige among the rationalist Jewish physicians of Castile (first third of the fourteenth century). The version of the *Canon* that was used among the Jewish physicians of Catalonia by the 1350s was in Hebrew.[100] However, the author did not tire of repeating that his work was addressed to the practising physician, and he insisted that the practising doctor had to be mindful of the peculiarities of what might be called the 'regional path-

[100] ACA, C., reg. 686, fol. 69r–v, 2 December 1355; reproduced by Rubio y Lluch, *Documents*, vol. II, p. 111, no. 117.

ology', in other words, the set of illnesses dominant in a given region, shaped by physical and psychical factors and in which astral factors were also significant.

The author strongly criticizes the lack of similar works which take as their starting point the clinical problems particular to any geographical area. In this respect, there is constant veiled criticism of the abuse of speculative medicine which relegates the specific patient to the background. The author clearly prefers medicine to be a practical activity based on biological knowledge given by a living Galenism. The physician should have a wide range in his practice; a range which is directly proportional to his knowledge and his clinical experience. The knowledge is acquired through study and reading – in this respect there are constant allusions to consulting and studying medical works and authors. The clinical experience is a matter of time, but it may also be transmitted – and thus learnt – by means of writings. Knowing how to communicate one's own clinical experience through the written word is considered to be the greatest expression of the physician's maturity. This communication should adopt a direct and specific style. Arnau de Vilanova – a Latin contemporary of this author – exemplified this by his aphoristic writing.[101] In this way it was intended to make the conceptual and intellectual complexities achieved by Galenism in the early fourteenth century, in the Latin as well as the Arabic and Jewish worlds, accessible to the practising physician.

The Jewish author of the *K. al-tibb al-qastali* therefore adopted a direct style. His text lacks conceptual solemnity, even though all the sophisticated conceptual complexity of early fourteenth-century developed Galenism underlies it. The Galenism is not presented as a uniform and immutable doctrinal block, but offers different options for interpretation, both at a doctrinal level and in the application of particular forms of treatment. In this work there is not the slightest trace of elements alien to Galenic rationalism. We believe it to be a good example of the Galenism practised by the Jewish rationalist minority in Castile.

The text exhibits a form of Galenism resulting from total intellectual tools and resources of its own, totally separate from the intellectual resources and doctrinal means that were being produced in the nearby world of Latin medical scholasticism in Montpellier or Italy. The author exhibits evidence of knowing some of the intellectual products of this Latin scholasticism, although he does not appear to have been aware (or at least he does not show it) of the intellectual products of the most recent medical scholasticism of these medical centres; neither does he show any interest in the scholastic technique of reasoning, nor in the background (the liberal arts) required by Latin university medicine, which converted medicine into a *scientia* with consequent practical repercussions. The sources of

[101] *Repetitio Arnaldi de Villanova s. canonem 'Vita brevis'*, ed. by M. R. McVaugh in AVOMO (Barcelona, in progress).

information were the same as those that the most demanding Christian university physician of the first third of the fourteenth century had access to, with the additional advantage of access to them directly through Arabic. During this period Jewish rationalists do not yet seem to be very attracted by Latin scholastic medicine, although this was to happen to Jewish rationalist physicians at the end of the fourteenth century in western Mediterranean countries.

The information that we possess on the state of the intellectual atmosphere of the Muslim and Jewish minorities in Castile at the turn of the thirteenth and fourteenth centuries indicates that only those scholars who were members of the Jewish minority used the Arabic medical sources in existence in Castile. These manuscripts circulated in Castile with sufficient freedom for Jewish physicians to have access to them without difficulty. The text also clearly reveals the existence of intellectual freedom, at least in those Jewish circles that the author moved in, together with a certain climate of intellectual exchange between Christian surgeons and physicians and their Jewish counterparts. All these points may be deduced from the repeated allusions of the author to problems that were the subject of debate both among Jewish physicians and between the latter and individual Christian surgeons and physicians, whom he refers to, though unfortunately not by name. This indicates a degree of communication between the practitioners of the two communities characteristic of the fourteenth century.[102] Nowhere in the text does there appear any reference to contact with contemporary Muslim professionals practising in Castile. From other sources we know that a relationship with Muslim colleagues living in the Kingdom of Granada, however, did occur.[103]

102 There is much clear evidence in fourteenth-century Catalonia and Majorca of professional collaboration between Jewish and Christian medical practitioners in the treatment of the same patient: see, for example, Regional Archive of Puigcerdá, notarial records, Joan Torrelles, *Lib. extraneorum*, 1361–2, fol. 45v, 18 March 1362. The collaboration was between the Christian Magister Anthonius de Capeyll, *physicus*, and Samuel Adday, *judeus physicus*, both living in Puigcerdá. See note 51 above.

103 See note 64 above.

VIII

Academicism versus empiricism in practical medicine in sixteenth-century Spain with regard to morisco practitioners

In this chapter I intend to examine the relationship between empiricism and academicism in Spanish practical medicine in the sixteenth century. In particular I shall concentrate on certain aspects of the relationship between academic (or university-based) medicine and the remnants of Arab medicine which still existed in Spain.

In sixteenth-century Spain medieval Arab medicine was still practised by a large part of the so-called morisco population.[1] This was mainly composed of Muslims who had stayed in Spain after the Christian conquests of the thirteenth to fifteenth centuries and who were all forced to convert to Christianity at the beginning of the sixteenth century. In spite of this compulsory conversion they retained their identity as a separate culture. This culture, as Islamic, came into open conflict with the dominant Christian majority which then attempted to suppress it in the name of supposed national unity. The conflict continued, however, and became one of the most serious problems in Spain in the later sixteenth and early seventeenth centuries. The Christians could only solve the problem by deporting the moriscos to other parts of Spain or finally by exiling them. In contrast to the moriscos, those who had always been Christians, without any conversion either from the Islamic or from the Jewish faith, were called 'Old Christians'.

I propose that medicine cannot be divorced from the political, religious and economic forces which form social groupings. Therefore morisco medicine, in all its aspects, was an integral part of the general process of the moriscos' alienation and final suppression.

Arab medicine, both as a medical science (Arabicized Galenism) and a practical system used by the Muslim or converted minority, broke down between the thirteenth and seventeenth centuries.[2] This dissolution was complex, for it was not the result of one change nor did it follow any set pattern. In fact, Arabicized Galenism was in a state of crisis throughout the sixteenth century.

However, we should not forget that this medicine and its practice were only small parts of the social scene in Spain between the thirteenth and seventeenth centuries. In Spain at that time, as in the rest of Europe, the proportion of doctors in the population was the same as in modern day Ethiopia or some of the most depressed areas of Vietnam. In Barcelona, for example, in the fourteenth and fifteenth centuries there were on average only one and a half to two doctors for every ten thousand inhabitants, whilst the figure in Valencia in the first third of the sixteenth century varied between five and seven doctors per ten thousand inhabitants.[3] If this was the situation in urban areas then we can only assume that in the country the figure was much lower. Unfortunately there is not any solid documentary proof of this. So what, then, was the medical service given to the Muslim, and later morisco, population? A population, that is, which in the Kingdom of Valencia in the sixteenth century comprised a third of the total population and in Granada almost half. And what actually was the medicine practised by the moriscos? I hope to answer these questions in this chapter.

Valencia was conquered by the Christians in the thirteenth century and Granada at the end of the fifteenth. Before the conquests, because of socio-economic and socio-medical conditions, the majority of the people in these areas received medical aid based on empiricism and non-academic belief and they were served by 'professional' practitioners. This situation continued after the Christian conquests. However, the influence of empiricism and belief on Muslim and morisco medicine was greatly increased by the general disintegration of Islamic culture and the gradual social alienation of Muslims and moriscos. Some examples of these beliefs were the use of scapulars (religious images worn over clothes), religious texts on the pregnant womb, spells, certain forms of judicial astrology, the occult, and others. Simultaneously the image of the professional doctor diminished, giving way to a flowery and picturesque world of quacks. This is not to say that the quacks would not have existed alongside scientific medicine, and together with these empirical practitioners would have been practitioners whose knowledge could be assessed against an academic 'corpus' of learning. Thus the population as a whole could have benefited from the dialectic between 'academic medicine' and 'empirical medical knowledge'. Actually in Christian Spain the majority of the Muslim, and later morisco, population was served only by doctors with empirical knowledge.

Morisco culture suffered by the disappearance of academically trained doctors, even though it favoured the scholastic model in medical science which was typical of the Christian majority. The morisco population was denied access to academic medicine, not for intellectual or academic reasons, but because the moriscos were of 'another caste'. Thus the dominance of empiricism in morisco medicine is another symptom of cultural confrontation.[4]

A general characteristic of the moriscos in the sixteenth century was their tight grip on the surviving Islamic culture of the Muslim population. Medicine, as an integral part of culture, gives us evidence for these strong links with Islam. By looking at archives and sixteenth-century Inquisition cases, we can see that in the morisco society of the mid-sixteenth century Muslim teachers (*alfaquí*) continued to play the versatile and diverse role they had always done in Arabic culture.[5] Their functions included working in the Civil Service, religious duties, and teaching both arts and sciences. Their work was confined to their own community. However, their professional standing changed from that of doctor to quack for many reasons. Their medicine was pulled away from its relationship with natural science; they were often reduced to the conditions of peasants; subject to all kinds of social, political and religious pressures. Academic teaching and academically trained scientists disappeared. Even the Old Christian high society and the Court tolerated and accepted quack doctors. However, while fulfilling an important role at the heart of the community they also came into open conflict with academic medicine.

The cultural solidarity amongst the moriscos of which I wrote earlier was not in fact common to all the regions where the moriscos suffered cultural oppression. There were appreciable differences between the moriscos in, for example, Granada, the Kingdom of Valencia and the Kingdom of Aragon. In Aragon the Castilian language replaced Arabic as the means of communication, even in religion and amongst heads of communities.[6] As we know, language plays a vital part in the cultural unity of a group. For example the cultural disintegration of the moriscos in Castile and Aragon before the expulsion of moriscos from Granada in the 1570s was so great that Arabic remained solely as a ritual and holy tongue – fragmentary and completely meaningless to those who used it.[7]

Andrés Laguna's Castilian translation of *Materia Medica* by Dioscorides became one of the morisco healers' source texts.[8] The morisco healers personified the mixture of Christian and Arab cultures; the former because they spoke Castilian and read medical texts written in Castilian and also in Latin, the latter because Arab medicine was passed on by an oral tradition. Moreover, because they could not read and write Arabic they had no access to texts from their own culture. The texts were in any case very difficult to obtain outside certain libraries in the second half of the sixteenth century. We shall also see that this contact with academic Christian medical science occurred frequently in an area which falls between empiricism and academic science: that is clinical therapy.

Muslim medicine finally disintegrated when it changed into healing which drew on both beliefs outside academic medicine and on empiricism. For this we have proof from Valencia, Aragon, Granada and Castile.

Among the Muslim and morisco minority the move from scientific to folk medicine was due to social changes which were taking place throughout the middle ages and which culminated in the sixteenth century. The healer, who counterbalanced the scientifically trained doctor, owed his social respectability to a complex series of socio-scientific and socio-economic reasons. Among these was the lack of a medical service by academic medicine to large sectors of the population; discrimination between rich and poor in treatment (both Christian and morisco); failures in academic medicine; the existence of chronic and incurable diseases, and the cultural vacuum following repressive measures.

Before we go any further, we must deal with a semantic problem: the concept of 'doctor' and 'surgeon' and what they both meant to the people and those with academic training in the sixteenth century. Unfortunately it has not been very thoroughly investigated.

Leaving the morisco with a university degree to one side, we refer here to the morisco who had picked up a certain knowledge on the fringes of mainstream academia and was practising it in a community (both morisco and Old Christian) which accepted him as having healing knowledge and techniques.

The morisco healer was the continuation of the school of Moorish medicine of the late middle ages. The Moorish scientific system was born of the Greco-Arab paradigm and upheld an open academic system which passed on knowledge freely. To say that the morisco doctor was a continuation of this system, however, does not mean that he preserved it. The evolution of the Moorish to the morisco doctor was more a degeneration than a progression, owing to a number of external factors. So great was the change that the links between the two forms of medicine virtually disappeared. Surprisingly enough it took only two or three generations to dismantle a type of medicine that had been alive and well, although stronger in teaching than in innovation, in the last decades of the fifteenth century. For example in 1494 the Muslim minority in Aragon was vigorous enough socially and academically to retain autonomous medical teaching and practice along Arab cultural lines. This teaching took place in the *madrasa* or Islamic university of Saragossa. The language used was Arabic.[9]

Both extremes of sixteenth-century Spanish society (disregarding the minority of intellectuals) were slow to recognize the change from Moorish to morisco medicine. Moriscos who were merely healers were still called 'doctors' and 'surgeons' in the sixteenth century, as their predecessors had been in the last third of the fifteenth century: it does not help here to draw clear lines between 'the middle ages' and 'the renaissance' or 'modern age' as if a narrow straight had been crossed and a new continent entered.

Things began to change in the last third of the sixteenth century. The reason for this was Philip II's creation of a bureaucracy which was felt at all social levels. We should bear in mind that the social relevance of a professional is closely linked to the creation and effectiveness of a bureaucracy, or rather to a radical and rigid separation of social strata. This tendency was very strong in fifteenth- and sixteenth-century Spain – possibly as a balance to the upward surge of classes in a young, developing society. What in fact happened was that the concept of 'doctor' came to be seen as being on the top rung of a ladder above the Latin surgeon, the barber-bloodletter and finally above the quacks, who were outside any legal category yet very widespread.

Nevertheless it should be said that despite the solidity of the medical profession in Spain during the sixteenth century, and particularly at its end, the categories within the profession were not fixed as they are today. There were still traces of that early medieval overlapping I referred to earlier. For example the morisco healer was called a 'doctor' or 'surgeon' by both the people and the Inquisition Tribunal, whereas today we would have no hesitation in calling him a quack. Today academic medicine and the social standing of its practitioners are such that nobody would refer to a quack (even though he might mend fractures and cure illness) as a 'doctor' or a 'surgeon', even in the least advanced parts of Spain. This lack of definition is important when we try to explain the prestige enjoyed by the morisco healer among the Christian aristocracy and the commercial bourgeoisie in Madrid or Valencia and the absence of social prejudice when it came to consulting one. The only clear case that I have found of censure against a morisco healer was that by Daza Chacón (1510–96), a leading figure in Spanish surgery during the renaissance, and some of his colleagues from the court.[10] Their reasons for censure were entirely academic, based on the methodology which related medicine to natural philosophy and which separated the academic healer from the empirical healer. Outside small academic circles the words used for these empirical healers were 'doctor' or 'surgeon', even though they had no qualification or licence to practise.

This last point is very important for realizing that we should not apply twentieth-century assumptions to sixteenth-century Spain. We must remember that a university degree did not have the same rôle as today. Our contemporary university degree came into being during the nineteenth century in line with the bourgeois mentality which produced it. Thus in the first half of the sixteenth century the presence or absence of a medical degree was not the vital factor in acceptance or rejection of the medical practices of healers or magicians. The reasons were more complex. A good example of the exchange of ideas in the first half of the sixteenth century is personified by the converted Jew, Andrés Laguna (*c.* 1510–59) who was a student at the Sorbonne, was connected with the University of Alcalá, was the Emperor's doctor, and was a leading figure in the movement towards medical humanism.[11] Laguna was not averse to consulting wizards and healers, learning from them, applying their remedies, noting their results and even going to them himself when he himself needed attention for a serious illness. From his point of view as an academic (and with the material available) he studied the healers' remedies, and with respect, not contempt. In one of these studies he identified some herbs which 'a little old German woman . . . who looked like a witch' had given him as being henbane (*Hyoscamus niger*) and then went on to describe its effects. In another case he studied the hallucinogenic properties of 'a certain green ointment' used by two wizards in Metz.[12] He used it in experiments on a patient and found that it contained 'extremely cold and soporific herbs, which were hemlock nightshade (*Atropa belladonna*), henbane and mandrake'.[13]

Morisco healers were never labelled as 'wizards' or 'enchanters' (as Laguna had described the healers of Lorena) by their academic Christian 'colleagues'. The social prestige of the morisco healer together with his deep integration into Old Christian society, was in sharp contrast to the growing alienation of the majority of moriscos. Not that the morisco healers did not have any problems with already established doctors who were protecting their established practices.

What is surprising, though, is the limited use made by Christian society (and therefore also by the morisco population) of the doctors who had academic training – those doctors who also claimed a monopoly over science and medical practice. As it was, people had no qualms about consulting morisco doctors, knowing full well that they had neither university degrees nor licences to practise. Not only did they consult the morisco doctor but they were also quite happy to talk about it publicly. The church tried to stop this use of morisco doctors right up to the end of the sixteenth century with prohibition after prohibition. The church's concern shows just how far the morisco doctor (meaning healer) had become integrated into society.

From what I have written I hope I have given some idea of some medically-related aspects of Spanish society in the sixteenth century.[14] It is a very complicated topic, but the major points of background to my theme I hope have been covered.

To continue, I would like to take five topics as the basis for an examination of the relationship between academic practitioners with their rational medicine and morisco healers with their empirical or non-empirical medicine.

The five topics are these:

1. Academic science's attack on empiricism using a so-called rational methodology.

2. The failure of the academic world and society to recognize medicine and its practice as signs of a living cultural group. In this case the group is morisco.
3. The refusal of academic medicine to assimilate the morisco culture peacefully. Moriscos were barred from medical faculties.
4. The identification of the morisco social group as a causal factor (that is aetiological factor) of 'social pathology'.
5. The designation of areas common to morisco empiricism and academic science.

First, in the last twenty years certain historians of medicine and technology have looked at attitudes to practical techniques in the sixteenth century. Paolo Rossi[15] and López Piñero[16] have analysed European thinkers' new appreciation of techniques in the sixteenth century. This appreciation was to be one of the most important factors of change in the new era. Practical technique was represented in medicine principally by surgery, the importance of, and interest in which, had been increasing all through the early middle ages within academic circles, having come to Spain from Italy. In Spain this new interest went hand in hand with the high reputation of surgeons.[17] One of these surgeons was Dionisio Daza Chacón, who practised in Emperor Charles I's army. He proclaimed, changing the title of the well known work of Galen, that 'the good surgeon is the true doctor'. One of Daza's aims was to emphasize the worth of scientifically-based technique over mere empirical practice. Accordingly he was at great pains to emphasize the importance of the university-trained surgeon.

When the Valencian morisco Pinterete was summoned to treat Charles, the son of Philip II and heir to the throne, Daza took the opportunity to attack the empirical nature of morisco doctors' treatment. Daza was quite categorical:

> Many times it was proposed that we doctors should cure his highness with the ointments of Pinterete, moor from the Kingdom of Valencia; there are two ointments – one white . . . another black . . . Most of us have rejected these ointments, first because we did not know their composition and it was not proper to use them without knowing what was in them, and secondly because it did not seem rational that the same medicaments were always used, whatever the time, and on all ages and patients.[18]

In spite of all this, the morisco healers' ointments were used on the prince and so Daza had to give an explanation. In his explanation he denounced the rôle of mere belief, which went more or less hand in hand with folk medicine, by saying: 'More in view of the faith which many had in those ointments . . .'.[19]

I suspect that these same reasons were used by Luis Collado (*c.* 1520–89), professor at the medical faculty of Valencia (incidentally the person who introduced the anatomy of Vesalius to Spain),[20] when he had violent exchanges with the morisco doctor Jerónimo Pachet.

Let us see how these events are recorded in the Inquisitorial summary:

> Item, this man (Pachet) also cured one Bautista Tridi eight or nine years ago, with the help of the devil. Tridi was being attended by doctor Collado and doctor Ardevol (Jaime Ardevol), and he had a diseased liver, a weak stomach, almost completely destroyed, and his intestines full of vapour, he was very sick, almost dead, and though the physicians visited him they gave him no medicines. So they sent for this man, and when he had come he argued with Collado and Ardevol, for they were dismissed immediately. *He understood the disease from experience*, but as it was in such an acute phase *and he did not understood the use of medicines*, he consulted with his 'familiar' (that is to say, he used the devil), and he showed him the medicines inside and outside. And the man was cured within two or three days. He was well paid, and he took both fame and money from the case, the other physicians hated him.[21]

In 1580 Pachet was tried by the Inquisition for practising the Islamic religion.

Second, the sixteenth century saw the gradual collapse of Muslim and Christian ability to live side by side. Due to the peculiar circumstances of the time and the nature of the two cultures involved, this break transcended merely religious or personal levels. It also brought out socio-economic and political conflicts.[22] Nevertheless, for neither the Old Christians nor the moriscos (converted from Islam) was religion a secondary factor. The introduction of the Inquisition at the end of the fifteenth century was to affect certain minorities greatly. Particularly affected were the Jews who had converted to Christianity and were more or less integrated into society, and also the moriscos who more by force than choice had embraced the Christian faith and recognized its baptism. For these people accusations of heresy loomed large.

Also, as Muslim theologians and institutional religion lost influence and control, popular morisco religious belief, which in Islam was very rich, had become flamboyant and superstitious. In the religious-theological field, then, there was the same process of disintegration that we saw in the medical field.

One of the most interesting aspects of this popular flamboyance was the belief in devils, with its roots in neo-platonic Islam. Along with their continued Mohammedanism after official conversion, this belief in devils and in their invocation was what brought morisco 'doctors' and 'surgeons' before the Inquisition. Here we see, once again, medicine as one of the manifestations of a living culture, in this case of the morisco community. All this, along with the diligence and detail of the Inquisition, has allowed us to penetrate the complex world of morisco beliefs and practices related to medicine. We can also examine, with solid evidence, its confrontation with academic science. Even though the richness of this world of belief is only partially expressed by documents, some of the books written in Spanish with Arabic characters (*aljamiado*) by morisco communities in Aragon (which Ribera studied and of which he translated large parts) have been crucial in getting a fairly accurate picture of popular morisco medical practices.[23]

The existence of these Inquisitorial trials against morisco doctors and surgeons raises a series of doctrinal and practical problems. We might ask why they were tried, and why invocation of demons was considered heretical. And what were the reasons for the Inquisition's persecution of the barbers and surgeons who performed circumcisions (*retajadores*), and of surgeons and midwives in general.

The crimes for which the moriscos were brought before the Holy Office were usually the following:

1. Crimes against the faith; accusations of Muslim practices and beliefs.
2. Crimes of superstition (witchcraft, sorcery and magic).
3. Offences against morality (for example sodomy and hermaphroditism).
4. Political crimes (alleged alliances with the Turks, Berber pirates and others).[24]

Almost all the cases against doctors seem to have fallen into the second category, allegations of being in league with the devil; whilst the proceedings against the surgeons who performed circumcisions fall into the first category.

The question of invoking demons was what worried the Inquisition officers more than anything else about morisco doctors. They considered it a very real possibility and a punishable one. However, diabolic belief meant quite different things to the inquisitor and the morisco. Both accepted its reality, yet each saw it from a different cultural point of view.[25] The inquisitor's view sprang from a scholastic conception of devil-pacts and invocation whereas the morisco's belief was based on his belief in semitic spiritualism and Alexandrine neoplatonism. They spoke a different language. Leaving aside the cases of deceit or mental illness which could have existed, the four or five trials which have been found (and the material provided by Ribera) leave no shadow of a doubt of the genuine belief in devils on both sides.

The entire universe, to a morisco, was not something static and lifeless, it was like a dynamic kingdom ruled by Allah's governors, or spirits of all sizes. These spirits ruled everything. It was necessary, therefore, to be on good terms with them, which meant knowing the words which pleased them, their categories, and the way to treat them. Knowing these things allowed the moriscos to call up spirits to protect them from illness, forecast serious illness, know about far-off events, and so on. Many spirits or demons had left signs by which they could be summoned by those who knew them. The signs varied a great deal: a drawn palm leaf, an iron, a figure drawn in saffron on spun cloth, etc. Each had to be combined with the necessary spell. There were, however, evil spirits which had to be cast out since they brought illness and bad luck.[26]

The invocation of demons was a common practice amongst morisco doctors. It was completely in keeping with the belief which ran through their whole society. It was also completely real for the Inquisitors. In the trial of the wretched morisco healer Román Ramirez (who worked in Aragon and Castile) we can see how the two worlds crossed. The public prosecutor said:

> And crime followed crime, by evil means and with the aim of enrichment, curing illness, he has been and still is in league with the devil, with whose help and advice in the month of June 1594, he cast an evil spell on a woman of Tajaguerce, near the city of Soria. This woman whose name was Ana Sanz, had married one Bartolomé de Ortega. On their wedding night he caused her to lose menstrual blood with many fits of melancholy which cut her desire to share her husband's bed. He also caused her a feeling of rejecting holy things and other outward signs of being possessed, loss of sanity and memory in such a way as not to recognize her parents nor remember their names.
>
> [The woman's relatives called the doctor] and when the woman saw the accused her condition worsened, she fainted and fell down. He treated her with the aromatic oil of juniper, made her rise, though not without great pain.
>
> So that he could communicate with and treat the demon within her, the accused gave the woman certain powders in an egg . . . And since on that occasion they gave him no more than 40 coins, he complained . . . swearing to God that they would need him again soon, as later happened.
>
> For, having treated her with aromatic smoke and ointments which he had left the said woman, she worsened, in such a way that the demons returned to possess her. She became sick of the head, her mouth twisted and her head fell onto her shoulder. She went for three days without eating or drinking. These were all obvious results of the threat the accused had made on underpayment.[27]

The prosecutor, then, accepts these notions of pacts, invocations and demonic possession quite seriously. What is noticeable is that having had a scholastic–rational education the Inquisitors did not apply their book-learning to everyday life. Instead they developed a gloomy belief system in order to deal with the practical, popular and ingenuous world view of the moriscos. Neither did the Inquisitors realize that it was quite different from their own. Three levels can be identified in the inquisitorial trials in relation to beliefs in devils.[28]

(1) The rational attitude of the Supreme Council of the Inquisition.
(2) The attitude of the provincial Inquisitors: they internalized and transformed the European belief about devils by integrating it

into a rational system based on medieval scholastic formulae. With this transformation they created a superstructure, of which they were completely convinced, and which they tried to impose on the people. They were thus upholding the *status quo* by using a belief system loosely based on the rational attitude of the Supreme Council.

(3) The morisco world of belief, in which demons were a reality, but a different reality from that described in the second level. This world of belief was shown through simple everyday practices by the humble peasants, some of whom were charlatans. In spite of this the Inquisitors took them seriously. Together with this was the religious problem and the rôle of the Inquisition as a destroyer of morisco social structures. We must not forget that medicine and medical practice were part of this social structure.

In the trial quoted above the accused doctor, Román Ramírez, gives a quite different version from the prosecutors. We shall see how he finally explained his experiences with devils. He only did so after three months in prison and under pressure from the Inquisitors. His first declaration made to the Christians was about popular methods of healing, and it is a mixture of folk beliefs and academic science. In the two declarations the dilemma of his existence comes through strongly: the pretences and repressions of a newly converted Moor in a life full of social and personal tensions. In the first declaration he says that he was called to Tajaguerce by the girl's family and on arriving found the girl:

> her neck was twisted, her chin thrust into her shoulder. The first thing he did to cure her was tell the parish priest to read the gospels to her . . . then, he asked the apothecary to send him certain herbs, mineral powders (sulphur) and juniper oil. He mixed them and made an ointment which he applied to the patient. He told the family that the illness was serious and that if the symptoms returned they should apply the ointment again, recite the Gospels and invoke the Virgin Mary . . . the family said that when the sick girl was better they would pay him well.[29]

Later I will deal at length with the interesting problems posed by this empirical use of pharmaceutical herbs and in particular that of the sources of his knowledge in this field. Usually these empirical doctors knew of these herbs through the oral tradition and personal experience. (We should not forget that they were mostly country people.) In Román Ramírez, however, a series of interesting features coincide: his ignorance of the Moslem tradition (he could not speak Arabic), a tradition of medicine in his family (his grandfather and mother both practised medicine) and his contact with the medical materials used by Christian doctors. He would have used Andrés Laguna's translation into Castilian of the work of Dioscorides.

Let us return again to the devilish world of our doctor Ramírez. His second declaration reveals the whole Islamic belief in the devil myth. This second statement was only made under great pressure. In it we can see the oral tradition operating – a tradition which preserved the mixture of practice and belief:

I was taught by Juan de Luna, my grandfather, who was a great doctor. When I was ten or twelve years old my grandfather, who was going to die, told me that if I needed anything, between eleven and twelve at night I should call out *Liarde*. He said he had ordered *Liarde* to come and help me. I understood that *Liarde* was a demon with whom my father had a pact. Later I heard my grandfather talking to him a few times from his bed at night. After a year I asked my grandfather who he was talking to. He said again that after he died the person he was talking to would come and help me whenever I called. Since my grandfather died I have called the demon *Liarde* many times between eleven and twelve at night, just as my grandfather told me. The demon has answered many times, although at other times he has not . . .[30]

The family nature of the medical profession (with its roots in the Judaic–Arabic medical tradition) was obviously influential when it came to decide on a future career. In spite of Ramirez's initial lack of enthusiasm for medicine he considered himself obliged to continue the tradition of his grandfather and his mother in medicine.

As we see, Ramírez attributes his own and his grandfather's medical knowledge to the demon *Liarde*. Jerónimo Pachet, the famous morisco doctor from Valencia, did the same. At his trial he said:

When I first worked with the demon, I often cured people with his help (since I did not have much experience). But after fourteen or fifteen years I stopped using him because I knew enough about the properties of herbs and medicines. I have occasionally called him, but only when the case was very serious and I did not understand it by natural means, and when university doctors had given up.[31]

This is a clear attempt to bring medical knowledge together with the Beyond, or the devil. A doctor who could boast of this connection in his practice was thus guaranteeing his knowledge in the eyes of the people. The sacred origins of his science put him above criticism. The morisco doctor thus embodies the rich and complex beliefs held by moriscos and even Old Christians, because the whole population, both Old and New Christians, had lived together for centuries. There was also the possibility of doctors dishonestly exploiting people's beliefs.

Apparently morisco healers were not always called to treat the higher reaches of society. Only when there was no alternative, that is when the (Christian) doctor left the patient 'in the hands of God,' were they consulted. 'Those morisco doctors only treated those whom the Christian doctors had said would die'.[32]

Chronic and incurable diseases were the usual reasons for the high classes and intellectuals calling for healers. As Malinowski has pointed out, magical and religious explanations usually replace natural or scientific ones when we move into the world of unpredictable events, where the human will sees its own inability to control events.[33]

As I have stated, the morisco believed in many kinds of demons. There were the medical specialists who advised certain healers and many others who were evil, who could cause illnesses. To get rid of the evil demons, people did not have to call in a specialist, for it was enough to carry around a piece of paper with a spell and a verse of the Koran written on it. A morisco document advises:

> If anyone wants to stop spirits entering the house and upsetting their peace and health, they only have to put the paper into a tube, seal the tube with fish and put it in the main door-way of the cowshed. Also it is good to put it in the roof and in the corners, always inside the walls, so that the spirits cannot find a way in through cracks in the walls.[34]

Now, in the 1980s, these charms can sometimes be found when old houses are demolished in Aragon or Granada or Castile. They can also be identified in Inquisition cases against the moriscos, for example, the young merchant's servant from Alcoy (Alicante) who was found to have a bag which 'was smooth and coloured, containing some rings and a little musk and a small piece of paper with writing on it . . .'.[35] This writing, which was Arabic, was translated by order of the Inquisition. It read:

> It is proven that the man carrying this about his person and writing four of the following will be protected and defended from everything. The words are, *Alguaco, Alguaca, Sogel, Sagel, Mosaguin, Johuage, Jahuage, Guaquimisi a la raig.*[36]

The Jesuit translator added: 'All these names are those of demons and especially *guaquimisi a la raig* which means "lame devil"'. The Inquisition accused the young servant of 'carrying demon's names in Arabic'. The trial was in 1620. Ten years previously, when his mother had to leave the young boy, she gave him the bag and entreated him to keep it to protect himself from all evil and sickness.[37]

A morisco reader of Arabic texts, made a comment in the margin of one text:

> The good Muslim should never be without charms for the person who goes without them is like a house which cannot be shut because it has no door. Without a door anyone can enter. Anyone who goes without charms can be entered anywhere by demons.[38]

Morisco doctors often used spells, charms, phrases from the Koran and similar things in their practices. An example comes from 1596 in the trial of the morisco Francisco de Córdoba in Toledo. One witness, an academic, told the story like this:

> Don Alonxo Mexía de Tovar, student of the University of Alcalá, after swearing in, said that the previous Lent, in the year 1595, in Villacastin (Segovia) his brother

Antonio Mexía de Tovar was ill. Some said that he had been bewitched. Don Alonso heard of a Morisco called Francisco de Córdoba who lived in Toledo . . . and heard that the said morisco could cure his brother's illness, so the doctor was brought. When he came the witness saw that the said morisco was administering some powders and was telling the family to scatter the powders in the patient's room and also to scatter powder in the room of the woman suspected of sorcery, and also in the eggs the patient was to eat. Each time he made certain signs with a feather and saliva. He also gave them some small written documents and ordered them to be soaked in the patient's wine or water.[39]

Later, when they had been translated by the Arabic professor in Alcalá, they were seen to be fragments of the Koran.

Leaving aside the empirical part of the morisco's medical practice, which was basically pharmacological, it is clear that his medicine was mixed very much with religious belief. Short prayers were common amongst the people. For example those which the abbot of the monastery of Valldigna (Valencia) found on a morisco and which he quickly sent to the Inquisition. Apart from being written in Arabic, 'they seemed to contain something against the Faith'.[40]

The documents which the diligent monk took show quite clearly the duality of empiricism and belief which I have previously indicated. One of them, for example, is a recipe against scabies, which could easily have been written by a medical faculty professor. It says:

Burn two ounces of sulphur and two ounces of alum together. Grind the residue and mix the powder with orange juice and olive oil. Make an ointment and rub it into the parts affected by scabies. Afterwards bathe with boiling water and rosebay and flax-leaved daphne.[41]

I do not think it is a coincidence that we owe the first descriptions of scabies to Arab doctors and that they possessed a richer pharmacological tradition. The above prescription was found with some short prayers for the sick. For example: 'To Our Lord, Healer of those who call him, listener to the dead, grant me what I ask'.[42]

Soon after the expulsion of the majority of moriscos from Granada in 1572, archbishop Pedro Guerrero condemned 'sorcerers' and anyone who used:

Any type of riddle, such as omens, birds, sneezes, so-called proverbs, lucky charms, spells and those who use water, glass, swords or anything which shines, or those who cast spells with metal or anything else, those who perform magic with the heads of corpses or animals or with children's or virgin's palms or bewitch with wedding rings, or who cut the mountain rose because it cures the sickness which they say comes from the mountains, and anything similar to gain health or worldly goods . . .[43]

This text, which was part of the conclusions of the Synod of Granada, sums up the richness and complexity of the baroque world of morisco belief.

Third, after the conquest of the Muslim Kingdom of Granada in 1492 the Spanish kings were left with a large number of people on their hands whose culture was Islamic. Even though their leaders, intellectuals and the better-off emigrated to North Africa in the following decades, there still remained a 'learned' morisco minority in Granada. This minority, which was linked to the royal bureaucracy, formed the centre of the morisco social structure, the members of which came ultimately to live on what were almost reservations. This minority, which hispanicized its names, tried to bridge the gap between itself and the dominant Christian power. The crown and the church began a carefully planned scheme to rob the moriscos of their culture. The intention behind the scheme was to try to turn morisco children into model Christian scholars, and in implementing it schools and later the University of Granada were founded. The scheme was to prove very useful to the Castilian crown during the conquest of the non-European cultures of the New World.[44]

For a number of reasons this scheme failed. The moriscos in Granada rebelled and were only put down after a bloody war (the 'war of the Alpujarras'). Philip II then had the idea of dispersing the moriscos of Granada throughout Castile. This was done between June 1569 and December 1571, but rather than providing solutions, it created new social and political problems in Castile.[45]

It is in this context that we should consider Pedro de Vesga's words when he asked the king in the Castilian Parliament to prevent 'the moriscos who recently revolted in the Kingdom of Granada'[46] and the old moriscos from entering medical faculties and also from practising medicine. Parliament stated that

> many moriscos study and practise in the universities of Alcalá and Toledo and others; we implore the king to find a solution because it is very likely that before long all or at least most of our doctors will be moriscos.[47]

The political and religious tensions between Old and New Christians and their old controversies played a vital part in the social alienation of the morisco doctor:

> After their rebellions and many other signs we can only conclude that morisco doctors hate the Old Christians, so who wants to be treated by his enemy? We must also say that judging by their confessions to the Inquisition that many doctors treated their own race properly whilst deliberately killing Old Christians and supplying medicines which induced abortion.[48]

The figure of the morisco doctor became a symbol of all the degradation and corruption of which medicine could be capable. Moreover, under the Inquisition's methods of persuasion, morisco doctors admitted to all kinds of professional misconduct. Thus the morisco doctor became something to be eliminated from a society made up of Old Christians. Only Old

Christians should have the right to enjoy the status of a doctor and surgeon, and the traditionally virtuous reputation of the good doctor.

If the moriscos are doctors they will have the status owing to a doctor, they will wear luxurious clothes, and travel by coach. The laws of the kingdom forbid the moriscos the use of these things and to hold honourable professions, and if the medical profession is the most honourable, why must they practise it?

Going into convents to cure nuns, and knowing how imaginative and curious they are, the moriscos could show them things harmful to their faith. There are few positions which require more virtue than that of a doctor, but instead the moriscos have bad tendencies. They do not confess, or if they do confess it is out of a sense of duty. They do not give alms. A doctor must send his patient to confession and heal the poor freely and with charity. How can those who do not call a priest when they are ill or never do good works fulfil the above conditions? With many medicines it is possible to kill secretly and subtly, without being asked, and we can be sure that we are correct when we presume that they use these medicines, and between them kill more people in this kingdom than the Turks, the English and others.[49]

The wickedness of the morisco doctor's practice is clearly shown in the confession forced out of a morisco surgeon by the Valencian Inquisition, 'the said man confessed to having malevolently left Old Christians with only one arm so that they could not carry weapons'.[50] The Old Christians would not allow the morisco doctor out of the social alienation in which he had been put. They blocked all his paths for rising socially, within both the Faith and the University. Their conversion was considered as insincere. We should remember here the important social rôle played by the Christian Faith. '[Morisco doctors] do not confess, or if they do confess it is out of a sense of duty'.[51]

The morisco's great biological vitality could be dangerously capable of shaking social equilibrium in his favour, an equilibrium which was unlawfully held by the Old Christians.

For some years now the moriscos who were expelled from Granada have enrolled their sons in the medical faculty, but then they were not admitted as apothecaries, clerks nor any position of confidence, and this caused many problems because the Old Christians and honourable people did not want to enroll at the faculty of medicine for this reason, since the moriscos who practised medicine could have got revenge on the Old Christians . . . and that before long the majority of doctors will be moriscos.[52]

It was necessary also to close the door to social elevation which the university presented.

For these problems and others which will be omitted for the sake of brevity, it seems advisable that His Majesty make a decree in which he orders the universities not to give degrees to those who cannot prove that they are not moriscos, and to punish the clerk, witnesses and examiners, those who give the degree and the doctors who have a part in it. All this should apply to doctors' diplomas as well as to graduates and bachelors.[53]

But it was possible to be a romanist doctor or surgeon, that is, to obtain a diploma to practise, without going to university; only being examined by the Royal Tribunal of *Protomedicato* on practical knowledge and capabilities.[54] This they also tried to stop.

Item: when they go to be examined at the Tribunal that included in the practical information should be the fact that they are not moriscos, neither old nor modern.[55]

This requirement was introduced into the rules and regulations of the University of Alcalá in 1565–6.[56]

This still leaves a loophole through which the morisco can gain medical knowledge – he can still practise in illicit competition in certain ways, because even though he does not graduate he can still listen to university lectures.

And because they can still practise in secret, even without graduating, we must instruct the university bedels and secretaries, under pain of punishment, not to allow moriscos to enrol, practise nor attend lectures . . .[57]

Fourth, the Kingdom of Granada was seriously affected by the 'war of the Alpujarras' and its major consequence, the deportation of moriscos to other parts of Spain. The university of Granada, and especially its weak medical faculty, collapsed. For example medical publishing in Granada was interrupted in 1580, not to begin again until 1640! As Bernard Vincent[58] has observed, there are hardly any investigations on the subject of moriscos in Granada and Castile between 1570 and 1619, when the moriscos were all finally exiled from Spain. What information there is still lies in general and municipal archives. The long year after the decision to expel them was a crucial one. We should not forget that already in 1569 moriscos from some parts of the kingdom and from Albayzin (a quarter in the city of Granada) had been expelled. The latter was depopulated when twenty thousand inhabitants left.[59] At this time the attitude of the population of Castile was vital to the chances of the integration of the morisco community.

Under what conditions did the move from Granada to Castile take place? How were the moriscos accepted in the different places? What ideas directed the different phases of expulsion? In short what solutions did the Spanish have in mind for the old conflict . . . which, whatever the policy, could disappear or break out again?[60]

We still cannot answer these questions properly and we hardly have any data to judge the repercussions on medicine of such a serious measure. For this reason I shall confine myself to an important piece of evidence which throws up a new problem in the relationship of morisco and academic medicine in Castile.

The dispersion of the moriscos was not only a punitive measure or one of internal security. It was also the only apparently feasible way of trying to integrate them into society . . . deep down the problem was not theological, but social.[61]

They had to be integrated in all respects 'into the society in which until then they had been a foreign body'.[62]

This was the aim of the intellectual Pedro de Valencia in his *Treatise on the Moriscos.*[63] It was written in 1605 and 1606 when the idea of exiling all moriscos from Spain was taking shape amongst the king's closest advisors. This terrible decision was taken in 1609. Ironically, the king who took the decision, Philip III, had been cured as a child of a very serious illness by a morisco doctor.[64]

In the way it was done the dispersion of moriscos through Castile was one of the most atrocious deportations in history. Lapeyre[65] established that 20.7 per cent of the 54 366 moriscos on the census died during the journey. Vincent,[66] however, from archive evidence, has put the figure higher, at 33.5 per cent, at least for six years in Estremadura. We can get an idea of the risk to life when we realize that it was during the exodus that one of the most serious epidemics of louse-borne typhus in the sixteenth century broke out. It is the illness typical of underdevelopment and poverty.

It is precisely this fact which brings out a new aspect of the relationship between moriscos and academic medical men. The latter saw the moriscos as the cause of a hitherto untraced illness: louse-borne typhus, called in Old Castilian *tabardillo*. With this a new problem is thrown up, not to be grasped until the beginning of the twentieth century, by social pathology: the social aetiology of illnesses. Let us look at it a little closer.

During the sixteenth century a number of 'new illnesses' were described. For example, 'English sweats', which flourished between 1485 and 1551, the *nuwe krenckte* of Dusseldorf, the *morbus gallicus*, a new diphtheria. Along with these there was a new form of fever. Although Girolamo Fracastoro in 1546 was the first to describe with any kind of clinical precision an epidemic of this fever and so permit its later identification as louse-borne typhus, the most conscientious study of the disease was by Luis de Toro who was a doctor from Estremadura (Castile).[67] We will leave to one side whether these diseases were all 'new' or if they were only the nosographic consequence of better observation. Luis de Toro's description of what now we know as louse-borne typhus is very correct and direct. His study was part of the contemporary renaissance scientific reach towards reality, which along with a great care to describe the patients he had, led him to distinguish new illnesses and to extricate them from the jumble of 'fevers'. His clinical description hardly differs from that which appears in any of today's medical manuals.

There are four things which I wish to emphasize here: first the rôle of illness in a consciousness of the morisco problem, second the dramatic nature of the illness, third contemporary doctors' own explanation of the social factors for example (cold, or poverty following war) which cause and aid the development of illness, and lastly the causal relationship between illness and the presence or absence of a social group in this case, the moriscos.

Like the majority of Spanish intellectuals and scientists in the second half of the sixteenth century, Luis de Toro saw himself as being involved in the morisco problem. His involvement was a consequence of the deportation of moriscos after the 'war of Alpujarras', which suddenly brought a problem straight under his nose. By carefully reading Luis de Toro's work we can make out an anti-morisco climate; a protest against these people on whose arrival a louse-borne typhus epidemic flared up again, straight on the heels of the previous one.

> They caused the disease to return and spread through large parts of Spain, being particularly cruel throughout Extremadura. The saracens were the source of the infection. All those who led and directed the dispersion, those who dealt with them or received them in villages and towns became infected and either died or came very close to it. At the same time those parts through which they did not go remained free of the disease. The disease was quite special amongst the moriscos, owing to the intense cold and poverty after the war in which they had to live.[68]

In all, in two years (1569–71) between seventy thousand and eighty thousand moriscos were dispersed in Castile, not counting those who were sent as slaves to the kingdom of Valencia. In the dedication of his book (1574) Luis de Toro talks of the cause of the disease as something insidious which has infiltrated and spread through Castile. He always refers to the moriscos pejoratively, as saracens (*sarraceni*) or moors (*mauris*).

Fifth, of all the morisco healers that we have found, very few could read or write, except those who were also teachers (*alfaquí*) or those who were trained as physicians outside the faculties of medicine. They were almost all farmers. Therefore, the training these healers received was limited to the oral tradition, usually taking place within the family itself. The lack of institutions through which this knowledge and wider culture could be passed and the repression which the moriscos suffered both contributed to the importance of oral transmission of information. The case of the morisco Román Ramírez, is typical of this situation. He was the grandson of Juan de Luna, 'who was a great doctor' and with whom he was brought up. Juan de Luna taught his daughter (Ramírez's mother) 'medical things' who then, says Ramírez, 'taught him everything he knew about herbs and curing illness'.[69]

Here we have, very clearly, the way in which medical knowledge was passed on. We could apply the same outline to the scientific teaching of surgeons. All this knowledge was based on a concise outline of traditional Galenic medicine which was still taught in the *madrasa* sixty or seventy years before. The *madrasa*, or Islamic university, was maintained by the Moslem community of Saragossa.[70] Alongside this system (or in fact mixed up with it) there existed a rich and complex belief world which had grown up in the absence of institutional control. The institutions had either disappeared with the conquest or led an increasingly difficult life. Their effect on the moriscos diminished or disappeared altogether, as they settled into lifelessness within a larger social structure. Along with this mixture of medical–scientific and belief systems, there existed a rich world of therapeutic knowledge. This knowledge largely centred on medical herbs. In all morisco doctors this is the most striking aspect of their medicine. What are more noticeable are not only the range of herbs they used, but also the complexity and extravagance of their prescriptions. Many ingredients were acquired at pharmacies.[71]

A new and interesting element is brought out in the interrogation of a morisco doctor. It is the use of Dioscorides translated into Castilian by Andrés Laguna. When talking about his mother's medical knowledge Román Ramírez says:

> I never had medical books, neither did she write down the medicines she prescribed nor have I had them written down. I only had Dioscorides' book, which I bought thirty years ago in Madrid.[72]

In spite of never going to school 'little by little I learned to read. Everything I read . . . I memorised'.[73] Moreover, we should remember that Ramírez did not know any Arabic.

These facts are clear evidence of how far the Islamic culture of the moriscos, in Castile and Aragon, had disintegrated. They also show the strong attraction of Christian culture; the extent to which science had been spread by printing and the use of romance languages; and also the great popularity of Laguna's *Dioscorides* which our morisco bought in Madrid in about 1560, that is to say, five years after the first edition was published in Amberes (1555). The use of Laguna's *Dioscorides* as the only teaching book and the fact that the tribunal made Ramírez read a medical book written by the doctor Huarte de San Juan (1529–88),[74] as proof of his ability to read Castilian, show an important step in the programme of morisco integration into Christian society, at least in the scientific field. The integration naturally took place at the expense of morisco cultural models. All this existed alongside circulating works written in Spanish with Arab characters (*aljamiado*), such as medical astrology and spells applied to medicine, deeply rooted in Judaic–Arabic tradition.

Even though in the kingdom of Valencia and in other Spanish communities, Arabic remained as a written and oral medium (in its dialect, *algaravia*), we can still ask whether books of Arab medicine circulated amongst the 'professional' practitioners. We will leave to one side the academically-trained morisco doctors' contact with Arab sources and the relative abundance of Arab scientific and medical manuscripts in Spain in the first half of the sixteenth century.[75] What interests us is seeing whether the morisco healer, who had not fitted into Christian society and its science, had any connection with his written scientific tradition. This is to say, how did information pass on outside the university?

While the available documentation makes it difficult to get near the reality of my subject (the morisco healer and the Christian society in which he lived), here we find even greater problems. The Inquisition was very careful to watch for circulation or mere possession of papers written in Arabic. In the second half of the sixteenth century it was enough to be caught with a brief note (even if it were a legal contract) to be charged by the Inquisition under suspicion of being part of 'the abject sect of Mahomet'.[76] Obviously, this has not helped to conserve such literature. Also we should not forget that almost all the moriscos were illiterate. This, despite a clandestine network of teachers (*alfaquies*) who taught people to read and write Arabic and who were thus centres of upkeep of Islamic tradition. In spite of the difficulties, I think we can be sure of the existence and circulation of a medical literature written in Arabic (even though fragmentary) among the morisco communities in Castile, Aragon and Valencia.[77] Obviously it was a literature which was practically reduced to prescriptions. For example, the papers which were intercepted by the abbot of Valldigna included prescriptions. One of them, a treatment for scabies, has been quoted above. During the trial of Jerónimo Jover, who we know could read, write and speak Arabic, and who lived in Valencia in the 1580s and 1590s it was said that

> when he left Valencia, (with the intention of enrolling at the Medical Faculty at Lérida, Catalonia) he took with him some books in Arabic. He left a different Arabic book at home, which the witness gave to the Holy Inquisition.[78]

Unfortunately, records do not speak of the contents of this book, nor has it been kept along with the court records. Were they medical books? It is very possible, since Jover was good enough for it to be worth his while going to the Faculty at Lérida to get a medical degree. His status was also high enough for him to marry the widow of the notary Pedro Fuster, an Old Christian. From the testimony of an apothecary friend of his we have been able to find out the names of some of the Christian books in his library. These books show the point to which these learned moriscos had become integrated, and the complex nature of the co-existence of the Islamic and scholastic Christian cultures. The apothecary said:

> The said doctor (the morisco Jover) auctioned all the Christian books he had; including a book by St Thomas Aquinas and a book by Friar Luis of Granada and a book called *Memorable Things of Spain*.[79]

In a farm of Ciudad Real, in Castile, about 1600, the Inquisition found a library owned by a morisco with fourteen books. One of them was a medical book in Arabic. The title was *Medical Prescriptions*. Unfortunately it was burned by the Inquisition.[80]

A recently discovered document permits us to trace with precision another channel for the circulation of medical knowledge among the morisco community and to establish, with documentary evidence, the existence of a form of medical training for the morisco doctor other than the empirical that we have seen Román Ramírez take. Ramírez belonged to the world of that medical sub-profession which is covered by the imprecise concept of 'quack', which is specially applied to a healer in sixteenth-century Spain. The morisco doctor we are going to deal with, however, stands within a medical tradition of medical education that still existed in the sixteenth century in which, we should once more emphasize, both medical professional models characteristic of the late middle ages coexist. The doctor in question, Gaspar Capdal, must have practised in the Kingdom of Valencia (Buñol, Requena and Valencia city). His testimony was recorded by the inquisitorial clerks as follows:

> He was born in Buñol; as soon as he could talk he became interested in learning how to read and write the language of the *algemía* [foreign language] which he was taught by a son of Martin Hernández, Old Christian, and the parson of Buñol . . . At the age of ten he moved to Requena and Valencia to study medicine . . . He knows how to read and write *algemía*, and not to read and write Arabic and he studied medicine with a doctor named Catalá at Requena and he studied through a book named Metiolosenes [Pietro Andrea Mattioli] and another named compendium of human health which is said to be written by the saints Cosmas and Damian and through another book named a practical manual (*practica*) by Pascual (Miguel Juan Pascual) and through the book by Fragoso (Juan Fragoso) on trees and *The Thesaurus of the Poor* (Spanish translation of *Thesaurus Pauperum* by Petrus Hispanus) and that he has not studied in any other place and has no books but only papers that he, from the cited books, has copied. After studying with Catalá he had conversations for two years with Master Damian, New Christian, resident in Valencia, at the apothecary Ynca's home.[81]

This text clearly shows how his own tradition had been forgotten (he could not read or write Arabic); if the interrogator had suspected him of doing so matters would not have been at all favourable for him. He was a morisco totally integrated in a society consisting of Old and New Christians in which the everyday act of living together with them was more normal and less tense than it appears through the narrow window of the inquisitorial processes. The fascination exerted by academic medicine and its obvious scientific and social prestige is something that shows itself throughout Capdal's testimony. He is proud of his knowledge of the new scientific languages (Spanish, Italian) which allowed him to acquire an adequate scientific training. This training proceeds according to the medieval model of open professional learning, away from the closed, institutional learning of the university. This model, still extant in the sixteenth century, and which was an important tradition in the Arabic and

Christian medicine of the late middle ages, is based upon a learning process, both theoretical and practical, that is carried out under one or several doctors. The learning period usually lasted several years. Through that time, the medical apprentice read medical texts, explained and annotated by his master, who gave him selected books. This period was completed with one or two years of practical medical training under the tuition and vigilance of an experienced doctor who had a licence issued by the authorities. In the case of Valencia this was a jury of doctors appointed by the Town Hall. After this training, whoever wanted to practise legally, obtained the necessary certificate from his masters and appeared before the jury who examined him on theoretical as well as practical aspects of medicine. The jury's judgements varied from rejection to admission, through to licences for a longer or shorter period of practice under an experienced doctor, or ones which did not allow their holders to treat certain diseases which required complicated therapeutics.[82]

Gaspar Capdal followed this model of professional training step by step. First of all, he learned Spanish (*algemía*), a relatively new tool for learning academic medicine; the term *algemia*, in its etymological sense, means 'foreign language'. As the Valencian moriscos remained very islamized they spoke, as their mother tongue, the *algaravía* or dialect Arabic language (which was very corrupt). For them, any other language, Spanish, Latin, Italian, was *algemia*.[83] From the medical literature handled by Capdal, we conclude that it was Spanish that he learned with 'Martín Hernández, an Old Christian, and with the parson of Buñol'. His knowledge of Spanish enabled him to read an Italian medical text. He studied under doctor Catalá, who practised in Requena (Valencia).

According to the cited works, the learning of Capdal had two sources: treatises of practical medicine (which we could call handbooks of internal and external medicine) and writings on medicinal therapeutics, basically on medical herbs. The first consists mainly of Vigo's *Short Practical Manual in Surgery* (1517) translated into Spanish by Miguel Juan Pascual (*c.* 1505–61), professor at the school of medicine in Valencia from 1542. The second, medical therapeutics, is represented by the work of Pietro Andrea Mattioli (1501–77) and Juan Fragoso (*c.* 1530–97).

Miguel Juan Pascual[84] did not, however, merely translate Vigo's handbook into Spanish; he added to it his marginal notes (*addiciones marginales*). To give an idea of the variety – and at the same time the complexity and subtlety – of the contents of this kind of work, it suffices to say that it deals in a more or less systematic way with anatomy, wounds, abscesses, ulcers, syphilis, fractures, simple medicines, mineral remedies, diseases of the different parts of the body, and so on. There are two elements in Pascual's translation that we should stress: one is the arabicized Galenism, whose main source of inspiration is the *Canon* of Avicenna; the other was the growing demand to convert direct contact with reality into a source of knowledge. This reflects a current of thought which originated and had its clearest development in Italian medical circles. Outstanding in this current was Berengario da Carpi (*c.* 1460–*c.* 1530), author, among other writings, of the book which brought up to date the *Anathomia* by Mondino de Luzzi (*c.* 1275–1326), a compendium of Galenist anatomy written in Bologna at the beginning of the fourteenth century (1316). The modern authors were frequently mentioned by Miguel Juan Pascual in his marginal notes. The traditional component is represented, above all, by Vigo's own work, which is more or less a simple compilation of that arabicized Galenism we mentioned above; on the other hand, many of Pascual's additions are intended to criticize or correct Avicenna's opinions. Where this aspect can be most clearly seen is in the sections on anatomy where Pascual gives priority to his own personal experience over the authority of Avicenna. His argument is quite simple: 'I have seen it myself'.[85]

If we have dwelt at some length on all these details, it is because we want to draw attention to the rich and complex world of medical thought and subject matter in which Gaspar Capdal (born *c.* 1579) was involved during his medical training in the Valencia of the 1590s.

The second of the sources around which our morisco doctor's learning evolved, was that of therapeutics. This was represented, as we have said, in his medical education and practice by the works of the Italian Pietro Andrea Mattioli (1501–77) and the Spaniard Juan Fragoso (*c.* 1530–97). The former became doctor to the Austrian Court (Ferdinand I and Maximilian II) in Prague. Right from the very start of his medical studies in Padua he showed a special interest in natural history and particularly in herbal medicine. This interest led him to publish in Venice (1544) the work which was to make him famous: his annotated translation into Italian of the classical treatise on therapeutics written by Dioscorides. The first Italian edition has as its title: *The five books by Pedanius Dioscorides of Anazarbus on Natural History and Therapeutics translated into the Italian language by M. Pietro Andrea Mattioli of Siena with extensive commentaries, notes and learned annotations and criticism by the translator himself.*[86] The Italian edition was the one the morisco Gaspar Capdal studied and later used in his pharmaceutical and medical practice. Indeed, when he tells the Inquisitors of the medical books that he handled, he refers to Mattioli's work in its Italian edition: 'And (I) studied through a book called Matiolosanes (=*Mathiolo Sanese*)'.[87] Ten years later (Venice, 1554) Mattioli was to publish the Latin edition of Dioscorides' work aimed at an academic and more-demanding public. The aim of the Italian translation was more modest but no less useful: he wanted to provide doctors and apothecaries with a practical manual which would enable them to identify, pick, store and supply medicinal herbs. The success of the Italian edition was so great that it was published in a fuller revised and illustrated edition in 1548, 1550 and 1552.[88]

Juan Fragoso (*c.* 1530–97) - the second of the authors mentioned from whose works the morisco doctor acquired knowledge of therapeutics – was surgeon to the Court of Philip II from 1570 onwards and he, too, was preoccupied by herbal medicine, which he summarized in a series of works written in Latin. In 1572 he did, however, publish a book in Spanish on simple medicines entitled *A Description of Aromatic Herbs, Trees, Fruit Trees, and many other simple medicines brought from the East Indies, which are of use in medicine*, which is based on the contributions of the naturalists García d'Orta and Nicolás Monardes.[89] This was the work used by Caspar Capdal.

To these sources we have to add a handbook, probably about hygiene, a sort of compendium that was a part of the artisan learning supported by the guild of barbers and surgeons under the protection of saints Cosmas and Damien,[90] and a *Thesaurus of the Poor*, supposedly written by Petrus Hispanus (*c.* 1277), a very popular handbook on therapy. He did not, probably, have sufficient money to acquire a necessary minimum of books, and this was why he resorted to the medieval procedure, which was completely normal by then among physicians and surgeons, of making a copy of medical writings, or the parts he was most interested in, for his medical practice. His training on patients and his expertise in the preparation of drugs he received from a morisco doctor, 'Master Damien, a New Christian', and the apothecary Ynca from Valencia.

As we have seen, this medical 'knowledge' which fed morisco healers outside universities circulated through identifiable channels: the oral tradition; empirical practice; training in which the medical doctor is seen as a craftsman and medicine as a craft; and the contact, however weak, with a double written tradition which, despite its academic origins, was popular. This tradition was linked, on the one hand, to the most interesting aspects of Arab therapeutics (like the treatment for scabies) and, on the other, to the therapy of the Christian academic world of 'medical humanism', such as the translation of the book of therapeutic pharmacology of Dioscorides into Italian and Spanish by Mattioli and Laguna respectively, or the current medical literature produced in the Christian faculties of medicine and written in non-Latin languages.

1 cf. my works 'Una Posibilidad Frustrada en la España del Siglo XVI: el arabismo como vía de acceso a las fuentes médicas griegas', *Cuadernos de Historia de la Medicina Española* (Salamanca), XIII (1974), 219–32; 'The Minority of Morisco Physicians in the Spain of the 16th Century and their Conflicts in a Dominant Christian Society', *Sudhoffs Archiv*, LX (1976), 209–34; *Medicina, Ciencia y Minorías Marginades: los Moriscos* (Granada, 1977); 'The Circulation and Use of Medical Manuscripts in Arabic in 16th Century Spain'. *J. Hist. Arabic Sci.*, III (1979), 190–213; *Los Moriscos y la Medicina* (Barcelona, 1984).

2 L. García-Ballester, *Historia Social de la Medicina en la España de los Siglos XIII al XVI* (Madrid, 1976).

3 L. García-Ballester, 'Los Orígenes de la Profesión Médica en Cataluña: el *Collegium* de dédicos de Barcelona (1342), in *Estudios dedicados a Juan Peset Aleixandre* (Valencia, 1982), II, pp. 129–49; *Arch. Mun. Valencia*, Tacha Real, K^3, 3–6.

4 L. García-Ballester, 'The Minority of Morisco Physicians. . .', 216–20.

5 *Arch. Hist. Nac.* (A.H.N.), Madrid, Inquisición de Valencia, leg. 552, no. 33.

6 J. Ribera, *Disertaciones y Opúsculos*, 2 vols. (Madrid, 1928), I,, p. 427.

7 A. Castro, *Sobre el Nombre y el Quién de los Españoles* (Madrid, 1973), p. 276.

8 C. E. Dubler, *La 'Materia Médica' de Dioscórides: Transmisión medieval y renacentista*, 6 vols. (Barcelona, 1953–5).
9 L. García-Ballester, *Historia Social de la Medicina* . . ., p. 65–9.
10 J. M. López Piñero, 'Daza Chacón, Dionisio', in J. M. López Piñero *et al.* (eds.), *Diccionario Histórico de la Ciencia Moderna en España*, 2 vols. (Barcelona, 1983), I, pp. 272–4.
11 *Ibid.*, I, pp. 502–5.
12 T. Rothman, 'Laguna's Commentaries on Hallucinogenic Drugs and Witchcraft in Dioscorides' "Materia Medica"', *Bull. Hist. Med.*, XLVI (1972), 562–7.
13 A. Laguna, *Pedacio Dioscorides Anazarbeo Acerca de la Materia Medicinal y de los Venenos Mortíferos* (Amberes, 1555), book IV, ch. LXXV, fos. 42–2.
14 cf. J. M. López Piñero, *Ciencia y Técnica en la Sociedad Española de los Siglos XVI y XVII* (Barcelona, 1979).
15 P. Rossi, *Los Filósofos y las Máquinas, 1400–1700*, Spanish transl. (Barcelona, 1965).
16 J. M. López Piñero, *Ciencia y Técnica* . . ., pp. 154–63.
17 L. García-Ballester, 'La Cirugía en la Valencia del Siglo XV', *Cuadernos Historia Medicina Española* (Salamanca), VI (1977), 155–71.
18 D. Daza Chacón, *Práctica y Teórica de Cirugía en Romance y en Latín*, two parts (Madrid, 1678), 2nd part, p. 195.
19 *Ibid.*
20 L. García-Ballester, 'Las Obras Médicas de Luis Collado (*m.* 1589). Nota a propósito de un manuscrito del British Museum (Sloane MS. 2489), *Asclepio*, XXIII (1971), 263–70; J. M. López Piñeiro, 'Collado, Luis', in J. M. López Piñeiro *et al.* (eds.), *Diccionario Histórico* . . ., I, pp. 234–6.
21 A. H. N., Inquisición de Valencia, leg. 840. The emphasis is ours.
22 cf. L. Cardaillac, *Morisques et Chrétiens. Un affrontement polémique (1492–1640)* (Paris, 1977); A. Domínguez Ortíz and B. Vincent, *Historia de los Moriscos. Vida y tragedia de una minoría* (Madrid, 1978).
23 J. Ribera, 'Una Colección de Manuscritos Arabes y Aljamiados', in *Disertaciones y Opúsculos*, 2 vols. (Madrid, 1928), I, pp. 417–33; 'Supersticiones moriscas', in *ibid.*, I, 493–527.
24 F. Pons Boigues, 'La Inquisión y los Moriscos de Valencia', *El Archivo* (Denia), II (1887–88), pp. 230–2, 251–8, 309–14.
25 C. Lisón, 'Breve Historical Brujesco Gallego', in *Ensayos de Antropología Social* (Madrid, 1973), pp. 165–226.
26 J. Ribera, 'Supersticiones Moriscas', I, pp. 512–13.
27 Archivo Diocesano de Cuenca (A.D.C.), Inquisición, leg. 343, no. 48–76.
28 C. Lisón, 'Breve Historical Brujesco Gallego', pp. 216 ff.
29 A.D.C., Inquisición, leg. 343, no. 48.
30 *Ibid.*
31 A.H.N., Inquisición de Valencia, leg. 840.
32 'Ysti (medici) Morischi medentur infirmis, de quorum salute desperarunt medici Christiani', cf. J. Bleda, *Defensio Fidei in Causa Neophitorum sive Morischorum Regni Valentiae* (Valencia, 1610), p. 368.

33 B. Malinowski, *Magic, Science and Religion and other Essays* (New York, 1955).
34 J. Ribera, 'Supersticiones Moriscas', I, pp. 512–13.
35 A.H.N., Inquisición de Valencia, leg. 549, no. 13.
36 *Ibid.*
37 *Ibid.*
38 J. Ribera, 'Supersticiones Moriscas', I, p. 512.
39 A.H.N., Inquisición de Toledo, leg. 192, no. 4.
40 A.H.N., Inquisición de Valencia, leg. 551.
41 *Ibid.*, leg. 551, no. 14.
42 *Ibid.*
43 *Constituciones Sinodales del Arzobispado de Granada hechas por el Ilustrísimo señor D. Pedro Guerrero . . . en el mes de octubre de 1572* (Granada, 1573), book V.
44 L. García-Ballester, *Medicina, Ciencia y Minorías Marginadas: los Moriscos* (Granada, 1977), pp. 22–3, 37–9.
45 A. Domínguez Ortíz and B. Vincent, *Historia de los Moriscos*, pp. 122–41.
46 *Actas Cortes de Castilla* (Madrid, 1607), November thirteenth, vol. XXIII, pp. 583–7.
47 *Ibid.*, p. 587. The French historian Le Flem in his researches on the Inquisition trial at Valladolid (1594) has found one morisco doctor and another morisco surgeon in Avila and only one morisco medical student registered in the faculty of medicine at the University of Valladolid. It is very difficult to find the name of a morisco student in the university registers because, as Le Flem says: 'the moriscos belonging to the upper classes resolved to conceal their "impure origin"'. J. P. Le Flem, 'Les Morisques du nord-ouest de l'Espagne en 1594 d'après un Recensement de l'Inquisition de Valladolid', *Melanges Casa de Velázquez*, I (1965), p. 233.
48 *Actas Cortes de Castilla*, p. 583.
49 *Ibid.*, pp. 583–4 and A.H.N. Inquisición de Valencia, leg. 840.
50 *Actas* . . ., p. 584.
51 *Ibid.*, p. 586.
52 *Ibid.*, p. 587.
53 *Ibid.*, p. 585.
54 L. S. Granjel, 'El Ejercicio de la Medicina en la Sociedad Española Renacentista', *Cuadernos Historia Medicina Española*, X (1971), 13–53.
55 *Actas* . . ., p. 585.
56 L. Alonso Muñoyerro, *La Facultad de Medicina en la Universidad de Alcalá de Henares* (Madrid, 1945), p. 152.
57 *Actas* . . ., p. 585.
58 B. Vincent, 'L'Expulsion des Morisques du Royaume de Grenade et leur Repartition en Castille (1570–1)'. *Melanges Casa de Velázquez*, VI (1970), 211–46.
59 B. Vincent, 'L'Albaicín de Grenade au XVI siècle (1527–87). *Melanges Casa de Velázquez*, VII (1971), 187–222.
60 B. Vincent, 'L'Expulsion . . ., p. 213.
61 A. Domínguez Ortíz, 'Los Moriscos Granadinos antes de su Definitiva

Expulsión, *Miscelánea Estudios Arabes y Hebreos* (Granada), XII–XIII (1963–4), p. 118.
62 *Ibid.*
63 *Tratado acerca de los Moriscos (1605–6)*, Bibl. Nac. Madrid, MS. 8888, fo. 54r.
64 'Quod autem hoc ita sit, constat de multis medicis, praesertim de illo Gandiensi Pachet (the Morisco physician), qui curavit dominum nostrum Regum adhuc infantulum'. J. Bleda, *Defensio Fidei . . .*, p. 368.
65 H. Lapeyre, *Géographie de l'Espagne Morisque* (Paris, 1559), p. 125.
66 B. Vincent, L'Expulsion . . ., p. 225.
67 L. de Toro, *De Febris Epidemicae et Novae, quae latinae puncticularis, vulgo Tavardillo, et Pintas dicitur, Natura, Cognitione, et Medela* (Burgos, 1574).
68 *Ibid.*, fos. 11v and 27r.
69 A.D.G., Inquisición, leg. 343, no. 48.
70 On the medical teaching in the Saragossa *madrasa* during the second half of the fifteenth century, cf. L. García-Ballester, *Historia social de la Medicina . . .*, p. 72–7.
71 On the relationship between morisco doctors and Christian apothecaries, cf. A.H.N., Inquisición de Valencia, leg. 551, no. 14 and leg 552, no. 9.
72 A.D.C., Inquisición, leg. 347, no. 48.
73 *Ibid.*
74 J. Huarte de San Juan, *Examen de Ingenios para las Sciencias. Donde se muestra la differencia de habilidades que ay en los hombres, y el género de letras que a cada uno responde en particular* (Baeza, 1575).
75 cf. L. García-Ballester, 'The Circulation and Use . . .'
76 J. Ribera, *Disertaciones y Opúsculos*, I, p. 228.
77 L. Cardaillac sustains the same opinion; cf. his book *Morisques et Chrétiens . . .*, p. 58.
78 A.H.N., Inquisición de Valencia, leg. 552, no. 9.
79 *Ibid.*
80 L. Cardaillac, *Morisques et Chrétiens . . .*, p. 58.
81 A.H.N., Inquisición de Valencia, leg. 549, no. 19.
82 L. García-Ballester, *Historia Social de la Medicina . . .*, p. 20 ff. and 'Los Orígenes de la Profesión Médica en Cataluña . . .', pp. 129–32.
83 L. Cardaillac, *Morisques et Chrétiens . . .*, p. 30.
84 Pascual's translation of Vigo's *Practica in Arte Chirurgica Compendiosa* appeared for the first time in Valencia (1537) entitled *Libro o Pratica in Cirurgia del muy famoso y experto doctor Juan de Vigo . . . Traducido de lengua latina en castellana por el doctor Miguel Juan Pascual, Valenciano.* The popularity of this translation is shown by the fact that it was reprinted three times in the sixteenth century (1548, 1564 and 1581). cf. J. M. López Piñero, 'Pascual, Miguel Juan', in J. M. López Piñero *et al.* (eds.), *Diccionario Histórico . . .*, II, pp. 144–5.
85 López Piñero emphasizes that Pascual, in opposition to those who denied the existence of the bile duct in the normal organism, states: 'This opinion is false because, whereas an abnormality is rarely found, we often see this duct. I, myself, have seen it'. M. J. Pascual, *Libro o Practica in Cirurgia . . .* (Valencia, 1548), book I: 'De la nothomia', ff. xiii–xiv.

86 *Di Pedacio Dioscoride Anazarbeo libri cinque. Dell'Historia, et Materia Medicinale tradotti in lingua volgare italiana da M. Pietro Andrea Mathiolo Sanese medico. Con amplissimi discorsi, et comenti, et doctrissime annotation, et censure del medesimo interprete* . . . (Venice, 1544). cf. B. Zanobio, 'Mattioli, P.A.G.', in Ch. C. Gillispie (ed.), *Dictionary of Scientific Biography*, 15 vols. (New York, 1970–80), ix, pp. 178–80.

87 cf. quotation above.

88 cf. B. Zanobio, 'Mattioli, P.A.G.', in DSB, vol. 9, p. 179.

89 *Discurso de las Cosas Aromáticas, Arboles y Frutales, y de otras muchas Medicinas Simples que se traen de la India Oriental, y que sirven al uso de la medicina* (Madrid, 1572). cf. J. M. López Piñero, 'Fragoso, Juan', in J. M. López Piñero *et al.* (eds.), *Diccionario histórico* . . ., I, pp. 355–6.

90 L. García-Ballester, 'La Cirugía en la Valencia del Siglo XV', *Cuadernos Historia Medicina Española*, VI (1967), 155–71.

IX

The Inquisition and minority medical practitioners in Counter-Reformation Spain

Judaizing and Morisco practitioners, 1560–1610

The medical history that we read and write today is still based mostly on the *writings* of an *élite* of medical men.

(E.H. Ackerknecht 1967)

Introduction: the problem of the minorities in sixteenth-century Spain

During the fourteen and fifteenth centuries, the Christian-controlled areas of Spain contained two substantial minority groups: the Jews, and those Moslems who had not departed for the lands still controlled by their co-religionists. The members of both minorities underwent persecution during these centuries at the hands of members of the Christian majority, and this became particularly intense from the late fourteenth century (1391) onwards. Many Jews therefore converted to Christianity. These 'New Christians' of Jewish origin were known by the name of 'Conversos'.[1] By contrast, mass conversion did not take place among the Moslem minority until they were forced to adopt Christianity at the beginning of the sixteenth century. After their conversion, the converted Moors were given the name 'Moriscos'.[2]

On a number of occasions I have considered the history of medicine among the Morisco minority in Spain in the sixteenth century and the first decade of the seventeenth century. I have studied the process of disintegration of their medical system, as well as the characteristics of their kind of medicine and of their medical practice.[3] Here I shall undertake a comparative study of the differing attitudes that the Inquisition held towards physicians of these two minorities: towards those who belonged to the Morisco minority, and towards those who were suspected of being descended from the old Jewish population. The different social circumstances of the two groups led to differing modes of action towards them on the part of the Inquisition. I shall concentrate on the period between 1560 and 1610, as these dates coincide with the peak period of the

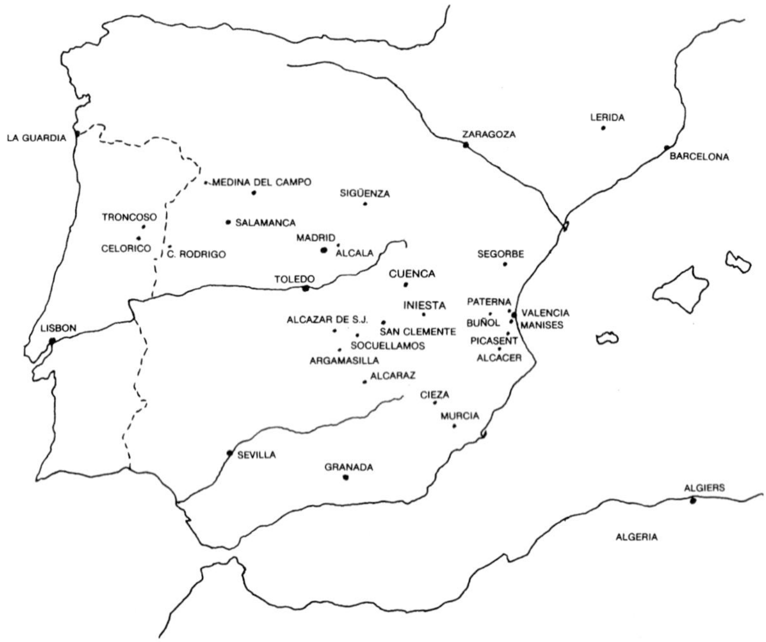

Illustration 8 Map of Spain, Portugal and North Africa, showing towns and cities referred to in chapter 8.

Counter-Reformation in Spain, and since the members of the Morisco minority were expelled from the lands of the Spanish monarchy at the end of this period.

The 'Judaizers' or 'Marranos'

Many of the converted Jews were sincere Christians. Many others believed that it would be possible to lead a double life with respect to their religious beliefs. This gave rise to a new social category, described by the legal and theological term of 'Judaizer' and the popular expression 'Marrano'.[4] As from the fifteenth century, converted Jews were suspected of 'Judaizing' or reverting to their original faith. This suspicion was based on purely ritual indications related to the Jewish religion (cleansing of the hands, washing of meat, rejection of pork, death rituals, among others), and also on forms of religious behaviour which were suspect from the point of view of what was subsequently defined as Catholic orthodoxy (for example, anticlericalism, particularly towards the religious orders; reticence towards the cult of saints, and to the status of the Virgin Mary, and certain forms of messianic expectation).[5]

The Conversos were the victims of riots and massacres in the fifteenth century. But this was not only due to religious reasons. The political complexity and economic difficulties of the Hispanic Kingdoms also played an important part. In 1478, the new monarchy inaugurated by the marriage of the so-called 'Catholic Monarchs' (Isabella, Queen of Castile, and Ferdinand, King of Aragon) introduced the Inquisition.[6] The same monarchs signed the decree expelling the Jews from Spain in 1492. In this way, the Jewish problem disappeared from Spain, although the Conversos continued to be suspected as possible Judaizers.[7] One of the purposes of the Inquisition was precisely to control the religious life of the Conversos.[8] In 1492 many of the Spanish Jews left for Portugal, where they were eventually forced to convert by a wide variety of methods. There was a long frontier between the two countries, and from 1580 to 1640 Portugal was incorporated under the Spanish crown.[9] This brought about a flow of Portuguese Conversos towards Spain, and the two Jewish communities were linked by many family ties as well as by intermarriage. Thus, as we shall see, it is somewhat artificial to separate Portuguese Judaizers (or suspect Conversos) from Spanish ones in the Counter-Reformation period.[10]

For Jewish physicians, conversion was something more than a personal or collective religious issue. For it also had repercussions in the field of medical practice. In effect, conversion to Catholicism carried with it the prospect of economic improvement for the members of Converso families, and this opened the doors of the universities for them; this was particularly attractive to them because of their traditional high regard for learning. This was a new situation which their ancestors, with their Jewish faith, had not been able to enjoy, for access to the faculties of medicine had been only open to Christians. As we shall see, all the trials of Converso physicians, held in the various Spanish inquisitorial courts (1560–1610), rested upon accusations of Judaizing. In none of them - at least in none of the cases from this half century - were accusations made against them of deviant medical practices, such as the invocation of devils, witchcraft, the use of charms and spells, and other such practices rejected by academic medicine. Almost all the Converso physicians who appeared in the Inquisition's courts had undertaken university studies (see Table 2).

Throughout the sixteenth century, but more especially in the first and last third, the so-called 'condition of purity of blood' was imposed on the 'New Christians' within the lands of Spain, and especially against the Conversos, probably because of the greater social prestige of the posts that they occupied. This measure, which aimed at preventing anyone who might be 'stained' with Jewish blood from holding any post in society (whether civil or ecclesiastic), was contrary to the principle of social unity applying to all those who had received baptism and it was therefore not accepted by Spanish Catholicism; hence it was an element of great social unrest.[11] The 'purity of blood' measures spread to the universities. An example of this movement can be seen in the constitutions of the University College of San Ildefonso (1519), which belonged to the prestigious new University of Alcalá:

> It is ordained that no one shall be admitted nor elected as a member of the college . . . without it first being ascertained that he is neither a son of, nor a descendant of, a Jew, or Moor, or 'Converso' . . . and if on any occasion, whether by error, or by fraud or by negligence, any such person should be elected, he shall be expelled from the College . . . The information should be drawn up concerning his parents and four grandparents.[12]

In spite of these measures to prevent the descendants of 'New Christians' from entering the faculties of medicine, the descendants of the Conversos found ways to get round these prohibitions.[13] The Converso physician, like the Converso population in general, intermingled with the 'Old Christian' population after 1492. They were not an identifiable social grouping. Yet the Conversos were hampered by the climate of suspicion towards them, which varied during the sixteenth century, but which became particularly strong during the Counter-Reformation, leading to an obsession on the part of the Inquisition with particular settlements and instititions, both civil and ecclesiastic, where accusations of Judaizing had accumulated against certain families or individuals.[14]

The Moriscos

By the beginning of the sixteenth century the Spanish monarchy had expelled those of its subjects that belonged to the Jewish faith, but it continued to have in its territories a substantial population which had an Islamic cultural background and practised the Moslem religion. This population was by no means uniformly distributed over the whole country. It hardly existed in the northern parts of the peninsula, nor in Catalonia, with the exception of the southernmost districts forming part of the Ebro valley, while the Moslems formed but a small minority in the extensive territories of Castile and western Andalucia (the Guadalquivir valley). By contrast, they represented a third of the total population in Aragon, Valencia and Murcia, and an even higher proportion in the areas of eastern Andalucia, which coincided with what had been the old Arab Kingdom of Granada. In Portugal there were also Moslems whose background was similar to that of their co-religionists in the other kingdoms of the Iberian Peninsula. Christian society would no longer tolerate the presence in its midst of non-Christians, and thus proceeded with the mass enforced baptism of Moslems. By the 1520s the vast majority of Moslems were officially Christians. These 'new Christians' were, as mentioned above, known as Moriscos. Between 1569 and 1571, the whole Morisco population of the former Kingdom of Granada was expelled, most of them settling in Castile. This expulsion was the punishment imposed on them for the revolt that they had staged against the so-called 'Old Christians' who had been oppressing them. Thus the dream of the first Archbishop of Granada, Hernando de Talavera, to count among his faithful an Arabic-speaking Christian population, was shattered once and for all.[15]

However, the water of baptism would not wash away the fact that they belonged to the Islamic culture, nor their old faith, which the majority of them continued to practise in secret, and which was transmitted - as in the case of many Jewish Conversos - by means of oral tradition. One manifestation of this was the continued survival and the use of the Arabic language (*algarabía*), especially among those living in Valencia, Murcia and Granada, as well as a series of rituals connected with everyday life (such as meals, clothes, and wedding and death rituals) that identified them as a group; an external sign of their continued adherence to Moslem tradition was the continued practice of circumcision, a custom which had a deep cultural significance rather than just a strictly religious one. Furthermore, when the Moriscos constituted a minority of the population of a settlement, then they clustered in particular districts. The 'Old Christians' and the Moriscos were in constant conflict throughout the sixteenth century. As the century progressed, and in particular after the decrees of 1566–7, the 'Old Christians' instituted measures to eradicate the defining differential characteristics of the Morisco population, with the clear aim of marginalizing them in both social and economic terms. One of these characteristics was the form of medicine they practised.[16] Ultimately, between 1609 and 1612, King Philip III decreed the expulsion of all the Moriscos from his realms.[17]

Unlike the Converso, who might be poor but never a serf, the Morisco had a social status typical of that of the serf in feudal society. With few exceptions their new Christian faith did not allow young Moriscos to enter universities in order to study medicine, whereas this was feasible in the case of members of reasonably wealthy Jewish Converso families (such as the sons of physicians, artisans or merchants). Moslem healers - and in general the whole system of medical attention available for the Morisco population - were affected by the general disintegration of their cultural way of life.[18]

The drama affecting the 'New Christians' (both Conversos and Moriscos), the growing tension that they experienced from the last third of the sixteenth century onwards, was the most serious social problem of

Spanish society. The expulsion of the Moriscos, hardly a hundred years after the expulsion of the other great minority – the Jews who refused to accept baptism (1492) – was the greatest social upheaval that Spain underwent during the period of the Counter-Reformation. The vast society ruled by the Spanish Crown (Portugal, Castile, Aragon, other European lands and the extensive overseas territories) may have gained in uniformity, but it lost in freedom and openness. In this process, the Spanish monarchy not only made use of all the political means available to it within secular society to control the life of its subjects, but also reinforced its position by using the authority of the Catholic Church. The ecclesiastical institution which pre-eminently supported this process was the Inquisition.[19]

The Inquisition, minorities and medicine

The role of the Inquisition was decisive in the twofold process of, on the one hand, destroying the Islamic culture of the Morisco minority, and on the other of attempting to assimilate the converted members of both the Moriscos and the Conversos within the orthodox form of Catholic Christianity which was imposed in Spain by the Counter-Reformation. The way this was achieved was by delving into all the acts of the everyday life of the Moriscos and Conversos, even at the most intimate level. The Inquisition made use of all available means, especially anonymous accusations. One of the most negative consequences of this was the introduction of fear and mistrust into human relationships and between social groups.[20] This led to situations like that of the wife of Enrique Leiton (*fl.* 1588), a graduate in medicine, who confessed that her husband was ignorant of her Jewish practices, such was her fear that her husband might be put on trial. Despite his wife's efforts, he was arrested and subjected to torture.[21] On other occasions, it was a wife who accused her own husband, as in the case of Luis Castro (*fl.* 1606), doctor in medicine, who was sentenced in his absence because he had managed to flee to France, abandoning his wife and the rest of his family to their fate.[22] Fear did not always destroy solidarity among those living through such dramatic circumstances. One of the accusations made against the physicians Mateo Nuñez (*fl.* 1595) and Felipe de Nájera (1560–*c.*1610) was that of 'having received into their homes fugitives from Portugal fleeing from the Holy Office'.[23] Mere possession of the medical works of Isaac Israeli came to be a motive for suspicion for the Inquisition 'because the author was Jewish'.[24] For this reason, it is not at all surprising that the Inquisition should have been perceived by Moriscos as the very symbol of repression, especially from the 1570s onwards, and that the Converso accused of being a Judaizer should consider it to be worse than 'the devil himself'.[25]

Table 1 Offences recorded by the Court of the Inquisition of Toledo (1575–1610)

Offences	*Number of cases*
Judaizers	174
Moriscos	190
For not considering fornication as a crime	264
Blasphemy	46
Witchcraft	18
Heresy	62
Soliciting in confession	52
Total	806

Source: H. Kamen, *The Spanish Inquisition*, London, 1965.

The Inquisition's state of near obsession with the Jewish and the Moslem minorities of medieval and Renaissance Spain becomes immediately apparent simply by reading and comparing the tables of those cases recorded by the court of the Inquisition of Toledo between 1575 and 1610, the period of the full social implementation of the Counter-Reformation in Spain (see Table 1).

As can be seen, trials of Judaizers and Moriscos amount to 364 (45 per cent); those of the Moriscos alone made up almost a quarter of the total.

While these figures are highly revealing, those referring to the numbers of healers (physicians, surgeons and barbers) are not so striking. Hardly a dozen Morisco healers can be traced in all the Inquisition courts (not only those of Toledo). Between 1560 and 1610, the number of Converso physicians, or members of their families, tried by the Inquisition (according to the material surviving from all the courts) is 36, nine of whom were of Portuguese origin (see Table 2).

It is true that the death sentence was in general hardly ever applied to Moriscos by the Inquisition courts. The ratio between death sentences/sentences in the courts of Zaragoza (Aragon), Cuenca (Castile), Granada and Murcia in the late sixteenth century, was in the region of 1 to 40.[26] For the Conversos, while no such ratio is available, it can be safely said that the Inquisition was much stricter and that Conversos were often condemned to death.[27] In the case of Judaizing physicians put on trial in the period 1560–1610, the ratio was 1 to 5. Generally speaking, the Inquisition preferred to impose fines, stimulated as it was by the increasing need for money to cover the expenses incurred by its own bureaucracy. For this reason, special contributions were agreed upon with Morisco communities, and in the case of Conversos sentences included the confiscation of their worldly goods and possessions. For example, of the 36 Converso physicians or members of the families of Converso physicians, 26 had their property confiscated, two were heavily fined, seven were acquitted and seven were condemned to death. The

Inquisition's greed for money was so infamous that one of the physicians put on trial, the bachelor of medicine Felipe Nájera (1609), at one stage of the interrogation, after undergoing torture,[28] said to the inquisitors: 'if you are doing this because of my estate, take it'.[29] In the case of physicians or healers, professional disqualification for life was added to the sentences (this is made explicit in the sentence imposed upon the Morisco healer Gaspar Capdal).[30]

As a result of all these measures those who were tried were reduced to poverty, together with their families. In the case of the Moriscos, the more numerous and better organized social group, this measure was deliberately taken into account as a means of preventing any improvement in their social status. The Archbishop of Valencia, Juan de Ribera (1532–1611), a typical eccclesiastical representative of the Spanish Church during the Counter-Reformation, was very clear on this matter: 'There is also a great advantage in this measure [punishing them with fines and imposing special taxes], which is that it makes them poor.'[31] The Dominican Friar Bleda, also from Valencia, maintained in the same vein: 'These dogs should not be given the bread of their children, but they must be expelled from colleges and assigned to the galleys, and never to the liberal arts [the step prior to the study of medicine].'[32]

The Inquisition kept up a relentless campaign of harassment against the Morisco minority. The aim was to try to bring about the disappearance of the Morisco cultural identity as such by means of judicial persecution. The magical forms of Morisco healers' medical practice attracted the hostile attention of the Inquisition. The confrontation between the Inquisition and Morisco healers was a confrontation between academic medicine and popular forms of medical practice steeped in magic and empiricism. The very system of medical attention that had been gradually created among the Moriscos (with their own healers), the physician–patient relationship when a Morisco was one of the parties involved, and the body of medical doctrine used by Morisco healers, which was considered to be effective by Morisco (and non-Morisco) patients, these were all carefully monitored and undermined by the Inquisition.[33] The inquisitorial trials in the courts of Toledo, Cuenca and Valencia, against Moriscos who practised medicine, increased in the last third of the sixteenth century and in the first few years of the seventeenth century: that is to say, in the final phase of the disintegration of the medical subculture in the Morisco community and in a Spain dominated by the Counter-Reformation. The Spanish monarchy linked its methods of political control to the Counter-Reformation movement, which was concerned with the preservation of Catholic dogma. Thus a mixture of political, religious and legal ideas was achieved, a mixture that clouded the life of the whole of Spain in this period.[34] What was collected by means of the Inquisition's interrogations demonstrates

Table 2 Medical training of the Judaizing practitioners prosecuted by the Inquisition (1560–1610)

University training	*No. of cases*	*Training unrecorded*	*No. of cases*
Doctors	4	Physicians	6
Licenciates	16	Barber surgeons	2
Bachelors	7		
Student of medicine	1		
Total	28	Total	8

Source: AHN, Inquisitorial records; J. Contreras, Database (personal information).

undeniably the increasingly desperate situation of the Moriscos, the fear and the mistrust permeating the whole of Spanish society, and the wish of the Moriscos to live unmolested and hence in freedom. Christian society in Counter-Reformation Spain was unable to integrate into itself the Morisco attitudes towards illness and medicine, and endow them with social dignity. Faced with these problems, it opted for the easiest solution, which was at the same time the most traumatic: to make the Moriscos disappear.[35]

The fact that Converso physicians were fully integrated within the medical system of the 'establishment' and that they practised the form of medicine that was usual among the Christian majority (I leave aside here the popular forms of medicine, as yet unstudied by historians) meant that the situation that affected Morisco healers did not arise among the Conversos. Converso physicians were tried by the Inquisition for being Judaizers, but not for medical practices deviating from what was considered 'normal' in the neo-scholastic Galenism that flourished in Spanish faculties of medicine in this period.[36] It must be remembered that as from 1559 Spanish universities and their members, both staff and students, were forbidden by Royal decree to maintain intellectual contacts with any other university centre in the rest of Europe. One year earlier (1558) strict control over intellectual publications (from theology to natural philosophy and medicine) had been introduced also by Royal decree; this in fact was the establishment of a proper censor's office, which had negative repercussions on Spanish intellectual life. This kind of measure was another consequence of the Counter-Reformation movement in the Spanish realms.[37]

The Conversos did not possess their own form of medicine, nor did they organize a system of medical care and attention specifically for their own community. The thirty-six Converso healers suspected of Judaizing who were put on trial by the Inquisition between 1560 and 1610, belonged to the medical establishment. Their medical training was as shown in Table 2.

Inquisitorial trials as a source for the study of Morisco and Converso healers

Any Morisco or Converso was liable to be prosecuted by the Holy Office simply because of his status; for this reason, he distrusted all those around him. Whereas civil courts only intervened in the ordinary circumstances to be found in contemporary civilized European society (including Spain), the Inquisition poked into the most remote corners of society without respecting the norms of other courts. Although the degree of strictness it employed was by no means the same in all regions, it was omnipresent. Because of its power and methods, it kept the Moriscos and the Conversos in a state of permanent worry and fear. The Inquisition even prosecuted Moriscos and Judaizers in the Americas and India (Goa), when Goa was incorporated into the territories of Portugal and finally into those of the Spanish Crown between 1580 and 1640.[38]

Paradoxically, the strictness and efficiency demonstrated by the Inquisition enable us to further our knowledge of the medical sociology of the Moriscos, Conversos and Judaizers, providing us with material on their healing activities which would otherwise be very difficult, if not impossible, for us to reconstruct. The same is the case with Converso and Judaizing physicians.[39] The zeal of the Inquisition has enabled us to discover the existence of a not inconsiderable number of general practitioners (the majority of whom were university-trained physicians) who were Conversos, many of them Judaizers, who served as town physicians throughout the length and breadth of Spain. They were the protagonists of a dramatic situation which led many of them into exile, in search of a place where 'they might be well received' and where they could live 'with freedom to be Jews', as a Judaizer confessed,[40] or in order to 'be able to renounce our Holy Catholic faith and apostatize and live in greater freedom in the sect of Mohammed', in the words of a Morisco healer.[41] According to the evidence of Conversos themselves (either directly from those on trial or indirectly from those who had fled), these places were: Italy, and especially Rome (because of the tolerance shown by the Popes themselves in their own territories), France (Bordeaux, Paris, Rouen), the Low Countries (Amberes), Germany (Hamburg), North Africa (Algeria), Turkey (Constantinople) and overseas territories (the New World and Goa).[42]

The current state of research does not allow us to quantify the number of Converso or Morisco physicians who had to go into exile, or to measure the effects that this movement must have had on the sixteenth and seventeenth century Spanish medical system. Even though we are aware that there were more, we have only traced one case of exile among the Morisco healers sought by the Inquisition: that of Jerónimo Jover, which will be considered below. More numerous were the Judaizers who opted for exile. We can instance, among others, the famous physician and naturalist Garcia d'Orta,[43] the pattern of whose life was to be repeated by many Conversos. The son of Spanish Jews who had been deported and who were converted while in Portugal, he undertook medical studies in the Castilian universities of Salamanca and Alcalá (between 1515 and 1522–3). In 1534, he left for Goa, where he died in 1568, without having been troubled, even though the Inquisition had been established there in 1560. His sisters were prosecuted by the Inquisition in Portugal; one of them (Catalina) was tried for a second time in 1568 and burnt at the stake the next year. The trial gave rise to suspicions about Garcia d'Orta, who was tried *post mortem*. On 4 December 1580, his remains were exhumed and burned. His work as a naturalist (*Coloquios dos Simples e Drogas da India*, Goa 1563) was permeated by the memory of his parents' expulsion from Spain (1492) and by his fear of the Inquisition because of his status as a Converso.[44] Another famous contemporary of Garcia d'Orta was Amato Lusitano or Joao Rodriguez de Castello Branco, who, after studying medicine in Salamanca, left for Italy and the Low Countries in 1534, where there was a sizeable colony of exiled Conversos, especially in Amberes.[45] We might also mention Rodrigo de Castro (born in 1548), who went into exile in the Low Countries and later in Hamburg, where he was still living in 1629.[46] To a later generation belonged Zacuto (born 1575), who also studied in Salamanca and who graduated from the minor University at Sigüenza. He was a descendant of the Spanish Jewish astronomer, Abraham Zacuto,[47] who was also exiled to Portugal in 1492. After practising in Lisbon, he went back to Castile in 1625, but subsequently his fear drove him into exile in Amsterdam. It was there that he wrote his history of the most important physicians, *De Medicorum Principum Historia* (Amsterdam, 1629), which is of great interest for this subject, since it informs us, by means of his medical correspondents, of the widespread network that the Conversos formed in the various lands of Europe (including Castile) and overseas, ranging from the Low Countries, Germany and France as far as Turkey and Goa. Their evidence allows us to gain an idea of the importance this continual gradual drain of exiled physicians meant, an outflow that was increased in the period of the Counter-Reformation.[48]

Heresy and minority medical practitioners

The theological and doctrinal justifications for the prohibition of the practice of medicine by Morisco or Converso practitioners were based on a puristic Catholic attitude which had its roots in the years when the early Christian communities had to ask themselves the question: who cures? is it Christ, or the pagan physician who is treating them?[49] Likewise, was it permissible for an 'Old Christian' to be treated by a 'New Christian' who was suspected of being a secret Moslem or Jew?

It is true that the Moriscos and many Conversos were Christians, even if only outwardly. Being constantly suspected by the Church and society of continual deviation, the Inquisition stigmatized them as 'heretics'. This was a very wide term which, according to the famous declaration of the University of Paris in 1398, included all forms of superstitious practice on the part of a Christian, whose results could not reasonably be explained either to be proceeding from God or from nature.[50] This was precisely the way in which the Inquisition attacked Morisco practitioners.

Explicitly or implicitly, it was considered that any cure achieved by a Morisco physician could be nothing other than the work of the devil, and consequently the result of a pact with him. Continuing the line of the theological authorities in Paris, in 1492, Bernardo Basin, a canon of Zaragoza, using a solid (!) scholastic argument, concluded that every pact with the devil, implicit or explicit, should be treated as if it were heresy, whether it was so or not.[51] In the same tradition, in 1552, Bishop Simancas declared that the devil entered all superstitious practices and charm rites, whether man so desired or otherwise.[52] In this way, everything was to be attributed to the 'arts of the devil'. Torreblanca, a Spanish theologian of the late sixteenth century, even suggested in his *Epitome Delictorum sive de Magia*,[53] that in any cure we have to assume the presence of a pact if recited or murmured words are used, even if it involved the merest touch, or the use of a simple piece of clothing with no special properties. There is also a suspicion of a pact if verbal imprecations against the disease are used; these are approved of by the Church but can only be used by those who are in holy orders. And in general, there is suspicion of a pact in any cure of a disease which physicians cannot explain. Consequently, all the activities of healers and charlatans fell under the jurisdiction of the Inquisition. These measures were finally endorsed by Sixtus V's Bull of 1585 (*Caeli et Terrae*).[54] The wide and unrestricted field in which the Inquisition moved meant that any cure carried out by Morisco practitioners which Inquisition experts (that is, physicians at the service of the Holy Office)[55] found difficult to explain was open to the suspicion of having been carried out by means of a pact with the devil. In the trial of the physician Gaspar Casal[56] - a Morisco physician who practised medicine in the town of Buñol, western Valencia, an area with a large number of Morisco inhabitants - the prosecutor concluded:

> 1. I accuse him especially of having an express pact with the devil, with whom he communicates freely, and from whom he knows the

> future and also many other things which human knowledge could not encompass, and in view of this it is very probable that he obeys, venerates and adores the devil. 2. . . . and in accordance with the contents of the preceding chapter, the said 'Morisco' is held to be a physician who carries out extraordinary cures, which could not be achieved by human art, nor by other physicians, and that many people come to him, drawn by his reputation. . . .[57]

To these arguments should be added those derived from professional competition with 'Old Christian' practitioners, in which money and prestige were involved. This is clearly stated by one of the Morisco physicians: 'And since the Morisco received both honour and money [from attending rich patients], he was hated by the [Old Christian] physicians'.[58] This sort of reason gave support to a feeling which we could call 'professional anti-Semitism', both against Converso and Morisco practitioners.[59]

Reasons of a religious/pastoral nature (i.e. those related to the care that religious authorities, as shepherds of their flocks, are supposed to take) gave support to the argument against both Morisco and Judaizing physicians: 'how can a Morisco or a Judaizing physician encourage a patient to confess his sins if he himself does not consider confession a sacrament, or receive Holy Communion either?'[60] If 'Old Christian' physicians were negligent in this respect, how much more probable was it that 'New Christian' physicians would be so? In view of this, Catholic moralists even rejected the consolation that every doctor could offer a patient - even a hopeless case - namely the possibility of a cure. The intransigent moralists of the Spanish Counter-Reformation did not hesitate to condemn one of the most venerable aspects of medical behaviour in the Western medical tradition:

> We must reject the advice of Galen, who taught that a physician should comfort a patient and promise him health, even though it is in fact impossible to save him. This is rejected by St Ambrose, who affirms that the medical precept, in this case, is contrary to the divine condition [i.e. to properly prepare the sick to go to the next life through confessing their sins].[61]

So, 'it is proper for the service of God and for good government that "New Christians" should be prohibited from curing and using the arts of medicine with "Old Christians" '.[62]

The members of the Inquisition courts took special care to establish the degree of Christian training possessed by suspect Converso physicians. They were interrogated about their fulfilment of the obligations to confess and to take communion at least once a year, about their knowledge of the prayers, especially the Lord's Prayer and the Creed, and the Inquisition carefully investigated whether they demonstrated the necessary external signs of pious behaviour (the cult of the saints and devotion to the Virgin Mary). All of these were practices which were encouraged in the Counter-Reformation, following the Council of Trent. Any relaxation on the part of a physician as regards the fulfilment of these practices - having totally or partially forgotten the necessary prayers, indifference towards or rejection of the external signs of devotion - strengthened the suspicions that were harboured about their being Morisco or Judaizing physicians. The evidence in this respect is particularly abundant. There is for instance the case of Felipe de Nájera, bachelor of medicine, who was accused of Judaizing in 1607 before the Inquisition in Toledo, two years after having been accused of homosexuality. He was observed by his cell-mates, who reported him to the Inquisition judges; they noticed that he did not pray in prison[63] - that he even made fun of his fellow prisoners who did[64] and nor did he know how to recite the Creed properly.[65] It was obvious therefore that the precept concerning the need to induce a sick patient to make his confession was not being fulfilled with the diligence that the Fourth Lateran Council (1215) had required.[66] The poorly defined frontier between the physician of the soul and the physician of the body was made use of by the Inquisition, who dusted off this old medieval precept.[67]

Morisco physicians, by contrast, were to be prohibited from treating their own Morisco patients at all. As there was no clearly demarcated professional status amongst Moriscos (which was characteristic of their culture), many of them were 'alfaquíes', meaning individuals practising as teachers, religious and political leaders, and also as healers. For this reason, according to Catholic moralists, 'under the pretext of administering physical remedies or drugs [they] were really spreading the impiety of Mohammedanism'.[68] For these same reasons, Morisco midwives were forbidden to practise in Granada (Synod of Guadix, 1554) and Valencia (1561) since, 'when the children are born, they usually circumcise them. They are only allowed to attend a delivery in the presence of a Christian [i.e. 'Old Christian'] physician or surgeon, who should prevent the rite of circumcision.'[69] Thus the physician was used not to improve medical conditions or to supervise the delivery, but to play a religious and political role. Non-Morisco surgeons who did not carry out this order or those who attempted to resist the pressure of the Church, backed as it was by Royal authority, were frequently prohibited from practising at all.[70] This kind of measure against Morisco practitioners was possible because the Moriscos were a minority who not only lived close together but who also possessed external cultural signs which were easily identifiable,

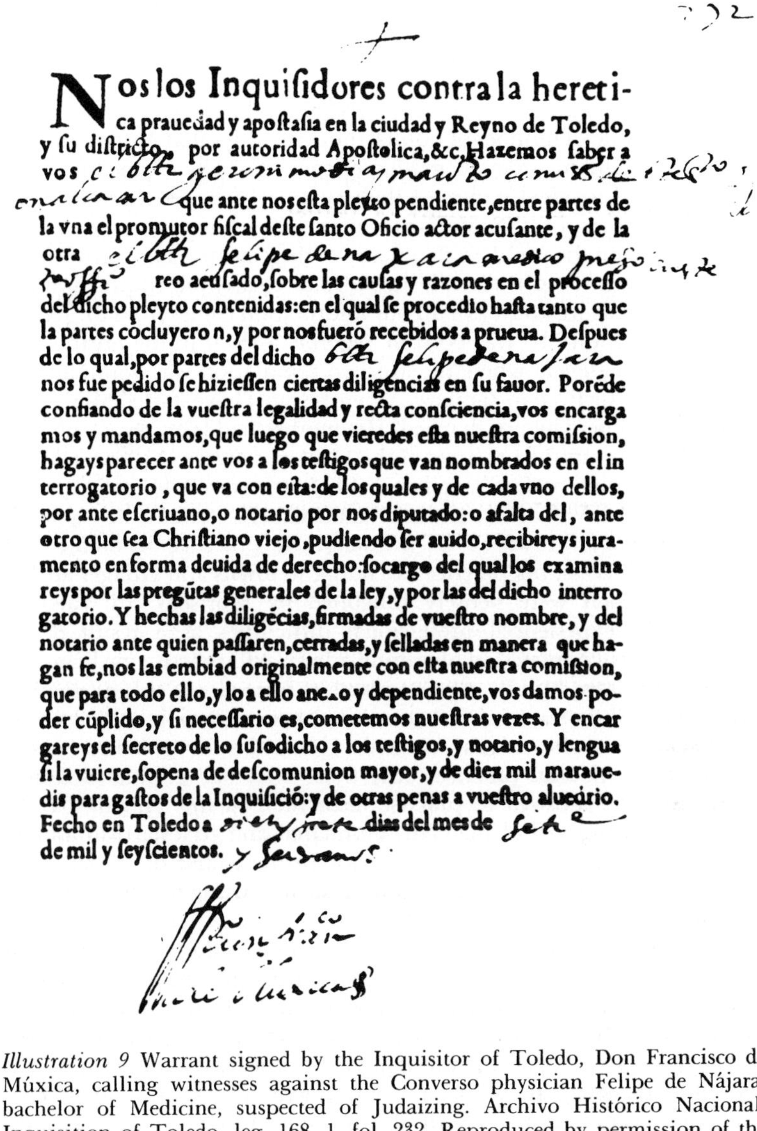

Nos los Inquisidores contra la heretica prauedad y apostasia en la ciudad y Reyno de Toledo, y su districto, por autoridad Apostolica, &c. Hazemos saber a vos que ante nos esta pleyto pendiente, entre partes de la vna el promutor fiscal deste santo Oficio actor acusante, y de la otra reo acusado, sobre las causas y razones en el processo del dicho pleyto contenidas: en el qual se procedio hasta tanto que la partes cócluyeron, y por nos fueró recebidos a prueua. Despues de lo qual, por partes del dicho nos fue pedido se hiziessen ciertas diligencias en su fauor. Poréde confiando de la vuestra legalidad y recta consciencia, vos encargamos y mandamos, que luego que vieredes esta nuestra comision, hagays parecer ante vos a los testigos que van nombrados en el interrogatorio, que va con esta: de los quales y de cada vno dellos, por ante escriuano, o notario por nos diputado: o a falta del, ante otro que sea Christiano viejo, pudiendo ser auido, recibireys juramento en forma deuida de derecho: so cargo del qual los examinareys por las pregútas generales de la ley, y por las del dicho interrogatorio. Y hechas las diligécias, firmadas de vuestro nombre, y del notario ante quien passaren, cerradas, y selladas en manera que hagan fe, nos las embiad originalmente con esta nuestra comission, que para todo ello, y lo a ello anexo y dependiente, vos damos poder cúplido, y si necessario es, cometemos nuestras vezes. Y encargareys el secreto de lo susodicho a los testigos, y notario, y lengua si la vuiere, so pena de descomunion mayor, y de diez mil marauedis para gastos de la Inquisició: y de otras penas a vuestro aluedrio. Fecho en Toledo a dias del mes de de mil y seyscientos.

Illustration 9 Warrant signed by the Inquisitor of Toledo, Don Francisco de Múxica, calling witnesses against the Converso physician Felipe de Nájara, bachelor of Medicine, suspected of Judaizing. Archivo Histórico Nacional, Inquisition of Toledo, leg. 168, 1, fol. 232. Reproduced by permission of the Spanish National Archive, Madrid.

whereas Converso individuals and physicians were scattered among the population as a whole and thus stood out less.

Two case-studies: the Morisco healer Jerónimo Jover and the Converso physician Felipe de Nájera

Jerónomo Jover

The case of the Morisco physician Jerónimo Jover (*fl.* 1577–80) quite clearly illustrates a number of points: the difficulties that Morisco healers were faced with in order to graduate from a faculty of medicine; the empirical and magical nature of their cures, which were basically used among members of the Morisco community, but also among 'Old Christians'; and the problem that many of these healers had to consider – whether or not to go into exile in order to escape the Inquisition and death.[71] As far as we know (for all our information comes from the records of the Inquisition), he was born in Segorbe, a town in the north of the Kingdom of Valencia where the Morisco population was dominant; for part of his life he lived in Zaragoza, where he must have started his medical activity and where he got married. His mother had been responsible for instructing him in the practices of the Moslem religion; he learnt Arabic and read Castilian perfectly, and probably Latin as well. He subsequently left Zaragoza for Valencia, where he remarried. His second wife was a rich 'Old Christian', the widow of a notary. He practised medicine with noteworthy success, his practice extending to towns and villages around Valencia, which were densely inhabited by Moriscos. In Valencia, however, he experienced professional difficulties as a result of the problems he encountered in obtaining a licence to practise medicine.

From the later Middle Ages, university-trained physicians – all of whom were Christians – aimed at uniting their monopoly of knowledge (for medicine could only be studied in faculties of medicine) with a monopoly of medical practice (only those who had graduated from a university were allowed to practise medicine). In this aim they could count on the support of the civil, municipal and ecclesiastical authorities. This double monopoly took shape in the course of the sixteenth century, and in Spain it was linked with the increasing bureaucratization carried out by Philip II (1527–98).

In the last third of the sixteenth century, one could gain access to the practice of medicine through such non-university institutions as the guilds of surgeons and barbers. Their medical practice was controlled and regulated by a state organization (the 'Protomedicato' council) and by the municipal bodies themselves, which could rely on the support of the tribunals which authorized (or not) practice of a profession after the necessary examinations.[72] Both the 'Protomedicato' council and the municipal tribunals were dominated by university-trained physicians and surgeons and became very sensitive to the practice of ensuring 'blood purity'.[73] In the case of Valencia, for example, the municipal tribunal was a jury of doctors appointed by the city council. Anyone who wanted to practise legally had to appear before the jury, who examined them on theoretical as well as practical aspects of medicine. The jury's decisions varied from outright rejection to admission. Licences were granted for a shorter or longer period of practice under the supervision of an experienced doctor, and in some instances licences were granted which did not allow their holders to treat certain diseases which required complicated therapy.[74] In the period under consideration, these tribunals and the university itself were not left unscathed by the social tension existing between 'Old' and 'New Christians'. For reasons which have already been explained, the Morisco healer lacked university education. In spite of this, his services were required, both by the Morisco population and by 'Old Christians' who were suffering illnesses. This gave rise to confrontations between university-trained physicians and Morisco healers. If we consider the documentary sources, the clearest and most explicit confrontations took place after the 1570s and the 1590s, and the motives were clear: '. . . and since [the Morisco] carried off the prestige and the money, the physicians bore him so much hate'.[75] Some of these Morisco physicians who had acquired an improved financial position wished to get round the conflict by obtaining a university qualification, which would protect their medical activity. Let us consider the difficulties involved.

The case of the Morisco healer Jerónimo Jover illustrates the monopoly of knowledge/monopoly of practice binomial very clearly, the first term being expressed by possession of a university qualification, and the second by medical activity which was derived from such a qualification. One of the witnesses of the inquisitorial trial to which Jover was subjected said:

> that the said doctor [Jover] endeavoured to go to Lérida [Catalonia] to graduate, for the physicians would not let him cure since he held no university qualification, because in fact the aforesaid doctor possessed no qualification at all.[76]

An 'Old Christian' from Paterna (a small town near the city of Valencia), an ex-patient of Jover's, pointed out the difficulties that these unqualified Morisco healers continually came across, and also mentioned that they were gradually driven into a corner by the pressure from professionals with a university qualification:

> [The witness] said that in the month of June in the previous year, 1577, doctor Jover, a 'Morisco' physician, went to visit his patients in Paterna and admitted that the physicians of Valencia were doing everything possible to make sure that he did not heal the sick, and that, as a consequence, he had considered departing for the Faculty of Medicine at Lérida to obtain a degree. For that purpose, he was

> carrying quite a substantial sum of money and [he hoped] that, if all went well, he would obtain it within three or four months.[77]

Why, when there was a Faculty of Medicine in Valencia, did he plan to go off to that of Lérida, in Catalonia? From other trials of the Inquisition against other Morisco physicians, we know that the Faculty of Medicine in Valencia was particularly hostile towards Moriscos and that its best-known professor, Luis Collado, a former student of Vesalius, indulged in public debate, and even came to blows, with a Morisco physician who mocked him in front of his patients on more than one occasion. Moreover, university qualifications could be obtained with greater ease in Lérida because of the corruption of its governing board. Certain universities are known to have been responsive to bribes and to the pressure of 'ties of relationship' on the part of 'New Christians' (especially converted Jews) when awarding university degrees,[78] and this seems to have influenced Jover. Another of the witnesses, the Frenchman, Père Cassot, a farmworker in Valencia, declared that Jover had asked him for 100 coins 'saying that he wanted them in order to go to Lérida to graduate'. Another witness stated

> that he heard him [say] that as the physicians of the [municipal] tribunal of Valencia would not give him a licence to practise medicine, he wanted to go to Lérida to be examined. He also heard him [say] that he had received a letter from Lérida in which he was informed that he should go before St John's Day [the end of the academic year], because on that date the examiners were changed, and those that there were at that moment were friends of the person who was writing the letter of recommendation. And that made the said doctor Jover make haste in his departure for Lérida.[79]

The letter of recommendation had been written by don Jerónimo Fajardo, an influential figure in the world of finance in Valencia and Catalonia.

Jover's difficult situation of being a Morisco and not having a university education led him to take the decision to depart for Lérida, taking advantage of the friendship existing between don Jerónimo Fajardo and the examiners. Nevertheless, the difficulties must still have been considerable by the time when, despite his evident professional success, he drew up a plan for going into exile in a country where he could practise the Moslem religion openly and where he would be allowed to practise medicine without the need to obtain a degree. Another witness stated:

> that the said Jover had a very wealthy brother in Constantinople and that he had explained to him that if the physicians here [Valencia] did not give him a municipal licence to practise, he was considering

> leaving; he wanted to go to Lérida to graduate, and that if he did not succeed, he would not return, but he would go to where his brother was . . .; his wife said that since the physicians ['Old Christians'] would not let him practise medicine, he should try to do so in those new lands, and that she would rent their houses and she would join him there.[80]

In the end he fled to North Africa, where he practised medicine. The route that he took in order to reach Algeria was, as in the case of many other Moriscos, via the ports of the south of France, principally Marseilles. Once in Africa, impatient and homesick, and anxious for news of his loved ones, he wrote a letter, in Arabic, to his family in Valencia, which was intercepted by the Inquisition. It was translated by a Morisco who was being held prisoner in the Inquisition's gaol. Among other things Jover wrote:

> . . . I shall tell you what heppened to me after I left Barcelona, whence I went to Marseilles by sea, whence I departed and went to Bône in the land of the Moors [near Tunisia]. The journey took twenty-one days, and I made it together with three other companions. My intention is to go to Algeria. But in Bône I found the mayor sick and I cured him of his illness. In payment he gave me a horse, a suit of clothes and ten gold coins. But I want to go to Algeria. Do not worry about me; the only thing that I lack is your presence.[81]

The Inquisition submitted the circulation or mere possession of books or papers in Arabic to strict control. In the second half of the sixteenth century, it was enough to be caught with a brief note written in Arabic - even if it was a matter of a legal contract or a medical prescription - to be put on trial by the Inquisition as suspected of practising the religion of the 'degraded sect of Mahomet'. Naturally, this has not aided the survival of this type of literature. However, we should not lose sight of the fact that, in spite of the existence of a true clandestine network of 'alfaquíes', who taught people to read and write Arabic and who thus acted as focal points for maintaining Arab learning, the vast majority of Moriscos were illiterate. Nevertheless there is evidence for the continued existence and circulation of medical literature in Arabic among the Moriscos.[82] In the trial of Jover, whom we know to have read, written and spoken Arabic, it was said of him that 'when he left Valencia [with the intention of enroling at the Medical Faculty at Lérida], he took with him some books in Arabic. He left another Arabic book at home, which the witness gave to the Holy Inquisition'.[83]

Unfortunately, the subjects of the books are not mentioned, nor are they attached to the trial documents, by way of proof, as happened in other cases, nor is there any mention of their contents. Were they medical volumes? This is quite likely, since he left for the Medical Faculty of Lérida and may well have already been contemplating going into exile. From the evidence of a Christian apothecary who was an old friend of his, we are able to ascertain that he read Castilian and probably also Latin, which was by no means usual. In fact, from this same testimony we know of some of the books to be found in his library: 'The said doctor [Jover] auctioned all the Christian books he had, including a book by St Thomas Aquinas and a book by Friar Luis of Granada and a book called *Memorable Things of Spain*'.[84]

We do not know how Jover acquired his medical training. From what we know of other Morisco healers, it could have been a question of family apprenticeship and learning, in which medical training was transmitted from father (or mother) to son by oral tradition. However, this does not seem to have been the case here, considering Jover's wide knowledge of other languages. He may have been trained in a tradition of medical education that still existed in the sixteenth century following what we might call an 'open' model, under which anyone who had medical knowledge to impart might pass it on, outside any institutional framework. In such an open system, teaching activity reflects the interests of an individual teacher, not the requirements of a set curriculum, and the success of education, a student's qualification for practice, can be tested only by his success at curing his patients; it is ultimately the patient who will judge who is a physician and who is not. Where books for medical instruction are relatively scarce, as in Morisco communities, the open system, built round the master-disciple arrangement, further encourages the oral transmission of knowledge and consequently a tradition of empirical and family medical practice.[85] The Morisco doctor Gaspar Capdal, a contemporary of doctor Jerónimo Jover, who also practised in the Kingdom of Valencia, followed this model of professional training step by step. He did not know Arabic and he learnt medicine from an 'Old Christian' doctor and was able to read medical books in Spanish; he received his training on patients and his expertise in the preparation of drugs from a Morisco doctor, Master Damian, a 'New Christian', and the apothecary Ynca of Valencia.[86] Both Jerónimo Jover and Gaspar Capdal were totally integrated within a society consisting of 'Old' and 'New Christians' in which everyday living together was evidently more normal and less intense than appears from the narrow perspective provided by the Inquisitorial trials. Their training and family lives allow us to obtain some small idea of the complex co-existence of different cultures in sixteenth century Spanish society.

From the evidence of other witnesses we know that Jerónimo Jover practised medicine and used to carry out blood-letting; this he did at the correct and proper points of the body in accordance with orthodox

Galenism.[87] His clients were numerous and consisted mainly of Moriscos, as another witness indicates: 'many Moriscos with their urine used to enter and leave Doctor Jover's houses, and they came from the towns of Paterna and Manises',[88] towns near Valencia which had a largely Morisco population. However, he was also visited by 'Old Christians', both from the towns and villages and from the city of Valencia itself, as another witness reminds us: 'those with whom he had most dealings were the Moriscos of Picasent, Alcacer, Paterna, Manises and Moriscos from all the Kingdom [of Valencia] would come, and many "Old Christians", as is public knowledge and well-known in this city [Valencia]'.[89] Individuals from all manner of trades visited his house (tailors, shepherds, merchants, students, farmworkers, servants, weavers, even members of the families of university-trained physicians!) and he maintained a good relationship with the apothecaries who made up his prescriptions. Another witness tells us that he spoke *algarabía* (the dialect of Arabic spoken in Valencia) with Moriscos and spoke in their own language (Catalan or Castilian) with 'Old Christians'.[90] He used standard cures on all of them, but he also made use of invocations and spells, as one of his patients testified.[91] Jover's prestige must have been great, for it spread to far-flung parts of the Kingdom of Valencia, and he formed partnerships with 'Old Christian' apothecaries, and with them he used to organize visits to these distant areas. All this work produced substantial profits, as one of the apothecaries who had been a partner of his testified.[92] 'Old Christians' and Moriscos thus consulted the Morisco healer. At the popular level, and given the levelling effect that illness imposes across society as a whole, it would appear that the condition of the Morisco – 'the most despicable caste in the world', as one Morisco healer said of his own status before the Inquisition judges[93] – did not point to any special differences. The Inquisition, however, was not of the same opinion.

Felipe de Nájera, bachelor of medicine

The proceedings against the bachelor of medicine Felipe de Nájera are of considerable length and provide information, not only about Judaizers, but also about many other aspects of the medical milieu in late sixteenth and early seventeenth century Spain.[94] The trial procedure of the Inquisition court, which allowed and encouraged anonymous accusations without proof, based only on the infomer's testimony, was used to settle personal vendettas of every type: these could range from those resulting from the poor relationship of a physician with his patients to sheer spite in a sentimental relationship.[95]

The particular economic conditions of medical practice were the cause of confrontations between Converso physicians and their 'Old Christian' clients. From the financial standpoint, the physician–patient relationship in this period might be based on one of three models: (1) the contracting of the physician by a municipal council to attend to the needs of the population or a part of it (normally the so-called poor, a concept which it is difficult to define by present-day criteria); (2) the fee agreed (*iguala*) between the physician and the potential client. This agreement gave rise to a wide range of casuistry - from specific agreements for a particular illness (whether or not of a surgical nature) to total medical cover for a limited period of time (six months, one year); this might also be personal, for a family or for an institution (for example, to satisfy the medical requirements of a religious community[96] or a cathedral chapter); (3) payment for a visit when a client called a physician with whom he had had no previous established financial agreement.[97]

In practice, many of the witnesses who presented themselves voluntarily before the court of the Inquisition to give evidence against the Judaizing physician did so, in fact, to avenge themselves for the problems that derived from the financial system upon which the physician-patient relationship was based.[98] The Converso physician took great pains to warn the inquisitor:

> Your Lordship should be aware that I have many open and declared enemies in this town of Alcazar and also in Argamasilla [two towns in New Castile], not only because my personality is somewhat violent but also because I collected the agreed fees and salaries that I was owed by means of judicial summons. This has meant that I have had serious arguments with many of my patients.[99]

Some of them took advantage of the Inquisition's zeal for acting against Conversos suspected of Judaizing in order to get their revenge for what they considered to be the physician's greed. On other occasions, those who testified were endeavouring to get their revenge for a poorly performed cure or a consequence that the patient attributed to negligence or error on the part of the physician and which the ordinary courts had not considered as such (for instance, becoming blind in one eye as a consequence of an eye disease treated by the physician Felipe de Nájera).[100] Another prosecution witness was unmasked by the Converso physician himself, who was able to demonstrate that the person who was accusing him of being a Jew in actual fact wanted to get his revenge on him because, as a physician, he had refused to certify falsely that a relative of his was insane in order to have him declared unfit and thus to obtain his inheritance.[101] Another gave evidence out of sheer spite 'because the physician did not want to marry a daughter of his and spurned her'.[102]

In the same way, the trial against Felipe de Nájera allows us to catch a glimpse of the social milieu of the medical profession in late sixteenth and early seventeenth century Spain. We might notice the standard evolution of a university-trained physician's career, which starts with his university qualifications as his one and only possession: from the hard beginnings in financial terms of the young graduate, at the age of 25 (in 1588), 'who could not change his shirt for two weeks, nor change his sheets, because he did not have the funds',[103] until the moment, some fourteen years later, when 'his position as a physician, and the large number of clients that he had to attend to, both in his city and the surrounding towns' allowed him to employ maidservants as well as a house of some standing.[104] A brief description of his goods and chattels offer further evidence of his social position - both from an economic and an intellectual point of view - especially the size of his private library.[105] The trial allows us to see a cash-orientated society,[106] and to note the greed of physicians who frequently resorted to the civil courts in order to be paid the so-called *igualas* in the form of their equivalent in consumable goods (normally wheat, which the physician subsequently traded)[107] or precious metals (most commonly, worked silver).[108] This gave rise to tense situations, quarrels and even violent confrontations (on one occasion swords were drawn by the physician and a furious client).[109]

In the previous case, that of the Morisco physician Jover, we saw how anti-Semitism was used in connection with 'professional' problems. In the trial of the physician Felipe de Nájera, such 'professional anti-Semitism' also appears, but on this occasion among healers who acted within the bounds of legality. More precisely, there was friction between him and a barber-surgeon who had felt humiliated by what he believed to be arrogance on the part of the physician in the exercise of his profession.[110] Such were the typical rivalries between members of two categories of doctor with a certain social position, but with rather poorly defined functions: those of the physician with his university background, and those of the barber-surgeon with training of a more artisan nature. The tensions were emphasized not least because the barber-surgeons were the ones who actually provided most of the medical service for the population.

Contemporary Spanish society accepted the Inquisition as just one more element in social interaction, to the point of having it placed at the service of private interests, including those of the physician-patient relationship itself, as far as financial matters were concerned. This relationship brought together a medical professional belonging to the social and university establishment, and clients coming from a wide variety of different social categories: clergy, merchants, farmworkers, artisans, noblemen, lawyers, physicians, notaries, civil servants of the royal administration, even institutions such as monasteries or municipal councils; they all passed through the Inquisition court as a consequence of the trial against the physician Felipe de Nájera.

By a rare stroke of fortune for us, Felipe de Nájera shared an Inquisition cell in Toledo for almost a year with a Morisco healer, 'doctor' Juan de Toledo. This enables us to be certain about the very different medical training that they had each received, as well as to observe the different charges that the Inquisition laid against the Morisco healer and the Converso physician, who was accused of Judaizing.[111]

Felipe de Nájera belonged to a family of Converso merchants and farmers related to 'Old Christians' of some wealth. As in the case of many of the Converso physicians, among his family there were some who had undertaken medical studies. His maternal grandfather, Antonio de Nájera, was also a bachelor of medicine, as was one of his brothers, Pedro Alvarez de Mezquita, a resident of Madrid. His father's family was related to Portuguese Conversos. He himself was born in Portugal.[112] His case illustrates the tight control the Inquisition exercised over Spanish society, not only concerning problems directly connected with what was generically called 'heresy', but also concerning those connected with the moral standards of society. As we shall see, this particular physician had his first confrontation with the Inquisition when he was accused of being a homosexual. This was a serious matter in a society considerably less permissive than the present day.[113]

As he himself explained, he was born in Trancoso (Portugal) in 1563, where he received his primary education. He then moved to a nearby town, Celórico, where he continued studying grammar, in preparation for university entrance. When he reached the age of seventeen, his family sent him to the University of Salamanca to study arts and medicine. Eight years later he obtained his bachelor's degree in medicine and he began to practise as a physician. For eighteen years he travelled around Murcia and New Castile, working as a physician.[114] His route was typical of such university-trained village physicians, who sometimes worked for themselves but on other occasions were contracted by town councils to give medical attention to their inhabitants. Municipal councils held university-trained physicians in high esteem and their offers of employment (which included salary, tax benefits and accommodation) made up the principal job market for young graduates. These contracts might be for widely varying periods of time: they ranged from periods of a few months to a year or more. They were normally renewed annually providing the financial terms were satisfactory.[115]

After leaving the Faculty of Medicine at Salamanca, Nájera spent his whole career in the Kingdom of Castile. He started in the city of Cuenca, where he formed part of the medical staff of the Hospital of Santiago, acquiring professional experience there. From there he moved to Cieza (Murcia) with a contract from the town council for just three months. He then moved on to the town of San Clemente and almost immediately afterwards to that of Argamasilla de Alba, where he held a six-year contract from the council. He returned to his home town, Trancoso, for a few months, probably for family reasons, before leaving for Ciudad

Rodrigo with a contract for a further year. He returned to his home town for several months again, and then went back to San Clemente for one year more. From there he went on to provide medical services in a nearby town, Iniesta, for a two-year period. He was taken on by the municipality of San Clemente once again, and from there he moved on to that of Socuéllamos, for two and a half years. His last six years were divided between Argamasilla and Alcázar de Consuegra (nowadays Alcázar de San Juan), where he was under contract to the respective town councils. He never married.[116] During this final period, prior to his stay in Alcázar de San Juan, and while he was in Socuéllamos and Argamasilla, a housekeeper, Agueda García, a 40-year-old widow, took care of him.[117] It was in these two settlements that he had problems with the Inquisition: first of all, he was accused of practising homosexuality and thereafter of Judaizing. His career as a physician thus took place in the region of La Mancha, so familiar to his contemporary Don Quixote.

Felipe de Nájera's first brush with the Inquisition was in 1605, during his last stay in Argamasilla, and it arose from a conversation that his housekeeper had with a neighbour, in which she expressed her suspicions about her master's possible homosexuality. During interrogation, Agueda García spoke of her suspicions as well as the fact that, in her opinion, her master did not show due respect towards the images of saints or to the image of Christ himself, which demonstrated a lack of religiousness. The hearing was relatively rapid: the witnesses and the accused himself gave their evidence between May and September 1605; the defence managed to refute the evidence and the judge of Alcázar de San Juan acquitted him.[118]

Two years later, in November 1607, the inquisitor of Toledo, Don Francisco de Múxica, appeared in Alcázar de San Juan in order to make inquiries about certain Converso families who were living in that town. The atmosphere in the town was one of great unease. Three Converso physicians of the town were suspected of Judaizing: Doctor Yepes, the bachelor Barroso, and Felipe de Nájera, who was also a bachelor.[119] A lawyer neighbour of Nájera appeared before the Inquisitor voluntarily and accused him of practising rites that were typical of Judaizers and of maintaining friendship with Conversos; at the same time, he recalled the hearing of two years earlier, in which Nájera had been accused of a lack of respect towards holy images. He claimed

> that he heard Alonso Sánchez de la Serna, a priest, say that he had seen the bachelor Nájera, a Portuguese physician, wash meat before putting it into the cooking pot. Similarly, that he had frequent dealings with Conversos and that there had been proceedings against the said physician in which it was established that he treated images [of the saints] badly, which makes him a suspect individual.[120]

This was the usual way of presenting an accusation against someone suspected of Judaizing: besides the washing of meat, immediately afterwards another witness claimed to have seen him, on occasions, rejecting pork, removing the fatty excrescences from a leg of lamb (*landrecilla*), changing his shirt on Saturdays and Sundays, and seeking books written by Jews (these were the medical works of Isaac Israeli).[121] All this was sufficient to have him transferred to the secret prison of the Inquisition in Toledo (March 1608). There he shared a cell for a year with a Morisco healer, Juan de Toledo. The confidential comments that the bachelor made to the Morisco healer were used to add further information about his situation as a Judaizer. On the basis of all this information, the prosecuting counsel formulated the definitive accusation of

> Heretic, apostate from our Holy Catholic faith and Evangelical Law, excommunicant and perjurer, a Judaizer descended from Conversos; that being a baptized Christian, with danger for his soul and to the great scandal of the Christian people, he has said and has believed . . . that he is a Jew.[122]

The interrogation started immediately afterwards: first in Alcázar de San Juan (18 Feburary 1608) and subsequently in Toledo. Nájera was then 46 years old. The first point that the Inquisitor considered was the problem of 'blood purity' as he asked him 'about his caste and about the identity of his parents, grandparents and other transversal and collateral lines, and whether any of them has ever been held prisoner, sentenced, acquitted or condemned by the courts of the Holy Office of the Inquisition'.[123] The physician's reply reveals something of the complex network of family relationships among Portuguese and Spanish Conversos. His father was a Castilian merchant, from Medina del Campo, a new convert from Judaism, who had fled to Portugal during the civil war (1520–1) which set the Castilian municipalities against King Charles. He had five brothers and sisters, one of whom, also a bachelor, Pedro Alvarez de Mezquita, was a physician and practised medicine in Madrid.[124] He too must have experienced difficulties with the Inquisition because from a later declaration by Felipe de Nájera (who used his mother's surname) we discover that he fled to France together with his father.[125] Another of his brothers, Enrique de Nájera, left for Angola, where one of his father's brothers, Diego de Mezquita, traded in slaves, 'buying and selling negroes'.[126] Another brother was a cloth merchant and his two sisters were both married to merchants, one of whom was settled in La Guardia (Galicia).[127]

Despite such a background, he did not recognize his position as a Converso, stating that he was an 'Old Christian' and that none of the members of his family had been prosecuted by the Inquisition.[128] The long interrogation of the Converso physician, which lasted almost two years, offers a good example of inquisitorial proceedings, involving the confidential remarks made by the Judaizing physician to the Morisco healer and the latter's accusations before the judges, the intelligence and dialectical cunning of the judges, the unfeeling use of torture as a standard technique,[129] plus the fear that the court and the torture itself induced, as well as the use of lies, intelligence and even irony as defensive weapons in a desperate defence in which the very real threat of being burnt alive constantly appears.

At the beginning of his interrogation, Felipe de Nájera was a man proud of his qualifications as a university physician and his current social standing:

> I am an educated man and a graduate of an approved university, from the faculty of medicine, and by the mercy of God, I have a good name and a good salary in the town of Alcázar and its neighbourhood.[130]

He conducted his own defence against the accusations that were based on his dietary habits, suspected of being Jewish rituals, by resorting to his knowledge of medicine:

> I gave up eating bacon some time ago when I was suffering from an attack of gout or another internal illness for which bacon and other salted meats are harmful, according to Galen's opinion, which is expounded in his work *De alimentorum facultatibus*.[131]

A fellow physician, Gaspar López, called by the Inquisition, confirmed the diagnosis.[132]

Eventually, after two prolonged sessions of torture, which were noted down in detail with dispassionate detachment by the Inquisition scribe, we find ourselves present at the collapse of a man 'full of fear and bewildered . . . with his arms and body destroyed',[133] who concludes by confessing under torture that he has been a Jew:

> I have been a Jew from time to time. If your Lordship wishes me to say more, I shall sign it; but if I state anything else, it is so that I do not have to undergo torture. Do not kill me your Lordship, I cannot withstand any more torture. If I have already admitted that I am a Jew, what else does your Lordship require?[134]

The accusation centred totally upon his situation as a crypto-Jew. What concerned the Inquisition above all else throughout the interrogation was to discover the names of Judaizers, to find out the network of relationships and assistance among the Conversos;[135] to investigate the contacts between the Conversos of Spain and Portugal and those in other countries, those who had fled to France, to Rome, to Germany, and with whom they were in correspondence;[136] to attempt to reconstruct the

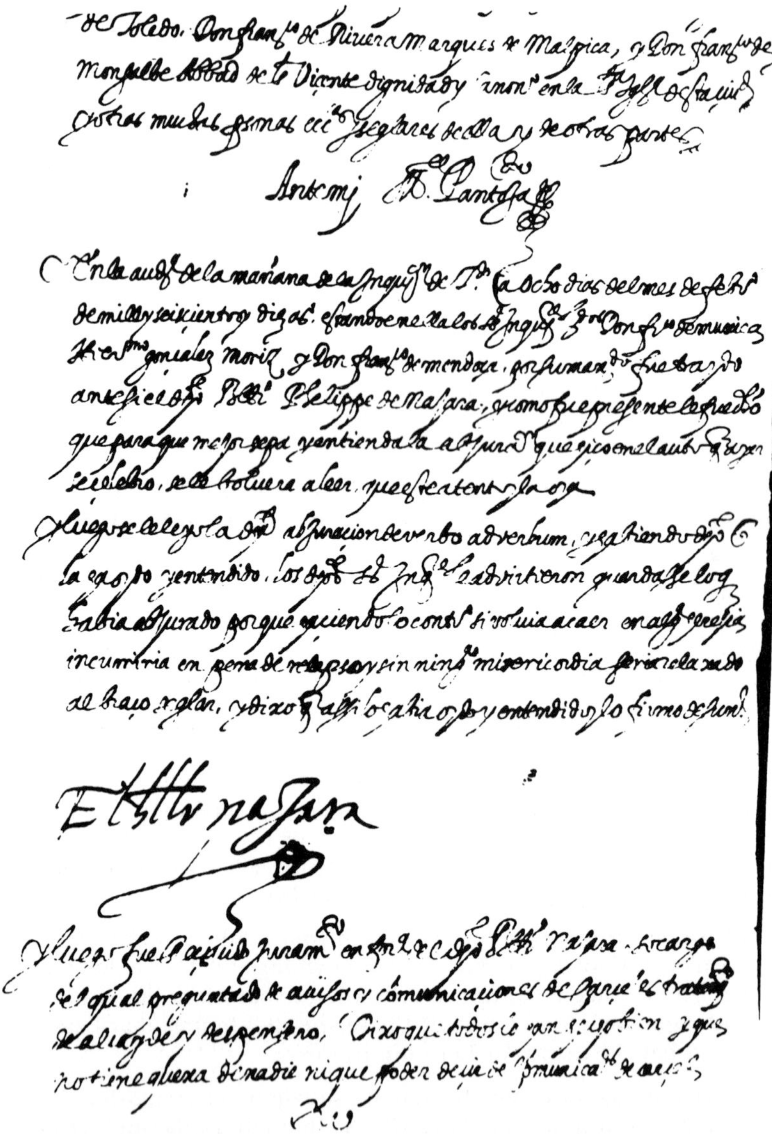

Illustration 10 Signature of the Converso physician, Felipe de Nájara, bachelor of Medicine, confirming that he was aware of the sentence on the morrow of auto-da-fe (8 February 1610). Archivo Histórico Nacional, Inquisition of Toledo, leg. 168, 1, fol. 365r. Reproduced by permission of the Spanish National Archive, Madrid.

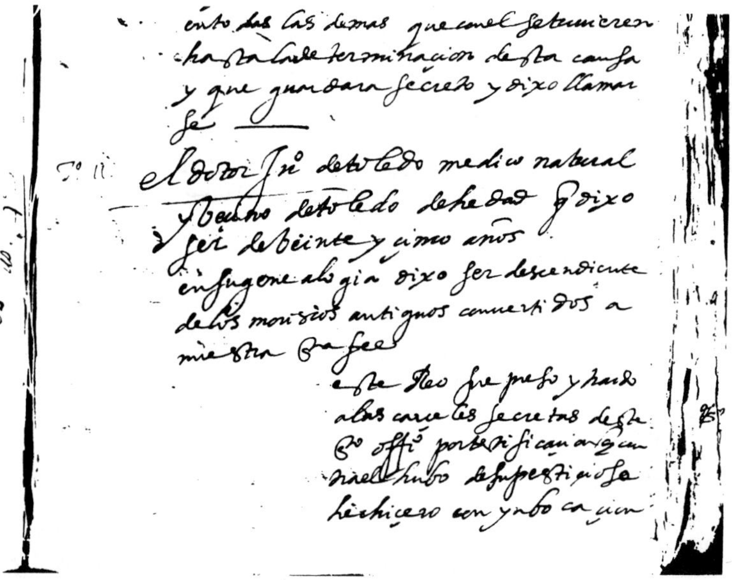

Illustration 11 Fragment of the Inquisition trial of the Morisco healer, Juan de Toledo, where he confesses that he is a descendant of Moriscos and that he is accused of superstitious behaviour and witchcraft with the invocation of demons. Archivo Histórico Nacional, Inquisition of Toledo, leg. 168, 1, fol. 172r. Reproduced by permission of the Spanish National Archive, Madrid.

crypto-Jews' clandestine system of religious education;[137] and, last but not least, to find out in as much detail as possible the financial situation of Felipe de Nájera the physician.[138]

Felipe de Nájera's skill in conducting his own defence, the dishonesty of many of the witnesses, and his insistence on stating after the sessions of torture 'that what I have confessed under torture has been said because I am much afraid',[139] was enough to cause disagreement among the five judges of the court of the Inquisition of Toledo: two of them condemned him to be burnt alive, but the other three opted for 'public exhibition in a habit in an auto-da-fe, life imprisonment, confiscation of his possessions, and five years at the oars in His Majesty's galleys, without pay' (1 October 1609).[140] Another way to be a condemned man.

The most compromising information for Nájera turned out to be that which he himself had told the Morisco healer with whom he shared a cell and secrets for a year. The difference in status and treatment by the Inquisition of the two cellmates, one a Judaizer, the other a Morisco, typifies the way the two minorities were persecuted. The Judaizer, Nájera, was a university-educated physician who found himself in trouble on what appeared to be purely ethnic/religious grounds. At no point in his trial was he accused of malpractice, superstition or other irregularities. His medicine appears to have been that practised by a traditional, university-educated Galenist. The Morisco healer, Juan de Toledo, aged 25, was called a 'physician' by the inquisitors and he himself stated that that was his title. When, of his own volition, he appeared to accuse the Converso physician of being a Jew, he began his statement by saying: 'I lived in Toledo and was a descendant of the old Moriscos who were converted to our Holy Faith'.[141] He had no objection to acknowledging that

> he was taken prisoner and brought to the secret prison of this Holy Court, having been accused of superstitious behaviour, of witchcraft with the invocation of demons and of making use of judicial astrology in his practice of medicine.[142]

These were exactly the same accusations as were hurled against all Morisco healers tried by the Inquisition up to the expulsion of the Moriscos from the Spanish realms between 1609 and 1612. They demonstrate that, as opposed to the Judaizers, the Morisco healers found themselves in trouble with the Inquisition particularly because of the way they practised medicine, and not only because of their supposed religious and cultural leanings.

Notes

I am indebted to Jaime Contreras and Ricardo G. Cárcel, who have allowed me to use their database of inquisitorial records. Thanks are also extended to Alvar Martínez-Vidal and Jon Arrizabalaga, who read the draft and made valuable comments, to Philip Banks who improved the English text, and to the editors for their help and kindness. Funding for the research was provided by CICYT grant number PB/89-0066.

1. See Y. Baer, *A History of the Jews in Christian Spain*, 2 vols. (Philadelphia, 1961).

2. L. Cardaillac, *Morisques et Chrétiens. Un Affrontement Polémique (1492-1640)*, (Paris, 1977); A. Domínguez Ortíz and B. Vincent, *Historia de los Moriscos. Vida y Tragedia de una Minoría*, (Madrid, 1978). The reality, at least at the intellectual level, was more complex; see L. García-Ballester, L. Ferre and E, Feliu, 'Jewish appreciation of fourteenth-century Scholastic medicine', *Osiris* 6 (1990), 85-117, and L. García-Ballester, 'A marginal learned medical world: Jewish, Muslim, and Christian medical practitioners faced with Arabic medical sources in late medieval Spain', in L. García-Ballester, R.K. French, J. Arrizabalaga, A. Cunningham (eds), *Practical Medicine from Salerno to the Black Death* (Cambridge, 1993); E. Gutwirth, 'Actitudes judías hacia los cristianos en la España del siglo XV: Ideario de los traductores del latín', *Actas del II Congreso Internacional 'Encuentro de las Tres Culturas', 3-6 Octubre 1983* (Toledo, 1985), 189-96.

3. See my work *Los Moriscos y la Medicina* (Barcelona, 1984); 'Academicism versus empiricism in practical medicine in sixteenth-century Spain with regard to Morisco practitioners', in A. Wear, R.K. French and I.M. Lonie (eds), *The Medical Renaissance of the Sixteenth Century* (Cambridge, 1985), 246-70, 338-42.

4. C. Roth, *A History of the Marranos* (Philadelphia, 1947). The dictionary defines 'Judaizer' as a person who conforms to the spirit, character, principles or practices of Judaism. See also H. Beinart, *Conversos on Trial. The Inquisition in Ciudad Real* (Jerusalem, 1981). This work, although focussing on fifteenth-century New Castile, is a very good survey of the relationship between the 'Conversos' and the Inquisition.

5. J. Caro Baroja, *Los Judíos en la España Moderna y Contemporánea*, 3 vols., 2nd edn (Madrid, 1978), II, 289-510; Beinart, *Conversos on Trial*, 237ff. Interesting evidence on these topics is to be found in Archivo Histórico Nacional, Inquisition of Toledo, leg. 168, 1, ff. 291v-292v, 334v-336v.

6. A good brief survey is in H. Kamen, *The Spanish Inquisition* (London, 1965). See also, H.C. Lea, *A History of the Inquisition of Spain*, 4 vols. (Philadelphia, 1906; repr. New York, 1966). Two recent accounts are, A. Alcalá (ed.), *The Spanish Inquisition and the Inquisitorial Mind* (New Jersey, 1987); and G. Henningsen and J. Tedeschi (eds), *The Inquisition in Early Modern Europe. Studies on Sources and Methods* (Dekalb, Illinois, 1986).

7. 'In the forced or voluntary conversion of the Jews of Spain, State and Church did not find a solution to the internal difficulties that beset the country in the 14th and 15th centuries. Nor did the establishment of the Inquisition and the Expulsion of the Jews of Spain provide the answer. For centuries Spain was to continue to grapple with the problem of the absorption within it of an entire population group,' Beinart, *Conversos on Trial*, 235-6.

8. Caro Baroja, *Los Judíos en la España Moderna*, I, 149; Beinart, *Conversos on Trial*, 25. See also Alcalá, *Spanish Inquisition.*

9. Good surveys are H. Kamen, *Spain 1469-1714. A Society in Conflict* (London, 1983); and J. Casey, 'Spain: a failed transition', in P. Clark (ed.), *The European Crisis of 1590* (London, 1985), 209-31.

10. Caro Baroja, *Los Judíos en la España Moderna*, I, 207-226.

11. A. Domínguez Ortiz, *La Clase Social de los Conversos en Castilla en la Edad Moderna* (Madrid, 1955), 36-73; Caro Baroja, *Los Judíos en la España Moderna*, II, 285ff.

12. *Constitutiones Insignis Collegii Sancti Ildefonsi . . .* (Alcalá, 1716), 10.

13. J.T. Lanning, *The Royal Protomedicato. The Regulation of the Medical Profession in the Spanish Empire*, ed. J.J. TePaske (Durham, N.C., 1985), 175-200.

14. A.A. Sicroff, *Les Controverses des Statuts de 'pureté de sang' en Espagne du XVe au XVIIe siècle* (Paris, 1960); Domínguez Ortíz, *La Clase Social de los Conversos*; and Caro Baroja, *Los Judíos en la España Moderna.*

15. On the Archbishop of Granada, see T. Herrero, *Vida y Obras de Fray Hernando de Talavera* (Granada, 1966).

16. See references quoted in note 2.

17. See Cardaillac, *Morisques et Chrétiens*; and Domínguez Ortíz and Vincent, *Historia de los Moriscos.*

18. García-Ballester, 'Academicism versus empiricism', 246.

19. The Royal decrees were published by P. Boronat, *Los Moriscos Españoles y su Expulsión*, 2 vols. (Valencia, 1901), II, 190-285. See the books mentioned by Cardaillac, Domínguez Ortíz and Vincent (note 2).

20. See the works of R. García Carcel, *Orígenes de la Inquisición Española. El*

Tribunal de Valencia, 1478-1530 (Barcelona, 1976); and *Herejía y Sexo en el Siglo XVI. La Inquisición en Valencia, 1530-1609* (Barcelona, 1979). The updating edited by A. Alcalá on the Inquisition, quoted in note 6, is useful.

21. Archivo Histórico Nacional, leg. 1988, case record 23, ff. 22r-3v.
22. Archivo Histórico Nacional, leg. 2106, 4, f. 10r-v.
23. Archivo Histórico Nacional, leg. 1988, 49, f. 16r; leg. 168, 1, ff. 283v-4r.
24. Archivo Histórico Nacional, Inquisition of Toledo, leg. 168, 1, ff. 124r-v.
25. Archivo Histórico Nacional, Inquisition of Toledo, leg. 2106, 9, ff. 41r.
26. García Carcel, *Herejía y Sexo*, 187ff.
27. Caro Baroja, *Los Judíos en la España Moderna*, II, 209ff.
28. On the use of torture, see F. Tomás y Valiente, *La Tortura en España* (Barcelona, 1973); on the rules of procedure of the Inquisition, see Beinart, *Conversos on Trial*, 105-94.
29. Archivo Histórico Nacional, Inquisition of Toledo, leg. 2106, 9, f. 46r.
30. Archivo Histórico Nacional, Inquisition of Valencia, leg. 549.
31. 'Ay también en este medio una gran conveniencia que es hacerlos pobres', Archivo del Colegio del Patriarca, Valencia, I, 7, 8, 275. The letter was written *c.*1590. See Boronat, *Los Moriscos Españoles*, I, 24ff.
32. 'Non igitur est dandus panis filiorum his cannibus, sed abigendi sunt ab illis seminariis et ad sordidas artes, aut ad triremes destinandi, non ad studia literarum,' Bleda, *Defensio Fidei in Causa Neophitorum sive Morischorum Regni Valentiae* (Valencia, 1610), 374.
33. See García-Ballester, 'Academicism versus empiricism', 251ff.
34. See Domínguez Ortíz, Vincent, *Historia de los Moriscos*, 129ff.
35. García-Ballester, *Los Moriscos y la Medicina*, 211-12.
36. On neo-Scholastic medicine in the Spanish faculties of medicine in the period we are considering, especially that of Valladolid, see J. Riera, *Vida y Obra de Luis Mercado* (Salamanca, 1968).
37. See, J.M. López Piñero, *Ciencia y Técnica en la Sociedad Española de los Siglos XVI y XVII* (Barcelona, 1979), 126-8, 140-8; J. Pardo Tomás, *Ciencia y Censura. La Inquisición Española y los Libros Científicos en los Siglos XVI y XVII* (Madrid, 1991).
38. See, Caro Baroja, *Los Judíos en la España Moderna*, II, 175ff.
39. See H. Beinart, 'The records of the Inquisition. A source of Jewish and Conversos history', *Proceedings of the Israel Academy of Sciences and Humanities*, II (Jerusalem, 1968), 211-16.
40. Archivo Histórico Nacional, Inquisition of Toledo, leg. 168, 9, ff. 42r, 44r.
41. Archivo Histórico Nacional, Inquisition of Valencia, leg. 552, 9.
42. All these places are mentioned in the inquisitorial records for 1560-1610. See also, Caro Baroja, *Los Judíos en la España Moderna*, I, 227-88; Beinart, *Conversos on Trial*, 209, and the references therein.
43. See a brief biographic survey in Caro Baroja, *Los Judíos en la España Moderna*, II, 189-93; see also, A.G. Keller, 'Garcia d'Orta', in Charles C. Gillispie (ed.), *Dictionary of Scientific Biography* (New York, 1980), X, 236-8.
44. It was edited by the Count of Ficcalho, 2 vols. (Lisbon, 1891-5). The passages I am referring to correspond to *Coloquios*, I, 24.
45. See, A. Hernández Morejón, *Historia Bibliográfica de la Medicina Española*, 7 vols. (Madrid, 1842-45; repr. New York-London, 1967), I, 100-1; M. Lemos, *Amato Lusitano. A sua Vida e a sua Obra* (Oporto, 1907); Caro Baroja, *Los Judíos en la España Moderna*, II, 193-4.
46. Hernández Morejón, *Historia Bibliográfica de la Medicina Española*, I, 107-8; Caro Baroja, *Los Judíos en la España Moderna*, II, 194.

47. See, L. de Alburquerque, in *Dictionary of Scientific Biography*, XIV, 583-4.

48. Hernández Morejón, *Historia Bibliográfica de la Medicina Española*, I, 104-6; M. Lemos, *Zacuto Lusitano. A sua Vida e a sua Obra* (Oporto, 1909); Caro Baroja, *Los Judíos en la España Moderna*, II, 195-8.

49. See, P. Laín Entralgo, *Enfermedad y Pecado* (Barcelona, 1961); O. Temkin, *Hippocrates in a World of Pagans and Christians* (Baltimore-London, 1991), 249-56.

50. See Lea, *A History of the Inquisition of Spain*, IV, 185.

51. Quoted by Lea, *A History of the Inquisition of Spain*, IV, 185.

52. D. Simancas, *Institutiones Catholicae . . .* (Vallisoleti, 1552), cap. 30, n. 10, 11.

53. F. Torreblanca, *Epitome Delictorum*, 2 vols. (Hispali, 1618), II, 9.

54. 'Statuimus et mandamus ut tam contra astrologos, mathematicos, et alios quoscumque dictae astrologiae artem, praeterquam circa agriculturam, navigationem et rem medicam inposterum exercentes, aut facientes iudicia et nativitates hominum . . ., qui supradictas damnatas, vanas, fallaces et perniciosas divinandi artes sive scientias exercent, profitenturet docent aut discunt, quive huiusmodi illicitas divinationes, sortilegia, superstitiones, beneficia, incantationes . . .', *Bullarum Diplomatum . . .* (Augustae Taurinorum, 1873), vol. 8, 650.

55. The collaboration between physicians (including Converso doctors) and the Inquisition has been studied by D. Gracia, 'Judaism, medicine, and the inquisitorial mind in sixteenth-century Spain', in Alcalá (ed.), *The Spanish Inquisition*, 375-400. He does not use the inquisitorial records, which form the basis of the present essay.

56. His medical training has been described in García-Ballester, 'Academicism versus empiricism', 267-70.

57. Archivo Histórico Nacional, Inquisition of Valencia, leg. 175, 1.

58. Ibid., leg. 840.

59. The concept 'professional anti-semitism' was first used in this way, but applied to Converso physicians, by Caro Baroja, *Los Judíos en la España Moderna*, II, 175ff.

60. 'Quomodo igitur monebit aegrotum peccata sua confiteri medicus, si Sacramentum Confessionis contemnit, et nunquam legitime confessus est, nec sacra communione refectus?', Bleda, *Defensio Fidei*, 366.

61. Bleda, *Defensio Fidei*, 367.

62. Cortes de Castilla's Proceedings, Madrid 13 November 1607, vol. 23, 583-7.

63. Archivo Histórico Nacional, Inquisition of Toledo, leg. 168, 1, f. 173r.

64. Archivo Histórico Nacional, Inquisition of Toledo, leg. 168, f. 187r.

65. Archivo Histórico Nacional, Inquisition of Toledo, leg. 168, f. 206r.

66. 'Quod infirmi prius provideant anima quam corpori. Cum infirmitas corporalis nonnunquam ex peccato proveniat . . .', J.D. Mansi, *Sacrorum Conciliorum Nova Amplissima Collectio* (repr. Graz, 1960-2), vol. 22, 1010-11.

67. See, L. García-Ballester, M.R. McVaugh and A. Rubio, *Medical Licensing and Learning in Fourteenth-century Valencia* (Philadephia, 1989), 42-4.

68. '. . . ac pretextu, et colere medicinae corporalis erunt seminatores Mahometanae impietatis', Bleda, *Defensio Fidei*, 365.

69. Ordenanzas de la Real Audiencia y Chancillería de Granada (Granada, 1610), f. 370.

70. Among the various pardons granted to the Morisco population of Granada, 'the surgeon who has practised circumcision' is specifically excluded. See Archivo de la Alhambra (Granada), leg. 159.

71. Archivo Histórico Nacional, Inquisition of Valencia, leg. 552, 9. A part of the extensive proceedings of his inquisitorial trial has been transcribed and reproduced (in Spanish) in García-Ballester, *Los Moriscos y la Medicina*, 179–89.

72. See, L.S. Granjel, *El Ejercicio Médico y Otros Capítulos de la Medicina Española* (Salamanca, 1974), 11–86; J.M. López Piñero, 'The medical profession in sixteenth century Spain', in A.W. Russell (ed.), *The Town and State Physician in Europe from the Middle Ages to the Enlightenment*, (Wolfenbüttel, 1981), 85–98.

73. *Recopilación de las Leyes, Pragmáticas Reales, Decretos, Acuerdos del Real Protomedicato . . .*, by Don Miguel Eugenio Muños . . . (Valencia, 1751; repr. Valencia, 1991), 71-3; see Lanning, *The Royal Protomedicato*, 175–200.

74. See a description of the procedure in García-Ballester, McVaugh and Rubio, *Medical Licensing and Learning*, 12–18.

75. Archivo Histórico Nacional, Inquisition of Valencia, leg. 840.

76. Archivo Histórico Nacional, Inquisition of Valencia, leg. 552.

77. Archivo Histórico Nacional, Inquisition of Valencia, leg. 552.

78. This was the case at the small University of Sigüenza, which is briefly described by V. de la Fuente, *Historia de las Universidades, Colegios y Demás Establecimientos de Enseñanza en España*, 4 vols. (Madrid 1884–89), II, 328ff.

79. Archivo Histórico Nacional, Inquisition of Valencia, leg. 552, 9.

80. Archivo Histórico Nacional, Inquisition of Valencia, leg. 552. 9.

81. Archivo Histórico Nacional, Inquisition of Valencia, leg. 552, 9.

82. García-Ballester, 'Academicism versus empiricism', 266; A. Labarta, 'Los libros de los moriscos valencianos', *Awrat*, 2 (1980), 72–80; *idem*, 'Textos para el estudio de la terapéutica entre los moriscos valencianos', *Dynamis*, 1 (1981), 275–310.

83. Archivo Histórico Nacional, Inquisition of Valencia, leg. 552, 9.

84. Archivo Histórico Nacional, Inquistions of Valencia, leg. 552, 9.

85. A description of this so-called 'open' model of medical teaching in the training of late medieval Jewish physicians is given in García-Ballester, Ferre and Feliu, 'Jewish appreciation of scholastic medicine', 93–7.

86. A description of the medical training of Gaspar Capdal is given in García-Ballester, 'Academicism versus empiricism', 267–70.

87. Archivo Histórico Nacional, Inquisition of Valencia, leg. 552, 9.

88. Archivo Histórico Nacional, Inquisition of Valencia, leg. 552, 9.

89. Archivo Histórico Nacional, Inquisition of Valencia, leg. 552, 9.

90. Archivo Histórico Nacional, Inquisition of Valencia, leg. 552, 9.

91. Archivo Histórico Nacional, Inquisition of Valencia, leg. 552, 9.

92. Archivo Histórico Nacional, Inquisition of Valencia, leg. 552, 9.

93. The Morisco healer was Román Ramírez, see Archivo Diocesano de Cuenca, Inquisition, leg. 343, 48.

94. Archivo Histórico Nacional, Inquisition of Toledo, leg. 168, 1, ff. 1–370; leg. 2106, 9, ff. 40v–46r. Caro Baroja used the first inquisitorial proceeding, see *Los Judíos en la España Moderna*, II, 211–20.

95. Archivo Histórico Nacional, Inquisition of Toledo, leg. 168, 1, f. 234r–v.

96. For example, Felipe de Nájera was the doctor of the Franciscan monastery at Argamasilla, Archivo Histórico Nacional, Inquisition of Toledo, leg. 168, 1, f. 28v.

97. The doctor-patient relationship has not been studied from the financial standpoint in sixteenth-and seventeenth-century European medicine, at least not in the Spanish realms. See L.S. Granjel, *La Medicina Española Renacentista*,

Salamanca, 1980. The three models we are summarizing were shaped in the late medieval centuries, see V. Nutton, 'Continuity or rediscovery. The city physician in Classical Antiquity and Mediaeval Italy', in Russell (ed.), *The Town and State Physician in Europe*, 9–46, repr. in V. Nutton, *From Democedes to Harvey: Studies in the History of Medicine* (London, 1988), no. vi.; also L. García-Ballester, 'Medical ethics in transition in thirteenth-fourteenth century Latin medicine: new problems with the physician-patient relationship, and the doctor's fee', in J. Geyer-Kordesch, A. Wear and R.K. French (eds), *A History of Medical Ethics* (in preparation).

98. Archivo Histórico Nacional, Inquisition of Toledo, leg. 168, ff. 228r–9v.

99. Archivo Histórico Nacional, Inquisition of Toledo, leg, 168, f. 226r.

100. Archivo Histórico Nacional, Inquisition of Toledo, leg. 168, f. 229v.

101. Archivo Histórico Nacional, Inquisition of Toledo, leg. 168, f. 234r.

102. Archivo Histórico Nacional, Inquisition of Toledo, leg. 168, f. 234v.

103. Archivo Histórico Nacional, Inquisition of Toledo, leg. 168, f. 230r.

104. Archivo Histórico Nacional, Inquisition of Toledo, leg. 168, f. 226r.

105. Archivo Histórico Nacional, Inquisition of Toledo, leg. 168, f. 22r–v. The library contained 121 volumes of different sizes. Unfortunately the scribe did not describe the incipits.

106. See, E.J. Hamilton, *American Treasure and the Price Revolution in Spain, 1501–1650* (New York, 1970), 73–103.

107. Archivo Histórico Nacional, Inquisition of Toledo, leg. 168, f. 228r.

108. Archivo Histórico Nacional, Inquisition of Toledo, leg. 168, ff. 228r–229v.

109. Archivo Histórico Nacional, Inquisition of Toledo, leg. 168, f. 229v.

110. Archivo Histórico Nacional, Inquisition of Toledo, leg. 168, f. 229v.

111. Archivo Histórico Nacional, Inquisition of Toledo, leg. 160, 1, ff. 172r–201v, 282r–302r.

112. Archivo Histórico Nacional, Inquisition of Toledo, leg. 160, 1, f. 205r.

113. Archivo Histórico Nacional, Inquisition of Toledo, leg. 160, 1, ff. 1–25.

114. Archivo Histórico Nacional, Inquisition of Toledo, leg. 160, 1, f. 206v.

115. See references cited in notes 94 and 97.

116. Archivo Histórico Nacional, Inquisition of Toledo, leg. 160, 1, ff. 205r–6r.

117. Archivo Histórico Nacional, Inquisition of Toledo, leg. 160, 1, ff. 50r–51v.

118. Archivo Histórico Nacional, Inquisition of Toledo, leg. 160, 1, ff. 3r–107r.

119. Archivo Histórico Nacional, Inquisition of Toledo, leg. 160, 1, f. 296v.

120. Archivo Histórico Nacional, Inquisition of Toledo, leg. 160, 1, f. 110r.

121. Archivo Histórico Nacional, Inquisition of Toledo, leg. 160, 1, f. 124r–v. See above on the large library Felipe de Nájera had in his house at Argamasilla, with a total of 121 volumes of different sizes; ibid., f. 22r–v. The subjects of the books were not noted down by the scribe. On the Jewish life of the Conversos see Beinart, *Conversos on Trial*, 237–85.

122. Archivo Histórico Nacional, Inquisition of Toledo, leg. 160, 1, f. 210r.

123. Archivo Histórico Nacional, Inquisition of Toledo, leg. 160, 1, f. 206r.

124. Archivo Histórico Nacional, Inquisition of Toledo, leg. 160, 1, f. 206r.

125. Archivo Histórico Nacional, Inquisition of Toledo, leg. 160, 1, f. 337v.

126. Archivo Histórico Nacional, Inquisition of Toledo, leg. 160, 1, f. 205v.

127. Archivo Histórico Nacional, Inquisition of Toledo, leg. 160, 1, f. 205v.

128. Archivo Histórico Nacional, Inquisition of Toledo, leg. 160, 1, f. 206r.

129. See the book by Tomás y Valiente, *La Tortura en España*, cited in note 28.

130. Archivo Histórico Nacional, Inquisition of Toledo, leg. 160, 1, f. 224v.

131. Archivo Histórico Nacional, Inquisition of Toledo, leg. 160, 1, f. 225v. See Galen, *Opera Omnia*, ed. C.G. Kühn (repr. Hildesheim, 1964), VI, 528, 661–3.

132. Archivo Histórico Nacional, leg. 230r, marginal note.
133. Archivo Histórico Nacional, leg. 230r ff. 332, 334v.
134. Archivo Histórico Nacional, leg. 230r f. 334r-v.
135. Archivo Histórico Nacional, leg. 230r f. 286v.
136. Archivo Histórico Nacional, leg. 230r ff. 292v, 294v, 297v, 309r, 337v; Archivo Histórico Nacional, Inquisition of Toledo, leg. 2106, 9, f. 42r.
137. Archivo Histórico Nacional, Inquisition of Toledo, leg. 168, 1, ff. 328-9v.
138. Archivo Histórico Nacional, Inquisition of Toledo, leg. 168, 1, f. 209r-v.
139. Archivo Histórico Nacional, Inquisition of Toledo, leg. 168, 1, f. 345v.
140. Archivo Histórico Nacional, Inquisition of Toledo, leg. 168, 1, f. 348.
141. Archivo Histórico Nacional, Inquisition of Toledo, leg. 168, 1, f. 172r.
142. Archivo Histórico Nacional, Inquisition of Toledo, leg. 168, 1, f. 172r-v.

ADDENDA ET CORRIGENDA

I

p. 195: The scientific encyclopaedia written by Juan Gil de Zamora has been edited with a full introductory study, Spanish translation and indexes by A. Domínguez and L. García Ballester, *Johannis Aegidii Zamorensis Historia Naturalis.* Introducción, edición crítica, traducción castellana e índices, 3 vols., Valladolid: Junta de Castilla y León, 1994 (Estudios de Historia de la Ciencia y de la Técnica, no. 11).

pp. 199–200: The corpus of Pedro Gallego's scientific translations from Arabic into Latin has been recently edited by J. Martínez Gázquez, *Petri Galleci Opera omnia quae extant (De astronomia, De animalibus et In regitiva domus)*, Firenze: SISMEL Edizioni del Galluzzo, 2000.

p. 200: To refer *Oeconomia (In regitiva domus)* to be 'probably based on the pseudo-Galenic Work' was my failure. It refers to the pseudo-Aristotle work.

pp. 200–201: The *Liber quaestionum medicinalium discentibus in medicina,* attributed to 'Huneyn filius Ysaac medici qui latine dicitur Johannicius', has been discussed by Marie-Thérèse d'Alverny, 'Marc de Tolède', in *Estudios sobre Alfonso VI y la reconquista de Toledo. Actas del II Congreso Internacional de Estudios Mozárabes (Toledo 20–26 Mayo 1985),* 4 vols, Toledo: Instituto de Estudios Visigótico-Mozárabes de Toledo, 1987–1990: vol. 3, 1989, pp. 25–59 (Repr. In *La connaissance de l'Islam dans l'Occident médiévale*, Aldershot: Ashgate, 1994. Variorum VII, p. 32).

p. 202: Any reader willing to find an answer to many of the questions dealing with medicine that I proposed at the end of my article, may turn to my book on medicine in medieval Castile (until c. 1525), *La búsqueda de la salud. Sanadores y enfermos en la Corona de Castilla, siglos XIII al XVI* to be published in Barcelona (Península Ediciones, in press).

IV

p. 91: On Meir Alguades and his translations of Aristotelian works, see Jean-Pierre Rothschild, 'Du Latin à l'Hébreu: Quelques problèmes posés par des traductions médiévales, in *Rashi, 1040–1990. Hommage à Ephraïm E. Urbach. Congrès européen des Études juives* édité par Gabrielle Sed-Rajna (Paris: Les Éditions du Cerf, 1993), pp. 695–712, and also also Lawrence V. Berman, 'The Latin-into-Hebrew Translation of the Nichomachean Ethics', in *Jerusalem Studies in*

Jewish Thought, 7 (1988), pp. 147–168 [Shlomo Pines Jubilee Volume on the Occasion of His Eightieth Birthday] (in Hebrew). Yolanda Moreno, Ron Barkai and myself are working in the study and edition of the clinical notes and recipes attributed to Meir Alguades and collected by one of his students (Parma, Biblioteca Palatina, MS 2474, iv, fols. 145–155v); the notes and recipes were written in *aljamiado* (Old Spanish written in Hebrew characters). The first results of our work have been incorporated to my above mentioned book on medicine in medieval Castile to be published in Barcelona (Península Ediciones, in press).

INDEX